Pregnancy

Gordon Bourne FRCS FRCOG

Consultant Obstetrician and Gynaecologist
St Bartholomew's Hospital, London

Pregnancy

New and revised edition

Pan Books London and Sydney

First published 1972 by Cassell Ltd
First Pan Books edition published 1975 (18 printings)
This edition published 1984 by Pan Books Ltd,
Cavaye Place, London SW10 9PG
29 28 27 26 25 24
© Gordon Bourne 1972, 1975, 1979, 1984
ISBN 0 330 28399 5
Printed in Great Britain by
Richard Clay (The Chaucer Press) Ltd, Bungay, Suffolk

Contents

Preface to the first edition

I have written this book for women before, during and after pregnancy, for their families and, indeed, for anyone with no specialized knowledge of medicine or midwifery who wants to understand pregnancy and childbirth. This is an educational book, not a textbook, and the occasional repetition is deliberate in order to provide a fluent narrative which is as clear as possible.

Even today, many women embarking on their first pregnancy know very little of what is happening to their bodies, why various changes occur, which symptoms are normal and which are abnormal. Fear of the unknown is very real and knowledge is half the battle in defeating this fear. By helping women understand what pregnancy is about I hope this book will remove any apprehension and give each one confidence in her ability to produce a normal baby and to enjoy this miraculous experience.

Every pregnancy is unique. The three phases of reproduction—pregnancy, childbirth and the puerperium, or period of time immediately after childbirth—involve many physiological, anatomical, psychological and emotional changes which differ, albeit slightly, in each woman. These three phases each have importance and labour must not be singled out as the only important event in the process. Pregnancy and childbirth are natural functions which may sometimes present physical discomfort and mental strain but which a healthy, well-balanced woman should accomplish with an immense sense of achievement and satisfaction.

It is undoubtedly true that the more a pregnant woman knows about pregnancy the more confidently can she enter each phase of the nine months before childbirth, the birth itself and the puerperium. At present there are so many gaps in the average woman's knowledge of pregnancy that she is extremely vulnerable to the many old wives' tales, horror stories and unfounded advice which continue to surround motherhood, and there is no comprehensive work to which she can turn to relieve her anxiety and answer her questions. This book is a genuine attempt to fulfil this need.

Modern antenatal care and the work of midwives and doctors, aim at avoiding complications and treating unusual conditions before they become dangerous. In this book I have described the course of normal pregnancy and also the abnormalities that may occur. The latter are included, not because they are common, but so that they are understood and the various precautions and treatments carried out by medical advisers are appreciated.

The final authority on any individual pregnancy is, of course, the doctor or midwife in charge of the pregnant woman. I have made every effort to be unbiased in presenting facts and have tried to be impartial about the various schools of thought and the different ways of coping with women throughout the three stages of reproduction. There are undoubtedly sections and statements in this book with which many doctors, midwives, pregnant women and mothers will disagree, but it is impossible, in one volume, to be completely comprehensive in dealing with the subject of pregnancy and the many different treatments used in its care. There will always be differences of opinion among doctors and midwives on certain topics, and if a mother receives advice or treatment differing from that which I have mentioned, she can rest assured that it is well considered and as efficient as any other.

It has naturally been necessary to include many units of measurement and those that will be most useful to the reader have been chosen; neither system, metric or imperial, has been used exclusively and conversion tables have therefore been included. Technical words and phrases are explained when they first occur in the text and again in the glossary for easy reference. I have stayed throughout the book with the conventional use of the word 'he' as the neuter pronoun for the baby merely to keep the book uncomplicated.

GORDON BOURNE

Preface to the 1984 edition

It is now twelve years since *Pregnancy* was first published. During this time many minor alterations have been made to the text and many helpful suggestions submitted by both men and women who have read the book have been included.

Repetitions within the text have not been altered because few people read *Pregnancy* from cover to cover. It is used by most people as a sort of reference book: to be read at different stages of pregnancy or as problems or questions arise.

This revision is quite extensive and includes a new chapter, 'Monitoring the Fetus'. The use of ultrasound, which is now an accepted part of antenatal care, has been recognized throughout the book, as have other advances in technology. New attitudes towards pregnancy and childbirth have also been included. Whilst every attempt has been made to be factual and impartial when describing those areas in which differences of opinion are very real, and to provide accurate information upon which the pregnant woman and her family may depend, the book continues to project the orthodox approach to pregnancy and labour.

The problems of intrauterine growth retardation are described more fully, as are some of the infections to which a new-born infant may be subjected. Changing attitudes towards labour itself and induction of labour, as well as alterations in management, are described. Epidural anaesthesia for Caesarean section is being requested more frequently and this is reflected in the increasing influence and participation of both husband and family, which are a welcome trend in modern maternity care. Prematurity and the onset of premature labour continue to be a major problem and this is discussed together with the ever increasing efficiency and success in the treatment of small babies. A small section is devoted to 'test-tube' babies, the use of prostaglandin, alterations in conception control, smoking and alcohol.

Chapter 16, 'Maternity Benefits', is based on Department of Health and Social Security leaflets MV.11 and NI.17A, and Department of Employment leaflet PL710, by kind permission of the Controller of Her Majesty's Stationery Office.

The increasing interest in pregnancy and childbirth over the past few years is to be encouraged and I hope that this book will go some way towards satisfying the demand for information and knowledge.

G.B.

1 Pregnancy

Importance of information

Pregnancy is associated with many complex and interrelated changes that occur throughout the entire body. These may be both physical and psychological and whilst some of them become obvious early in pregnancy, others do not become noticeable until pregnancy is well advanced. It must also be remembered that there are many minor alterations in bodily function of which the pregnant woman is completely unaware. Doctors and midwives can understand only some of these changes, many are inadequately understood and there are still some, mostly minor, about which very little or nothing is known and doubtless others as yet unrecognized even by medical science. It is all the more confusing because one woman will demonstrate one particular change more than another and any one woman will nearly always experience different phenomena during subsequent pregnancies and labours. You frequently hear a woman saying 'I feel much more tired in this pregnancy than in the last one' or 'During my first pregnancy I felt sick in the morning and during my second pregnancy I had no nausea at all and during this one I feel sick in the evening.'

There is a very close relationship between the physical and psychological reactions to pregnancy and, although it is a normal physiological process, it must also be accepted that some women will undergo a profound change in their emotional state as well as in their psychological balance.

It is important to appreciate that neither the physical nor the psychological changes end with the onset of labour or even with delivery. From a purely legal point of view it is accepted in Great Britain that psychological changes associated with pregnancy may continue for at least six months after delivery, and it is probably true that the physical and psychological equilibrium of the mother does not return to normal until up to a year after delivery, particularly if she breast-feeds for several months.

To understand what is happening during pregnancy is half-way towards enjoying a happy and successful pregnancy, but it is important that your husband and your family should appreciate why you are asked to attend the antenatal clinic. There is little point in trying to restrict your weight if the rest of the family insist on making you eat 'food for two'.

The importance of information is paramount. If you understand about your pregnancy and what is happening to your mind and body you will have more confidence in yourself and in your ability to produce a baby

Furthermore, you will not be afraid of the unknown, of your labour or delivery.

Doctors and midwives can only do a certain amount to guide and help you. The more you know about the whole process of producing a baby, the easier will be their important duty of caring for you, because you will understand what they want you to do and why.

Don't read medical textbooks

There is nothing secret in medical textbooks. You can see them in your local library or bookshop, or if you happen to be near a university you will nearly always find that there is a specialized bookshop which sells educational books. Most textbooks on obstetrics, midwifery and gynaecology deal with the abnormal: they are written for medical students and pupil midwives who must be taught how to prevent complications from occurring as well as how to deal with them should they arise. The great art, indeed the whole basis, of modern midwifery is one of preventive medicine and early treatment, designed to stop any complication from developing. Do not settle down to some good solid reading about a rather frightening complication that you imagine might be affecting you. British medical textbooks have a very wide circulation throughout the world, especially in countries where medical services are less developed and places where antenatal clinics are unknown. Our own doctors and midwives often visit such countries, and have to know how to cope with many of the complications not normally seen in Britain. Similarly, our medical schools and hospitals have to teach doctors and midwives from these countries how to deal with their native problems when they do arise. Many complications of pregnancy and childbirth are, however, no longer seen in this country except in those now mercifully rare instances where a patient refuses any form of antenatal supervision. Complicated obstetric operations and forcible delivery involving danger of damage to the baby (or his mother) have now been eliminated by the safety of Caesarean section, and the appropriate instruments for performing those outdated procedures will be found only in the museums of our medical schools.

Emotional changes in pregnancy

A woman's basic personality will not be changed during her pregnancy, but subtle and minor alterations will certainly occur. All women tend to become emotionally unstable at times when their hormone levels are either changing or at their highest, such as puberty, pregnancy, the menopause and also immediately before the onset of each menstrual period. It is well known that the majority of impetuous actions and crimes committed by women occur during the week immediately before menstruation.

The idea that your child is growing inside you is sufficient to create a degree of emotional instability, and the rapid rise in hormone levels during the first three months of pregnancy is a valid medical reason for all the emotional changes that may occur during this time. It is common for a girl who is highly delighted with her pregnancy and has few worries to burst into tears without the slightest provocation and to recover her normal gay personality a few minutes later. Women who are normally vivacious may be given to periods of depression, irritability, anxiety and ill-temper and those who are usually placid and quiet may have bursts of emotional irritability or even anger of which they are normally considered to be almost incapable.

In early pregnancy nausea and vomiting may produce a mild state of anxiety or depression. These are relieved when the nausea and vomiting cease at about the 14th week of pregnancy, but in the earlier stages most women require assurance that the abnormal amount of nausea and sickness is perfectly normal and will not harm either them or their baby.

The management of her other children my prove particularly difficult for the newly pregnant woman. Especially in the early stages, their annoying habits and characteristics with which she can normally cope quite adequately will irritate her beyond her self-control. If she is not very careful, her attitude towards her children will change into something that they consider to be completely unreasonable and she will find they associate her irritability and anger with her pregnancy; they will resent the new baby long before it arrives.

For similar reasons, even the most highly competent and efficient woman may find that her judgment is impaired. She may be inclined to make hasty decisions, her reasoning may not be as rational as it would normally be and her conclusions may be inaccurate and incorrect. It would, of course, be wrong to suggest that pregnant women are incapable, but a word of warning about emotional instability should make them consider things more carefully and may prevent them from doing things and making decisions which they might subsequently consider to be unwise.

At the end of the 14th week of pregnancy, the nausea and sickness, as well as some of the lethargy, usually disappear. The appetite returns and with it there is frequently a complete change in attitude. It is at this stage that the characteristic good looks of pregnancy appear and with this also comes a more tolerant and understanding attitude.

The baby will first be felt moving somewhere between the 16th and the 20th week. For the first time the woman is aware of the presence of a baby inside her uterus with which she can associate her pregnancy and all her symptoms. Her baby is now a reality for whom preparation must be made and over whom care must be taken. Her judgment will return to normal and although her personality may show a certain amount of emotional fluctuation, this will be less marked than previously.

The 28th week of pregnancy marks the date of viability, after which the baby is theoretically capable of leading a separate existence. In this last part of the pregnancy the mother is often anxious about the normality of the baby as well as apprehensive about its arrival. As the weeks progress the enlargement of the abdomen, together with a natural lethargy and tiredness, will often make her feel clumsy and irritable. She will become more dependent upon those around her.

As the expected date of confinement draws near she may well be subject to what is known as 'the nesting instinct'. This is a very real phenomenon in which the pregnant woman will spring-clean the house and check that everything is ready for the new baby. She will be visiting the antenatal clinic more frequently and establishing a much closer relationship with the doctors and nurses who are to take care of her during her labour. This gradually creates a confidence which is of the utmost importance as it will go a long way towards allaying her fears and apprehensions.

Unthinking friends and relations may well regale her with unpleasant or even horrifying stories of their own experiences during pregnancy and childbirth. These will undoubtedly result in some increase in anxiety about her own welfare and she should have no hesitation whatsoever in asking as many questions as she wishes when she visits the antenatal clinic. Most of her fears will be absolutely groundless but it is very difficult for a woman so far advanced in pregnancy and feeling so intimately involved with the symptoms to differentiate truth from fiction.

The natural tiredness and clumsiness associated with the last stages of pregnancy will affect the mother's mental outlook. She will tend to become bored with the continuation of the pregnancy and may become mildly depressed as a result of her inability to wear nice clothes or engage in her usual social activities. The last month of pregnancy frequently requires quite a lot of gentle encouragement as well as firm assurance. Depression often results from disappointment if labour does not start on the expected day, and as time passes with no sign of labour this is not helped by well-meaning friends, neighbours and members of the family who want to know why the baby is not yet born. 'Are you still there?' is a kindly question calculated with infinite finesse to depress any anxious and long-suffering woman who is one or two weeks past her expected date of confinement.

Apart from these special times, it is well known that a pregnant woman's personality becomes fragile, particularly in labour. An enquiring comment made with intended kindness may be misinterpreted as severe personal criticism and the reaction is a flood of tears.

But some of the emotional changes experienced during pregnancy are simply the result of boredom. This may be automatically corrected towards the end by the natural 'nesting instinct' which seems to overtake most women, and they busily clean and prepare for the new baby. Earlier in the pregnancy, if they are not working at their normal job, it is often very beneficial to take up some occupation or part-time work.

Taking tranquillizers during pregnancy is not usually necessary nor is it desirable. They should never be taken without first consulting the doctor. If a state of anxiety or depression persists the doctor and midwife should be notified. Reassurance is usually all that is needed but a small dose of a mild and innocuous antidepressant drug over three or four days can easily reverse a quite marked depression and anxiety can be relieved by a small dose of tranquillizer.

Since time began it has been the custom to consider that a baby is affected by his mother's emotions during pregnancy—that strange things might happen if she is frightened by peculiar sights or particular thoughts. This is untrue, but some authorities do argue to the contrary. There is no evidence that emotional disturbances of any sort can affect the welfare of the baby in the uterus, or that distressing sights or thoughts can affect the baby either mentally or physically. Excessive crying or sobbing cannot adversely affect a baby.

However, some women who suffer from a severe and profound shock, or who are involved in accidents which entail a physical shaking but do not suffer any severe or specific injury, may either miscarry or start premature labour. But it is seldom that even quite severe accidents have any effect on a pregnancy.

Old wives' tales

The problem of 'old wives' tales' is really one of confidence, simply because the majority of old wives' tales are essentially destructive or demoralizing. It is all rather like the old magpie proverb 'One for sorrow, two for joy', because anyone who believes in this ancient adage is bound to have an unhappy time. The chance of seeing one magpie is infinitely greater than the chance of seeing two. So we find that all the old wives' tales concerning pregnancy or the unborn baby are invariably messages of gloom and, because of this, there is no intention here of repeating any of them in detail.

The majority of people today realize that these old wives' tales are a cartload of rubbish but even so they leave behind them an unhappy legacy that is not difficult to understand. The pregnant woman is in a somewhat unstable emotional state and incredibly sensitive. She frequently has fears and apprehensions concerning not only herself but also her unborn baby. Any suggestions that something might happen to affect adversely either her or her baby will automatically arouse a little ripple of anxiety or fear. If the suggestion is repeated several times and perhaps with increasing conviction, then the anxiety becomes very real and the fear tends to become accepted.

One can easily imagine a comparatively short girl of 5 ft 2 in in height who is married to a comparatively tall man of 6 ft 2 in being told on repeated occasions 'My dear, you'll have such a big baby and you will have such a difficult time.' Eventually the poor girl comes to believe that she is going to have a huge baby and is going to have a very difficult labour and even when she is assured that this is completely untrue it may not entirely relieve her anxiety. In fact, women grow babies to suit themselves and not to suit anybody else, and a small girl in this country behaves in exactly the same way as a small girl in Japan. She produces a baby appropriate to her size. Furthermore, the size of a baby at birth has no relationship to his eventual size as an adult. This trivial example is given just to illustrate how easily people's fears can be aroused and how difficult it is to allay them.

Old wives' tales and their disastrous effect may even begin a long time before the onset of the first pregnancy. Most doctors have had to reassure comparatively young girls of fifteen or sixteen that just because they happen to have painful periods this does not mean that they are going to have painful labours inflicted upon them, or that someone who has a tilted uterus is going to suffer from disastrous infertility which may in turn be followed by recurrent miscarriages.

If you have heard some story or tale that has caused you any apprehension, then mention it the next time you see your doctor or midwife.

Old wives' tales are one thing, but the wicked tongue that tells nothing but stories of doom, disaster and death is entirely different. There must be precious few women who have gone through their first pregnancy without being told some horrifying story by one of their 'friends' or 'elders and betters'. Why do women have to recount such stories to one another, especially when the majority of them are blatantly untrue? Even the most sensible of pregnant women seldom have the presence of mind to tell the purveyors of these wicked stories to be quiet, and however much a woman may laugh about the story it nearly always sows a tiny little seed of doubt in her mind; doubt about herself, or her baby, or perhaps even the ambulance service, or the nurse or doctor or some other member of the staff of the hospital, or some aspect of the hospital itself. Such a comparatively simple remark like 'My dear, I suppose there is nothing that can be done about it at this late stage, but they did leave Mary Jane alone for hours' is the type of comment that it is impossible to disprove and will require massive reassurance to correct. If it is not corrected, even just a niggling thought two or three times a day that perhaps one might be left alone for hours in labour is detrimental to the trust and confidence a woman should have at this time. Probably more is done by wicked women with their malicious lying tongues to harm the confidence and happiness of pregnant women than by any other single factor.

Why do they do this? Perhaps it is some form of sadism or as a revenge payment for an unhappy experience of their own that they wish to magnify and share with someone who cannot answer back.

The mother's attitude to pregnancy

Pregnancy, particularly when it is your first baby, will bring a feeling of happiness and satisfaction which may be mingled with mild apprehension. Perhaps the most remarkable thing about human nature is that, being individuals, we are all different in our mental and physical make-up, so that we all react in different ways to altering circumstances. Some women are eager to meet the challenge of motherhood which, for them, brings immense fulfilment and is the ultimate process whereby they become complete human beings For others pregnancy may be unexpected or unwanted, or it may be just an inconvenience, and in such circumstances mental attitudes will show a wide range of variation. You will have to consider making slight adjustments in almost everything you do during the different stages of your pregnancy. The immense advantage of plenty of encouragement and support cannot be overemphasized.

It is not unnatural for most pregnant women to experience vague misgivings or anxieties from time to time and no matter how ridiculous these may appear they do nevertheless create a very real problem. A lot of fears about pregnancy and labour are triggered off by old wives' tales and half-truths which have little relation to reality. These stories are certainly either grossly exaggerated or blatantly untrue but may still create a state of anxiety about the pregnancy. Your own experience of pregnancy and childbirth will make you realize how unfounded were your fears.

A woman's attitude to pregnancy cannot be defined. The emotional changes alone are far from being understood and every sentence in this book has a bearing on her approach to childbirth. Small wonder that there is no simple answer to all her problems though many are readily solved. You are indeed a lucky woman if those around you make an effort to appreciate the problems that beset you during your pregnancy.

The mother's attitude to labour

The word labour as a synonym for the process of delivery is unfortunate and it is equally unfortunate that as far back as recorded evidence is available it has been associated with pain, fear, anxiety and sometimes disaster. Modern medicine has ensured the welfare of a woman in labour as well as that of her child, even when complications arise, but in the vast majority of labours which are free from complications modern medical aids not only ensure the safety of the mother and her child but also ensure that she will receive all the help and assistance that she requires. Apprehension of labour is often a fear of the unknown. There is no point, however, in saying to a woman who is in the advanced stages of pregnancy that her labour will be simple and easy if, since childhood, she has been indoctrinated with the idea that labour will be long, painful and tedious.

Every woman must understand what is happening to her during pregnancy, in order to appreciate the changes that are occurring and not be afraid of them. But it is even more important that she should be carefully instructed about the later stages of pregnancy and labour, for it is only by this means that she can recognize the normal processes of her body and gain confidence in her own ability to produce a child without undue pain or discomfort. Once this confident state is achieved the whole process of pregnancy and labour becomes immeasurably easier, not only for the mother but also for the doctors and midwives who are looking after her.

The emotional distress which may accompany pregnancy, labour and the puerperium is nearly always the result of ignorance, and this distress can be alleviated by careful understanding of the processes that are occurring, as well as by the quiet reassurance of those in attendance.

It is equally true to state that emotional strain causes physical tiredness or even distress. The importance, therefore, of instilling confidence and reassurance into the pregnant woman cannot be overemphasized.

The creation of life and the growth of a baby within a uterus is indeed an incredible, wonderful and extraordinary event. Anyone who has actually seen a baby delivered will never cease to marvel at the myriad factors which must have taken place all at exactly the correct time to produce this fabulous new-born creature. That this chain of events can proceed normally, naturally and to its final culmination with the natural delivery of a normal infant is by far the greatest wonder of the world, and it is right that a woman should always have a twinge of anxiety concerning not only the welfare of her unborn or newly born child but also his normality. This is natural motherhood.

Most women are endowed with a natural confidence in their own ability to produce perfectly normal children as and when they require them but during an actual pregnancy fears and doubts may cloud or override the confidence of prepregnant days. It is hoped that by reading this book carefully the woman, her husband and her family will learn what her pregnancy, delivery and the puerperium are all about, and that with this knowledge the pregnant woman will gain confidence in her own ability to proceed naturally through her pregnancy, delivery and the post-delivery phase assisted and helped by her family. It cannot be stressed too strongly that confidence comes directly from knowledge, and confidence in your ability comes from knowledge and reassurance.

The father's role in pregnancy

The attitude of many potential fathers to pregnancy and labour has undergone a dramatic change over the past few years. This has been brought about by several factors. Firstly, the press, radio and television have discussed pregnancy, labour, delivery and breast feeding much more openly. This has been the result of a demand for knowledge by the public as well as a general feeling that part of the secrecy and mumbo-jumbo should be swept away from the process of childbirth. This desire for knowledge which at first affected only the women did in fact spread very quickly to their husbands and partners so that an increasing number of men are now taking an interest in pregnancy and even more are being encouraged to do so. In the past, pregnancy and child-bearing have been regarded as a private part of a woman's life in which the men in the family have been encouraged to take very little interest. Many of the changes that take place in a woman's body during pregnancy are not confined to the reproductive organs, and almost every tissue and organ responds to the stimulus of pregnancy. An understanding husband or partner who knows about these changes can give much help and support to his wife at this time in her life. Pregnancy is not an illness and, despite the fact that many women become emotional and irritable while they are pregnant, it is amazing how well equipped they are to meet the increased demands which pregnancy imposes. However, it is an immense comfort to have a husband or partner who understands.

A second, but no less important factor, was the feeling of all who look after pregnant women that it was high time that they understood more about themselves, their pregnancies and their labours, because good ante-natal care, which is preventive medicine, can only be conducted really efficiently with the full cooperation of all concerned. The more the woman can be instructed, the more easily will her full cooperation be obtained.

Thirdly, and again not in order of precedence, came the influence of 'natural childbirth' and 'psychoprophylaxis', both of which imply, and indeed demand, a certain amount of knowledge concerning pregnancy and labour. The women who were learning and being taught in classes started talking to their husbands and partners who gradually became interested, so that slowly a situation has evolved in which nearly all the courses of antenatal instruction include a fathers' evening, which men are encouraged to attend and at which they may be shown a film and are certainly given instruction in, and encouraged to ask questions about, pregnancy and labour.

Today it is becoming increasingly common for a father to be present during his wife's labour and delivery. If you intend to be present you should learn as much about pregnancy, labour and delivery as you possibly can and should try to become as knowledgeable as your wife. If you do not intend to be present for her delivery but wish to be present during part of her labour, this still applies. If you do not wish to be present during any part of her labour she will still require your help and support throughout the whole of her pregnancy and to achieve this you must know what is happening to her both physically and emotionally so that you will be better able to help her.

Here are set out a few facts concerning the father's approach to pregnancy, labour and delivery, but if you are really serious in your desire to help your wife you must read most of this book and seek special instruction elsewhere.

The emotional aspect of pregnancy is a very complex subject. There is no doubt that the nervous system is more sensitive during pregnancy making women sometimes seem almost unreasonable and occasionally they will not even respond to logical argument. They may also have vague fears of pain, fear of the process of birth and fear of the unknown, and it is for these reasons that every woman needs the stabilizing influence and sympathetic understanding of her husband or partner. The expectant father has a very important role to play and a great deal of satisfaction and happiness can be achieved by sharing some of the problems and helping to solve some of the difficulties that his partner will encounter.

Modern family planning is so efficient that you should be able to sit down with your wife and plan not only the number of babies that you would like to have but more or less the exact time of their arrival. If your wife or partner is working then her present earnings, together with her future prospects, will be an important consideration in reaching your decision. Providing a pregnancy is normal (and there is no reason to suppose it will not be), there is no reason why your wife or partner should not continue to work up to the 32nd week of her pregnancy. Of course the decision to continue working depends on how far she has to travel, what work she has to do and how her pregnancy progresses.

Probably the first indication she will have of the possibility, or likelihood, of pregnancy is when a period does not arrive on time. The absence of the period may or may not be associated with other symptoms such as early morning sickness. The earliest time that a diagnosis of pregnancy can be established satisfactorily is about twelve days after the first day of the missed period. A urine test performed at this time is the commonest and the easiest way in which an early pregnancy can be confirmed. A special blood test (see page 100) will confirm the presence of a pregnancy as early as five days after fertilization or on the nineteenth day of a regular 28-day cycle.

The various changes your wife or partner may undergo are discussed under their different headings in this book. You should try to understand the emotional changes that occur in early pregnancy and look after her accordingly. She may suffer from severe symptoms of nausea and early morning sickness and may be increasingly tired, especially during the daytime. Such symptoms which make her irritable and lethargic are quite understandable and you should do your best to help her, even if some of your social engagements and parties have to suffer. If she 'goes off' alcohol or coffee, or anything else, do not be surprised. Alternatively, you may find that there is very little in the way of symptoms of early pregnancy and in fact very little change takes place either in her emotional state or in her daily life. Even so, please try to remember the physiological changes that are inevitably taking place in her body and that minor emotional changes are also occurring although they may not seem obvious.

Providing the pregnancy is normal and there has been no earlier history of miscarriage, sexual intercourse can continue as usual during early pregnancy, although you should treat your wife or partner particularly gently and remember that her breasts may become painful and tender.

The morning sickness and other symptoms of early pregnancy disappear at the end of the 14th week and the three months of middle pregnancy are the time during which your wife or partner will feel at her best.

During the last three months of pregnancy you should be prepared to accept more responsibility for day-to-day management around the house and home. You must make sure that all the necessary arrangements have been made for the new baby's arrival and that all other arrangements are complete and satisfactory. If your wife or partner is going into hospital you must make sure that she has everything ready and packed, that the ambulance number is readily available beside the telephone or, if you do not have a telephone, that you have made arrangements to use a neighbour's or that you have some coins put away to use in the local phone kiosk. If you are taking your wife or partner to hospital by car, make sure that you know the best and the most direct route and that you know the correct entrance at the hospital to which to take her. Make sure that you always have enough petrol in the car for getting both to and back from the hospital.

Your wife or partner will probably be attending a course of antenatal classes which will include classes in mothercraft and relaxation. If there is a fathers' evening, you should attend it. Plenty of other fathers will be present and you will find all the staff helpful and anxious to answer any questions that you may have. Incidentally, the evening before you go to the fathers' class it is a good idea to sit down with your wife or partner and make a note of any questions that you may wish to ask.

When your wife or partner attended the booking clinic she was probably asked, or she has herself enquired, about your being present during her labour or delivery. You and she will by now have reached a decision about this and if you have decided to be present during her labour and delivery you may have some additional questions to ask when you attend the fathers' class. Most maternity units allow fathers to be present during both labour and delivery, and in some hospitals fathers may be present for forceps delivery or during Caesarean section. If you are reading this book, then you will have a considerable interest in understanding all about pregnancy and you will have sufficient knowledge to realize that delivery can be a most exciting experience. Some women like their husband or partner to be with them, whilst others prefer that they should not be. Whatever decision you reach do not let the horror stories put you off. If your wife or partner wants you to be with her, then your presence while she is in labour will do more to help her than any other single factor and there is very little that can give her greater joy and happiness than that you should share this unique experience with her. Whether you are present or not is entirely up to you and your wife or partner. Do not be persuaded by other people's stories or by current trends in fashion.

The father's approach to labour

Your approach to labour will already have been decided by the time your wife or partner goes into labour. Even if you plan not to attend the labour or the delivery you should learn about the signs of the onset of labour (Chapter 24). If you plan to be with your wife or partner during her labour and delivery then you may have already attended one or more of the antenatal classes and learnt a considerable amount about what to expect, but more important you will have been told what is expected of you and will have received instruction during the classes accordingly.

When the expected day of confinement arrives, it is only natural that everyone should expect labour to start, but this does not always happen because the expected date is only an approximate or average calculation of the expected time of delivery. Try to prevent your wife or partner from building herself up to a psychological climax for the great day, because the great day may easily come and go without any sign of labour commencing, and when this happens it tends to be followed by a period of depression and disappointment. Of course the eager enquiries of neighbours and friends like 'Oh Mrs Jones, haven't you started yet?' or 'Mrs Jones, are you still here?', while they are meant very kindly only serve to deepen the depression. It can sometimes be helpful to be a little bit misleading and to suggest to people that the baby is due a week later than, in actual fact, it is expected.

When labour begins you should telephone the hospital to inform them that you are bringing your wife or partner and to let them know her condition so that they will be prepared. They will also give you any advice over the telephone you may require. Your arrival at hospital will be expected and your wife or partner will be taken by a midwife for her routine admission, while you are asked to wait. After a while you will be invited to join your wife or partner either in the ward or in the room reserved for patients during the first stage of labour.

Every hospital is slightly different and the routine in every hospital or maternity unit is also slightly different. It is not possible, therefore, to describe in detail what may be required during the first stage of labour. You will have been instructed about this during the antenatal classes or you will be told after your arrival in hospital. If you are staying with your wife or partner then she will probably be quite happy to have you just sitting in the room with her although she may want to talk for a bit, may want you to read to her or may just want you to be there while she goes to sleep. The essential thing in early labour is companionship.

As labour advances she will want more encouragement and support, together with help with her exercises if she has been taught how to do them. Even if you have not been specifically instructed you can easily encourage her to relax during contractions and make soothing kindly remarks when the contraction has ceased. You must help your wife or partner with any specific instructions that she has received from the midwife or the doctor and make sure that she has as much mental support as you can possibly supply.

During the second stage of labour and when your wife or partner is moved into the delivery room, if you are going to be present at the delivery you will go with her and having been properly gowned will probably be given a seat close to her head so that you can either hold her hand or help her with her breathing or analgesia. Some form of pain-killing drug may have been given earlier in labour so that she is not quite as alert as she would normally be and during the second stage of labour not many women have much time for the niceties of behaviour. You are not in the way; someone will tell you exactly where to sit, but if no one seems to take any notice of you this means that all is quite satisfactory and everyone is happy with your presence. You can repeat the doctor's or midwife's instructions to your wife or partner and make sure that she does her best to obey them. When the moment of delivery arrives you will be just as overwhelmed as your wife or partner and will be able to share with her that extraordinary moment when you hear your child cry for the first time. A woman's emotions at the time of delivery are extremely complex and frequently very upset. Do not be surprised if you find your own emotions also somewhat disturbed and disorganized.

Your other children's attitude to your pregnancy

Older children in the family may suffer from the arrival of the new baby who becomes the centre of attention and not only does he take up all mother's time but father also shows a greater interest in him and may unintentionally neglect the other members of the family. The other children may develop feelings of resentment and jealousy particularly when relatives and neighbours call especially to see the new baby and to bring him presents.

It is small wonder that if these circumstances exist the older children rapidly become jealous of the new arrival. When such jealousy does occur it makes life much more difficult for the mother since the management of the jealous older children as well as of the new-born baby is not only a difficult but a most time-consuming task. This jealousy can be avoided in

the majority of instances if a little careful thought and planning are introduced fairly early in the pregnancy and it is well worth any time and effort
that may be spent in trying to ensure that older children are not jealous
of the new baby. The idea of a new baby should be carefully introduced
to the mind of the older child and the stage in pregnancy at which this is
done will vary according to age. The older the child, the earlier it should
begin, but the general idea is to stimulate the child into wanting a brother
or sister. Once the desire has been created then he should be told in
simple terms that the baby is growing in mummy's tummy so that he will
gradually accept the enlargement of mummy's tummy as being his brother
or sister. This is particularly important since the pregnancy may limit the
mother's activities with her child. Similarly, the child may accompany her
to the antenatal clinic, in which case some explanation will be required for
the attention of the doctors and nurses, or alternatively the child must be
looked after by someone else whilst the mother goes to the clinic. Some
simple explanation should be easily and readily given, such as telling the
child that the doctors and nurses are seeing that his brother or sister is
growing satisfactorily and keeping quite well. He should be encouraged
to help with all the preparations for the baby and a short time before the
expected date of confinement should go with his mother to buy a present
for the new baby.

Perhaps the most important moment in introducing a new baby into a
home is the time when the older child first sees his mother after her
delivery. Let us assume that you have had your baby in hospital and that
your child is coming to visit you the day after your delivery. Most maternity hospitals nowadays allow children to visit their mother and the sooner
your child can visit you the better. You will be sitting up in bed ready to
receive your visitors and your baby will be in a cot either at the end of
your bed or in the nursery. You should not have your new baby in your
arms or on the bed or immediately beside you, and your baby's cot should
contain no presents or toys whatsoever. Your child will come in with his
father and you should greet him as usual. His curiosity may get the better
of him immediately and he will either demand to see or go and look at
the new baby and give the baby his present. If he does not do this
immediately, do not worry. You can gently tell him about the new baby's
arrival and very soon his curiosity will overcome his shyness and he will
ask to see the baby. It is unlikely that he will be able to hold or cuddle
the new baby while you are in hospital, but a little touch perhaps on the
forehead will go a long way to establishing brotherly love.

A return present from the baby to the older child or children is also
essential. This may be given at their first meeting or when you return
home but it must be stressed that it is from the new baby.

The older child must be encouraged to do as much as possible for the
new baby and it must be impressed upon him that it is his baby as well
as yours. The new baby should not interfere with the regular routine of

the older children and of course love and affection must not only be divided equally but must be seen to be divided equally. It is surprising how much pleasure, joy and satisfaction will be derived from 'now please take Auntie Jane upstairs and show her your new sister'.

If the older child has been well prepared, his acceptance of the new baby will be much easier. It is inevitable that there be a twinge of jealousy occasionally and at such times you must give him special attention and reassurance of his importance. Every encouragement should be given to him in caring for the new baby, so that he rapidly loses any resentment that might initially have been present.

Discipline

The management of pregnancy and labour is no different in principle from most other things in life. If something is to be done well it requires careful thought, meticulous planning, a great deal of practice or training and the certain knowledge that imperfections can be corrected. Since it is impossible for your first pregnancy to be preceded by appropriate training, a certain amount of knowledge, understanding and discipline is an essential part of your welfare. After all, a baby requires care during pregnancy as well as after delivery. A careful pattern of behaviour will help you not only during pregnancy but especially during labour and also after delivery.

You will learn to adapt to the difficulties and to accept the changes that occur. You will learn to cooperate with your professional advisers, which becomes easier if you understand the reasons for the advice they give you and for the restrictions they place upon you. Adequate rest is important and you must not expose yourself to undue danger. Excessive weight-gain is not only damaging to yourself and your baby but is detrimental to the preservation of your figure. You will learn about the factors leading up to the onset of labour and what to expect during labour and delivery; you will then be able to exert self-discipline and control not only on your emotions but also on your reactions, and face delivery with a minimum of fear or distress, understanding and obeying instructions given to help you.

Professional help

The National Health Service provides a wide and comprehensive range of professional people and services to give you adequate help before, during and after your pregnancy. A great deal of careful thought and planning has gone into the provision of the necessary services and expert help is available not only for everything to do with your pregnancy but also for the care of your new-born baby. These facilities fall into one of three main categories. Firstly your general practitioner, secondly your local authority, and thirdly the hospital service.

Your general practitioner

Consult your general practitioner as soon as you either believe or know that you are pregnant. He may or may not deliver babies, or even look after women during their pregnancies, but these facts do not matter. Whether it is your first or your tenth baby the prime consideration is the early diagnosis of your pregnancy and a discussion with your doctor so that a decision can be reached, after due consultation, on which particular aspects of the National Health Service facilities are most suitable for the management of your own particular pregnancy.

You and your doctor may decide that he will look after you or, if he does not personally look after maternity patients, one of his general practitioner colleagues will do so. Should you decide to have your baby at home, you will be under your doctor's supervision and direction throughout your pregnancy, labour and puerperium. Many general practitioners, especially those with group practices, organize an antenatal clinic at their own surgery where your care and supervision will be shared with your community midwife.

General practitioner maternity units. One of these units may be situated in your area and if you are to have your baby in that unit your doctor will supervise your antenatal care and your confinement. These units are nearly always attached to a large hospital maternity unit and every facility, together with consultant advice, is readily available should it be required.

Shared care. If you are going to have your baby in hospital it may be decided that your antenatal care should be shared between your doctor and the hospital. When your doctor has diagnosed your pregnancy, you will visit the hospital booking clinic and thereafter visit either your doctor or the hospital according to an agreed plan which will be explained to you. If you are having 'shared care' you will be given a maternity cooperation card to be filled in by both general practitioner and hospital doctors as a record. Always keep it with you.

Local authority services

The community midwife works in close cooperation with your doctor and if you are going to have your baby at home she will share with him responsibility for your management throughout your pregnancy, delivery and for ten days after your delivery. In some areas she will be responsible for your care if you are to be delivered in a general practitioner maternity unit, or even if you are to have your baby in a consultant maternity unit.

Local authority clinics. Your local authority runs a clinic which is attended by your community midwife and a community medical officer, or perhaps your own general practitioner. You may be asked to attend this clinic for your antenatal visits if you are going to have your baby in hospital or if your own doctor does not undertake maternity care. It also provides extensive facilities for advice after your baby has been delivered and you should have no hesitation in visiting the clinic if you have any cause for worry or anxiety.

The health visitor is a trained nurse, employed by the local authority, who has undertaken specialist training in the care and development of young children. If you have your baby in hospital the health visitor will call and see you shortly after your return home. Many people do not seem to realize the lengths to which the health service goes in order to provide a complete and comprehensive service for its patients. Whether you have your baby at home or in hospital, your delivery is specially recorded and a form of notification is sent to the local medical officer of health, who in turn notifies the appropriate health visitor on his staff. In due course she will call to see you and enquire if there is any help or advice she can possibly give. She will also provide information concerning the local authority clinic where you will find her and other experts in the management and care of new-born and growing babies. If she is attached to your general practitioner's health team she will tell you when to attend his clinics and how to get help and advice whenever you need it.

The hospital service

The hospital maternity service provides for your delivery in hospital. You may attend the antenatal clinics at the hospital throughout your pregnancy or your antenatal care may be shared either by your own doctor or your local authority clinic. Following delivery you normally remain in hospital for approximately six days or, if everything is satisfactory and appropriate arrangements have been made, you may return home earlier under a system known as 'planned early discharge'. If you wish to go home shortly after your delivery you must discuss this with your community midwife and the hospital because early discharge is only possible if your community midwife can look after you at home when you have left the hospital.

Obstetric emergency service. This is a special service provided by some maternity hospitals which may be used in an emergency. It consists of a team of doctors and midwives who travel in an ambulance from a maternity unit to visit women at home if complications suddenly occur They are 'on call' for 24 hours every day.

Use the services that are available to you. If you need help or advice, ask for it. The majority of the complications of pregnancy are preventable but they can be diagnosed earlier and prevented more easily if you cooperate fully.

Inherited factors

What will your baby inherit? What will he be like? Will he be fat or thin? Will he be tall or short? Fair or dark? Will he have blue eyes like you or the athletic prowess of his father? As they sit and think and let their minds wander over the whole range of combinations that may affect, and therefore alter, the appearance and character of an unborn baby, there is usually a time when both the mother and father become more serious and perhaps a trifle anxious. Will he be normal? Will he be perfect? All mothers and certainly most fathers experience this apprehension at some time during a pregnancy and for the majority it remains a lurking anxiety that is only satisfied after the safe delivery of a healthy, normal baby. Despite the fact that 97 per cent of babies are perfectly normal, anxiety over the normality of your own child is understandable. Some people, however, cannot stop worrying about the health of their unborn child, usually because there is some disease or disorder somewhere in the family. A relative may have suffered from a nervous breakdown; a grandfather may have been a diabetic, or someone may suffer from tuberculosis or someone else from cancer. Even such minor abnormalities as colour blindness, bat ears or a crooked toe can occasionally cause immense worry and distress to a woman throughout her entire pregnancy.

A great deal of information is now available on hereditary factors, or genetics, and genetic counselling is becoming a rapidly expanding part of the medical services available to anyone who wishes to enquire into the chances of any trait, good or bad, being handed down to their baby.

Very few, if any, of us ever pause to think why we are who we are, and why we have developed into our present unique, physical and mental personalities. Few people appreciate that an average number of 400 million spermatozoa (sperms) may be deposited with each ejaculation and that most of these 400 million sperms are capable of fertilizing an ovum. The first and perhaps the greatest battle for survival is fought amongst these 400 million sperms only one of whom may succeed in fertilizing the ovum. It seems reasonable to suppose that this is one of nature's ways of eliminating both the weak and the unhealthy, for only the strongest sperms can survive the journey through the cervix, up the uterus and along the Fallopian tube to arrive in a sufficiently fit and healthy state to have the power to fertilize by penetrating the outer cell membrane of the ovum.

Each sperm, as well as every ovum, contains 23 tiny rod-shaped chromosomes, every one being formed in a chain-like structure by thousands of smaller beads known as genes. Every single detail of a person's anatomy and personality is dependent upon a specific factor present in the genes so that, at the moment of conception when the 23 chromosomes of the sperm join with the 23 chromosomes of the ovum to form the 46 chromosomes which are normally present in a human cell, a complete 'working drawing' of the subsequent human is laid down to the ultimate detail. Environment and environmental changes in the uterus, as a baby, a child, an adolescent and later throughout adult life, may change certain aspects of anatomy, physiology or personality, but nevertheless the precise form of the future is decided exactly by the genes carried within the chromosomes of both the sperm and the ovum. Half the chromosomes, including therefore half the genes, have come from the mother and half have been produced by the father. Thus a person may inherit or develop characteristics from either parent. It is this choice of inheritance from two people which gives a certain amount of latitude and variation to nature, allowing hereditary trends to develop within a species which may gradually change certain aspects of that species.

All human beings develop from one ovum and one sperm each containing half the adult number of chromosomes, so that when fertilization occurs they weld together to form a single cell containing the correct number of chromosomes required to be present in each cell of the adult body. The fortune of one's biological inheritance is even greater when one considers the process of natural selection which has also been taking place in the ovary prior to the production of a single ovum. At the time of birth the ovaries in a female baby already contain all the ova that she will produce during her adult life. The ovaries do in fact contain many more than she will require, since they each contain approximately 500,000 ova. The average woman starts to ovulate (produce ova or eggs) at about the age of 13 and thereafter ovulates once with each menstrual cycle until the age of approximately 45. Some menstrual cycles may not be associated with an ovulation, whilst others are suppressed by either pregnancy or lactation. Most women will ovulate for about 25 years, so the number of ovulating cycles will be 13 per year for 25 years—that is 325 ova, or eggs, will be produced throughout the life of the average woman. At the beginning of each menstrual cycle somewhere between 100 and 150 ova will start to ripen in each ovary but only one will be successful. Each ovum will have a slightly different gene pattern, although the number of chromosomes will be the same.

The arrangement of the genes within the chromosomes is known as the genetic pattern. Each ovum, when it starts to mature at the beginning of the menstrual cycle, will have a slightly different genetic pattern, so that when the possible variations of genetic pattern amongst the ova and the sperms are considered it is easy to realize how variations in the final form of the eventual individual may arise. Each ovum has a chance of about 1 in 150 of being selected and each sperm, 1 in 400 million, so that the overall chance of obtaining a particular genetic pattern is in the region of 1 in 100,000 million.

Genetics

Genetics is the study of heredity. Every aspect of physical appearance, emotion, character and intellect is inherited from our parents and indelibly recorded in every cell in our body in the genes that are individually characteristic of every person. They record everything in the minutest detail from the size of our ears to our ability to be a great pianist.

Genes are a miracle of nature. They form an incredibly complex computer that is built into every cell and are made up of a chemical combination of protein and nucleic acid which is able to store and classify the most complicated information. The genes are stored within the chromosomes each of which contains many thousands of genes. The chromosomes themselves are so small that they are only just visible when enlarged by a very powerful microscope.

The newly fertilized egg has 23 pairs of chromosomes of which half come from the mother and half from the father, thus creating a new individual with his own particular blueprint of genes which every cell in his body will contain for the whole of his life. In a woman each pair in the 23 sets of chromosomes is identical but in the male one pair is different and it is on this particular pair of chromosomes that the whole differentiation of sex depends. When you realize that all the differences between male and female are the result of the information stored in one pair of chromosomes, you can only imagine the amount of information stored in the remaining 22 pairs.

The genes and chromosomes are responsible for the growth and development of the baby in the uterus and throughout his childhood. They will direct his development into adult life and even into old age, making him in many respects similar to his parents but also giving him a particular combination which renders him a unique individual.

The sayings 'like mother, like daughter' and 'like father, like son' are 50 per cent correct. For every child has 50 per cent of his genes from one parent and 50 per cent from the other. Brothers and sisters on an average have half of their genes alike and may grow to be very similar, or external influences and environment may make them develop into very dissimilar people. Twins on the other hand are very special. Identical twins, who come from the same egg and the same sperm, have exactly the same genes and any differences that develop between them are due to external environment and influence. Dissimilar twins who develop simultaneously from two separate ova and two separate sperms are no more alike than any other two brothers or sisters from the same parents.

The genes in the chromosomes determine those factors such as blood groups which cannot be altered by external influence or environment, and as such they may be used in determining the possible parents of a particular child. Similarly, eye colour is unaffected by outside influences, so that parents who both have blue eyes can be almost certain of having blue-eyed children, but if they both have brown eyes then they have a small chance of having a child with blue eyes. If one parent has blue eyes and the other has brown eyes then the chances of the children having blue eyes are 50–50.

Build and personality are also inherited factors, although both of these are subject to a great deal of influence by external environment. At the end of the scale is the long, lean, quiet, nervous type of person, while at the other end is the short, square, cheerful, sociable person. While talking of build it is interesting to note that the eventual weight of a person is in no way related to his size or length at birth. Height is determined by genes (again subject to external environment) so that eventual height and build are in no way related to the length or weight of the baby at birth.

Intelligence and the ability to reason, which are supposed to make man unique among the animals on earth, are certainly inherited assets. There are many examples of the way in which brilliant brains will run through brilliant families, but it is equally true that intelligence requires training, stimulation, encouragement and opportunity to develop. Intelligence is often something quiescent or latent and requires quite a lot of encouragement to develop to its fullest possible extent, and this is where parents, relatives and school-teachers play a most important part, for it is certainly true with each and every one of us that we never really achieve our full intellectual capacity. It is also true that the more care and attention you pay to your own child's intelligence and character, then the greater will be his intellectual ability.

What about physical beauty? There is no gene for beauty alone since beauty is made up of many things and in any event is only 'in the eye of the beholder'. But it is undoubtedly true that beautiful women will probably be blessed with beautiful daughters and that handsome men will frequently have handsome sons.

How then can you know what your baby will be like? The simple answer is that you can't. He will be a mixture of you and your husband or partner and yet will be a unique individual. He will inherit some of your characteristics and some of your husband's or partner's and the combination will create an entirely new person, both physically and mentally. If there are no inherited abnormalities or diseases in your family or that of your husband or partner, your baby stands more than a 99 per cent chance of being absolutely normal. If there are inherited diseases or abnormalities, then you should read the section on genetic counselling on page 445–6 to obtain further information.

How can you affect your baby's development? On the one hand there is very little you can do to affect the development of your baby while he is still in the uterus; on the other hand, there is a great deal that you can do to help him develop normally. A baby will develop properly and grow normally provided the pregnancy is normal. You should only take those drugs that have been prescribed by your doctor or by the clinic. You should keep away from people who have infectious diseases. You should attend the antenatal clinic and do as you are instructed. You should avoid gaining too much weight and you should report abnormal symptoms as detailed in Chapter 11. You should have as much rest as possible and certainly avoid becoming overtired. Modern antenatal care is designed to ensure that you will have a normal baby and that you yourself will be fit and healthy afterwards, and if you obey these principles you can rest assured that nothing will harm your baby.

Different methods of reproduction

Many different methods of reproduction are used throughout the animal kingdom. Each is efficient for the procreation of its own particular species within its own environment. Very primitive organisms containing only one cell have no sexual apparatus, so that in order to multiply, either the cell divides down the middle, becoming two new organisms, or a small part of the cell is broken off and then develops into a new organism. A sexual reproduction of this type is extremely common, resulting in very rapid multiplication, but it lacks the great asset of selectivity and variation that are essential to evolution because each offspring is an exact replica of the parent and, with the exception of freaks which may themselves reproduce, it is difficult to develop a new strain of the organism.

The paramount asset of a species possessing two sexes is that each offspring possesses a part of two parents and it therefore allows for variation and evolution. The human method of reproduction is by no means perfect and has many theoretical disadvantages. It has evolved, however, from systems which are comparatively inefficient and it does possess the outstanding merits of selectivity combined with the protection of the progeny *in utero* for approximately 1 per cent of its natural life.

In certain forms of marine life the discharge of the ova by the female and that of the spermatozoa by the male are completely unrelated. There is no physical contact between male and female and there appears to be no awareness by either one of the other. Fertilization is not only haphazard but very uneconomic and depends for its success upon both a large number of sperms and a large number of ova. A further development leads to a definite awareness between the sexes of each other, and while there may be no physical contact, the emission of sperms and of ova occurs at the same time and in relative proximity, so that the chances of fertilization are vastly increased. External insemination during physical contact is seen in the common earthworm, where sperms are discharged into direct contact with the ova. All these methods preclude the natural selectivity of spermatozoa and ova as well as exposing both to external dangers.

Internal insemination as practised by mammals and the human is not only efficient but provides ideal protection for both the ova and the sperms.

By this method the sperms are deposited deeply in the female genital tract. This has led to the development of a specialized male organ, the penis, and a female receptive organ, the vagina. The penis is capable of penetrating into and depositing sperms within the vagina. This mechanism is highly efficient in its practical use as well as being most effective in its protection of the sperms, which are nurtured at the correct temperature under ideal environmental conditions. Its efficiency may be gauged by the fact that although the male produces many millions of spermatozoa, the female produces only one ovum, well knowing that fertilization is very likely to occur if insemination has taken place at the correct time.

Sexual desire

If a particular species is going to survive, then the vital functions performed by that species which are important for its survival must give a certain amount of pleasure; thus we find that human beings find pleasure in eating, pleasure in drinking, pleasure for the male in providing for his female and pleasure for the woman in looking after her man, and pleasure also in reproduction or in the act of sexual intercourse which leads to reproduction. The desire for sexual intercourse is known as libido. Libido varies from person to person, just as it varies with age, tiredness, health and the menstrual cycle.

In many respects, mating by humans obeys all the basic biological laws of the jungle. During the process of evolution different types of men and women have been produced. The basic type of male or female depends not only upon natural physical attributes but also upon mental outlook, with personality being perhaps the most dominant intrinsic sexual attribute. Thus there are females who range in femininity from the intensely feminine to those who are almost masculine; similarly, there are men who range from the intensely masculine at one extreme to the most effeminate at the other.

The intensely feminine female ought to be the ideal human reproductive machine and such a person will usually attract and also be attracted to the masculine type of male, so that by a process of natural selection at a biological level the ideal reproductive female is mated with the ideal reproductive male. This particular phenomenon is observed throughout the world whether it be in developing countries or in so-called civilized society, and although it is entirely subconscious it nearly always follows that, regardless of social class, the feminine female marries the masculine male and the less feminine female marries the less masculine male.

From a purely biological aspect the masculine type of female and the effeminate type of male are not good vehicles for reproduction and the procreation of the human race. Nature caters for these phenomena by introducing female homosexuality, or lesbianism, which is the association of woman with woman and is partly confined to the masculine type of female. Male homosexuality is the association of man with man and is usually, but not always, confined to the effeminate type of male. Associations of this nature are, of course, reproductively sterile which is the obvious biological solution to the problem in so far as it automatically eliminates such particular human types from procreation.

Libido is under the control of hormones and, generally speaking, the greater the production of sex hormones the greater will be the libido and, therefore, the sexual desire. As people reach the age of fifty or sixty and their hormones decline in quantity so does their sexual desire or libido. The fact that libido exists as a physiological and biological function, which varies very greatly in its intensity from person to person, is sometimes overlooked by those who criticize other people because they fail to obey the restrictive conventions which are judged necessary by modern civilized society. There can be little excuse for promiscuity, but society must appreciate that it is much more difficult for some people to remain celibate than it is for others.

It nearly always follows that libido is greater amongst more feminine females than it is amongst the less feminine variety. The same argument also applies to men. It becomes, therefore, easy to understand why it is more difficult for the feminine woman, with a high libido, to obey the restrictive conventions of modern society than it is for the masculine female, who has less libido. The feminine female must exert a greater restraint in order to obey the rules of modern civilization, whereas the less feminine woman finds obedience to these laws much more easily accomplished.

Libido in the human female is dependent upon the hormone oestrogen. The action of oestrogen among lower mammals produces oestrus which is the symptom of the mating season. Oestrus may be restricted to a short time, occurring once each year (cattle, deer), or it may occur on several occasions during the year, as seen in domesticated animals and rodents such as cats, dogs, rats and mice, etc., and also in rabbits. The third type of recurrent oestrus is that found in the higher primates (humans, monkeys) in which there is an almost continuous willingness or desire to mate and this is particularly exemplified in the human female, who exhibits a monthly cycle or a recurrent oestrus which occurs thirteen times in each year. Even during the menstrual cycle, however, the libido of the average woman will vary, usually being greater immediately before and immediately after the menstrual period. Biologically it is difficult to understand why a woman should have her times of greatest libido (or oestrus) when she is least fertile, the human female being most fertile on the 14th day of a normal 28-day menstrual cycle.

2 The Female Reproductive Organs

The pelvis

The differences in the shape of the male and female body are the result of a great many complicated factors and a whole host of minor changes which begin to take place even before birth. They affect not only the primary and secondary sex characteristics, but also the construction of bones, muscle and the various positions in which fat may accumulate. They extend to include the differences in outlook and personality.

We are here interested mainly in the bony structure of the skeleton of the woman rather than in the other distinguishing features that make her different from her male counterpart. Fig. 1 is a very simple drawing to illustrate how the bones form what is known as the pelvic girdle to join the upper part of the leg to the lower part of the spine. It would be

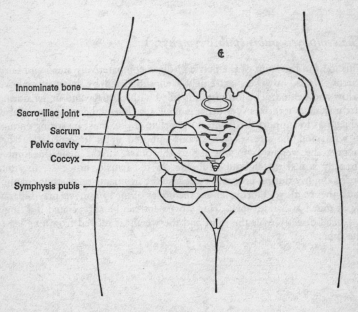

Fig. 1 The bone structure of the female pelvis

comparatively simple to design a mechanism whereby both the legs were jointed immediately to the lower end of the spine, but in order to provide a birth canal the bones are formed in the shape of a circle. The upper parts of the legs are inserted into the lower and outer portions of this circle and the upper and rear portion is attached to the spine, so that weight is transmitted from the legs, round the pelvic girdle, to the spine. The shape of the cavity of the pelvis is important because the baby must pass through it during delivery, and hence it is known as the birth canal. In the female the cavity of the pelvis is round and smooth, whereas in the male it tends to be more heart-shaped and distorted by several bony protuberances.

The pelvic girdle is made up of three bones—the sacrum at the back and two innominate bones, one at each side. The innominate bones join in front at the symphysis pubis and they join the sacrum at what are known as the sacro-iliac joints. The coccyx is the rudimentary tail at the lower end of the sacrum.

The size of the cavity of the pelvis has to be sufficiently large for the baby's head to pass unimpeded and at the same time to accommodate the pelvic organs. Fig. 2 illustrates a side-view of the pelvis. The cavity is not a straight tubular structure as so many people imagine, but is short in front and long at the back, so that once a baby's head has entered the pelvis it has to turn through an angle of 90° before it is delivered.

The symphysis pubis (pubic symphysis)

This joint in the front of the pelvic girdle is comparatively small and fairly narrow. It is, however, extremely well supported by ligaments above, below and behind. The joint itself is filled with cartilage and under normal circumstances it moves very little, if at all. Obviously the symphysis pubis, which has to support the front of the pelvic girdle, must be strong enough to withstand the stresses and strains imposed upon it, especially when moving the weight from one leg to the other. In the male the joint is virtually sealed throughout adult life. In the female, however, the joint opens slightly during pregnancy because the ligaments relax, thus enabling the bones to move. During labour the bones of the symphysis may separate by as much as half an inch. This movement can be appreciated if a finger is placed directly over the joint and the weight is moved from one leg to the other.

The sacrum

The sacrum is the curved bone which forms the rear part of the pelvic girdle. It consists of five vertebrae that have been fused together and joins with the spine itself above and the coccyx below. On either side it is attached to the innominate bones by means of the sacro-iliac joints. The size of the brim or inlet of the pelvis depends on the breadth of the sacrum, while the size of the cavity depends on its curvature. The sacrum should be broad, well curved and tilted well backwards in order to form a generous pelvic cavity. If it is unduly narrow then the size of the brim of the pelvis is restricted, or if it is flat the cavity of the pelvis itself is reduced.

The coccyx

The coccyx is the human's vestigial tail. It is of no real importance and is deflected backwards when the baby's head passes into the outlet of the pelvis during delivery.

The sacro-iliac joints

The long and complicated sacro-iliac joints which are situated between the sacrum and the innominate bones on either side are held firmly together by ligaments and fibrous tissue. The whole weight of the body is transmitted through them since they connect the spine and the legs, and it is for this reason that they do not permit any movement to occur after adolescence, except during pregnancy, when their supporting ligaments and fibrous tissue soften and lengthen to allow the symphysis pubis in the front of the pelvis to open slightly and increase (at least temporarily) the size of the cavity of the pelvis. This movement is comparatively small and takes place only during the latter part of pregnancy. The joints fuse again shortly after delivery.

The ligaments

There are obviously a large number of very strong ligaments supporting the joints in the pelvis, because they have to transmit the whole weight of the body to and from the legs. The ligaments that support the symphysis pubis and the sacro-iliac joints are of the utmost importance but there are also strong ligaments that bridge the spaces on the side wall of the pelvis between the lower part of the sacrum and the innominate bones

The birth canal

The birth canal extends from the inlet or brim of the pelvis to the pelvic outlet (fig. 2). Its direction changes through one complete right angle as

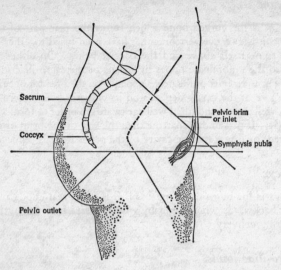

Fig 2   The birth canal

it travels through the pelvic cavity, the symphysis pubis being very short and the sacrum long, and it necessarily follows that the baby himself has to turn through a right angle as he passes through the pelvic cavity during labour. If the pelvic brim were at right angles to the mother's spine, so that the baby could fall directly downwards out of the abdomen, it would mean that the support of the pelvic floor would be very inefficient, whereas the mechanism of having the pelvic brim tilted on the spine ensures that all the contents of the abdomen do not drop straight out as if through a trap door when the baby is delivered.

The pelvic floor

The pelvic floor consists of a layer of muscle and fibrous tissue which extends across the lower part of the bony pelvis from the lower edge of the symphysis pubis to the tip of the sacrum. It is a complicated and important structure permitting the passage of urine and faeces and is perforated in front by the urethra leading down from the bladder, and behind by the rectum and anal canal. The vagina perforates the pelvic floor at approximately its midpoint. It would be difficult to design a man-made structure to be perforated by the urethra, vagina and rectum and yet to be strong enough to prevent all the abdominal organs from falling out of the bottom of the pelvis. It must also be remembered that the pressure within the abdomen, and therefore on the pelvic floor, increases to quite

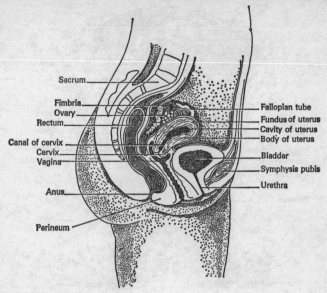

Fig. 3 The female pelvic organs

an extraordinary degree during coughing or sneezing, as well as during exercise and especially when straining to open the bowels.

The main structure of the pelvic floor is a pair of muscles called the levator ani. These stretch from each side wall of the pelvis, joining together in mid-line to form a type of hammock or sling across the pelvic outlet, and are supported by layers of fibrous tissue both above and below. During the actions of coughing and sneezing the levator ani muscles actually contract and thus give a special support to the pelvic outlet. The fact that these muscles can relax in order to allow the baby to pass through the pelvis is truly remarkable. As the baby's head passes through the pelvic floor the levator ani muscles and their associated fascia are folded sideways against the walls of the pelvis and, providing they are not badly damaged, they will rapidly return to their normal and natural state after delivery. Postnatal exercises are, however, most important in restoring the tone and strength of the muscles.

The vulva

The external genitalia are collectively known as the vulva which consists of the labia majora, the labia minora, and the clitoris, together with the perineum behind and the pubic pad of fat covered by pubic hair in front. The labia majora, forming the major protection to the vaginal entrance,

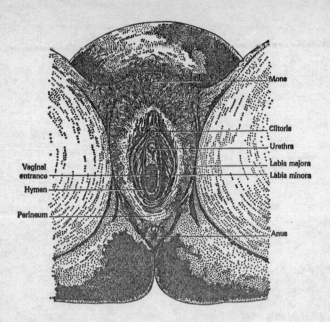

Fig. 4 The vulva

contain fat and are covered by normal skin containing both hair follicles and sweat glands. The labia minora are folds of delicate, sensitive skin which contain no fat, hair or sweat glands. The clitoris is situated in front where it is entirely protected and covered by the skin at the junction of the labia minora. It is a small cylindrical-shaped organ approximately half an inch in length, at the end of which is situated the highly sensitive glans rendering it the most delicate and sensitive part of the vulva. Being composed almost entirely of erectile tissue, similar to the penis, it becomes engorged and swollen under the stimulus of sexual excitement. The glans is normally covered by a fold of protective skin which can be retracted to expose it. The clitoris is the female's most erotic organ and it has no function except to enhance the woman's sexual excitement and response.

The perineum

The perineum is the triangular area of skin between the back of the vagina and the front of the rectum or anal canal. The importance of the perineum is not the actual skin but the muscles and fibrous tissue that lie beneath the skin. These are known as the perineal muscles and they extend from each side of the pelvis to join together in the mid-line. The muscles vary in strength from person to person and under normal circumstances they strengthen the posterior wall of the vagina and close the vaginal entrance, giving support to the vagina and the pelvic floor.

The perineum is stretched and may be injured, damaged or torn during the delivery of a baby. To avoid this tearing, or perineal laceration, an incision may be made in the perineum to enlarge the vaginal entrance during delivery. This is known as an episiotomy. Any tear or incision in the perineum is repaired immediately after delivery.

The vagina

The vagina is the passage that leads from the uterus above to open at the vulva below. It is approximately three to four inches in length and widens at its upper end to be attached round the cervix which is the neck of the uterus.

The wall of the vagina is a muscular tube capable of considerable stretching. It is lined on the inside by the vaginal skin which covers the cervix above and the vulva below. Because the vagina is a distensible organ and the vaginal muscular wall is capable of considerable stretching, the vaginal skin is thrown up into folds or ridges and the extra skin allows the organ to stretch when required. This particular property is utilized during sexual intercourse and especially during labour, when the baby's head passes down the vagina. The skin of the vaginal entrance is pinched up to form the hymen, a fold which partly seals the entrance.

The hymen varies considerably in shape and in size but even in the young it usually has a small opening through which the menstrual blood may pass. Many girls find that the opening is large enough for them to use internal tampons but in others it is too small to allow them to use this modern advance in female hygiene. The hymen may be ruptured or simply stretched during the first act of sexual intercourse. If it is ruptured there may be a small amount of bleeding which is unlikely to be severe and usually ceases spontaneously within a few minutes or a few hours. If it is lacerated or torn the hymen itself and the vaginal entrance are sore and tender until the injuries heal. Sexual intercourse may then cause discomfort or actual pain for one or two days and it is unwise for a woman to have intercourse again until the lacerations have healed. Painful intercourse does not give any pleasure and, as a result, a woman may easily develop an actual dislike of intercourse. Many instances of true frigidity can be traced to painful sexual intercourse, especially that which follows rupture of the hymen.

On rare occasions there is no opening in the hymen. This condition is known as imperforate hymen and although the girl may commence to menstruate the menstrual blood is dammed up in the vagina for several months until such time as the hymen either ruptures spontaneously or is opened surgically.

The vagina is normally and naturally moist. The moisture is secreted from the cervix and the walls of the vagina and forms a natural lubrication. It should not be sufficiently profuse to constitute a vaginal discharge.

Bartholin's glands are situated one at each side of the vaginal entrance and they respond to sexual stimulation by a dramatic increase in their secretion. Sexual excitement results in a rapid increase in all the vaginal secretions, but those coming directly from Bartholin's glands are the most profuse and important.

The uterus

The uterus, or womb, is a hollow organ situated within the pelvic cavity. It is rather like an inverted pear with the sharp end (cervix) pushing down into the upper end of the vagina. The uterus consists of two parts, the body and the cervix.

The body of the uterus, containing the uterine cavity, constitutes approximately two-thirds of the uterus, and the cervix comprises the other third. The upper part of the uterus is known as the fundus. The cavity of the uterus is triangular in shape with the Fallopian tubes entering at the upper and outer corners of the triangle.

The cervix, or neck of the uterus, protrudes into the vagina where it can be felt as a firm, hard, fibrous dome-shaped structure which varies in diameter from half to one and a half inches. Through its centre the cervical canal extends upwards for about an inch until it enters the cavity of the uterus.

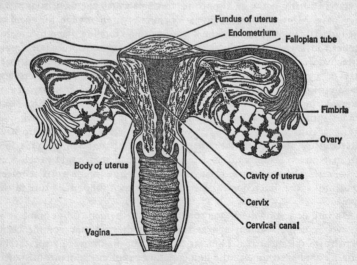

Fig 5 The female reproductive organs

The uterus is composed almost entirely of special muscle, together with a small quantity of fibrous tissue. There is no voluntary control over the muscle of the uterus. It is known as involuntary or smooth muscle, and is similar in this respect to the muscle of the intestine, of the blood vessels and to the highly specialized muscle of the heart. You can move your arms and legs by exerting control over the muscles in your limbs, but you have no conscious influence over the involuntary muscle of your heart, intestine, blood vessels, or of your uterus. The walls of the body of the uterus are approximately half an inch thick and the muscle fibres themselves are arranged in three different directions. Some encircle the uterus, some extend up, over the top and down the other side, while others are oblique and spiral. Because the cervix contains more fibrous tissue than the uterine body, it is much firmer and harder than the body of the uterus.

The cavity of the uterus is lined by a mucous membrane called the endometrium. This is a highly specialized layer of glandular tissue which is shed at menstruation (see fig. 5) and which is converted under the influence of hormones to form the decidua that is essential to the preservation and continuation of pregnancy.

It must be clearly understood that all the pelvic organs are freely movable. The uterus and cervix can be moved painlessly not only up and down but also sideways and from front to back. The uterus normally lies tilted forwards in a position that is known as anteversion with its fundus, or upper part, against the bladder. When the bladder fills the uterus is pushed upwards and backwards so that it comes to lie in direct line with the vagina.

If the uterus is tilted backwards it is known as retroversion, sometimes called twisted uterus, tilted uterus or upside-down uterus. A great deal of mystery surrounds the retroverted uterus. Approximately 20 per cent, or one in five, of all women have a uterus that is tilted backwards. This is known as a congenital retroversion and is absolutely normal. It has been in this position from birth and it will remain in this position (unless operated upon, or during pregnancy) for the duration of life. It does not cause any difficulties during menstruation or problems of infertility; nor does it predispose to miscarriage or lead to complications in labour.

The problem occurs if the uterus becomes retroverted as a result of disease or infection. This is known as acquired retroversion and may give rise to symptoms that are caused by the predisposing disease or infection.

The uterus is supported firstly by the pelvic floor and secondly by the tri-radiate ligament attached to the upper part of the cervix. This ligament consists of three parts. One runs forwards to the back of the symphysis, the second runs laterally to the side wall of the pelvis and the third goes backwards to be attached to the front part of the sacrum. All the outer ends of the tri-radiate ligament are attached to the bony pelvis and they form a type of hammock, suspending the uterus in the centre of the pelvis above the pelvic floor and allowing it considerable freedom of movement.

The blood supply to the uterus comes from the main blood vessels in the pelvis. This blood supply is very good and ample, and has an ability to increase to many times its volume during pregnancy.

The nerve supply to the uterus is very complicated. The muscle contracts rhythmically, especially during labour and during menstruation. Sensations coming from the uterus are similar to those that emanate from the intestine; in other words, the uterus only responds to stretching and this alone will cause discomfort. It can be cut or the cervix burnt as in cauterization of an ulcer on the cervix without any pain or discomfort. Stretching, however, of either the cervix or the uterus may cause quite severe pain. Some details of the nerve supply to the uterus are given in Chapter 24.

The Fallopian tubes

The Fallopian or uterine tubes are a pair of ducts which are attached to the upper and outer corners of the uterus. Each is approximately four inches long and about a quarter of an inch thick, although the size varies in its different parts. The ampulla or outer end of the Fallopian tube forms a funnel-like opening where the wall divides into finger-like processes called fimbriae. These not only guard the opening but, being close to the ovary, they also help to sweep the ovum into the canal of the tube itself. Fertilization occurs in the outer part of the Fallopian tube in the region of the fimbriae.

The Fallopian tubes consist of a fairly thick muscular coat surrounding a very complex inner lining, or mucous membrane, which secretes special material to nourish both the sperms and the fertilized ovum.

The function of the Fallopian tube is essentially twofold in nature. Firstly, it forms a route whereby the sperms migrate from the uterus to the ovary, and it possesses certain vital characteristics which enable it to nurture and look after sperms. It is commonly believed that sperms remain alive and capable of fertilization for two or even three days in the outer fimbriated part of the Fallopian tube and they are thus readily available when ovulation occurs Secondly, the Fallopian tube is the home of the newly fertilized ovum for the first seven days of its life. If the ovum is not fertilized it can only survive for 12 or perhaps 18 hours. Fertilization occurs on the 14th day of a 28-day menstrual cycle at the time of ovulation. Immediately after fertilization the ovum enters the fimbriated end of the Fallopian tube (or fertilization actually occurs within the Fallopian tube) and it does not reach the cavity of the uterus until the 21st day. The Fallopian tube supplies the newly fertilized ovum with all its nutrition and requirements during these seven days. On the seventh day after fertilization the ovum will have developed chorionic villi which are special protrusions on the outer side of the fertilized egg which enable the pregnancy to embed within whatever maternal tissue is nearest or most convenient at the time.

It is, therefore, vital that the journey of the fertilized ovum along the Fallopian tube should take precisely seven days, no more and no less. If the ovum arrives in the cavity of the uterus before the seventh day it is unable to embed itself and therefore dies, or conversely if it fails to arrive in the cavity of the uterus by the seventh day it embeds itself within the Fallopian tube and forms an ectopic or tubal pregnancy.

The ovary

The ovaries resemble large almonds in shape and size, and are situated one each side of the uterus just below the fimbriated end of the Fallopian tube. They are therefore quite close to the side wall of the pelvis and are protected from damage by the bones which form the pelvic girdle. They are extremely tender if pressure is exerted upon them. In a young girl the surface is smooth and pink, but later it becomes grey and rather puckered due to the formation of repeated tiny scars which are caused by the process of ovulation. After the menopause when there are no more ova remaining, the ovary becomes small, rather shrivelled and wrinkled. The ovaries have two main functions: the production of hormones and the production of ova.

Production of hormones

The formation or the production of hormones from the ovary is vital to the female throughout her reproductive life. The ovary produces two hormones, oestrogen and progesterone.

The production of oestrogen commences relatively early in life and is responsible for the development and the maintenance of all the secondary sex characteristics, such as the breasts and body contour as well as the maturation of the vulva and the growth of the vagina, uterus and Fallopian tubes. Oestrogen is also partly responsible for the regulation of the menstrual cycle. At the time of the menopause when the ovaries cease to produce the required amount of oestrogen, the periods stop and symptoms of the menopause develop. If the level of oestrogen falls very low post-menopausal symptoms develop.

Progesterone is produced from the corpus luteum, which is the small gland that forms in the ovary after ovulation has occurred. This hormone is essential for the maintenance of pregnancy and also for the development of many symptoms during early pregnancy. It is also responsible for ripening the endometrium, or lining of the uterus, during the second half of the menstrual cycle, and is one of the major factors responsible for a regular menstrual period as well as a normal menstrual flow.

The functioning of the ovary is under the direct control and command of the pituitary gland. This is a small gland situated in the base of the brain and is responsible for controlling most of the glandular secretions throughout the entire body. It not only controls the normal menstrual cycle but is also responsible for the onset, rhythm and eventual cessation of menstruation. The pituitary produces a small amount of an extremely powerful hormone called follicle stimulating hormone (FSH) which is released into the bloodstream and circulates to the ovary, within which it provokes the formation of follicles. The developing follicles manufacture oestrogen. One of these follicles ripens and bursts liberating an ovum—ovulation. This process is induced by FSH. Another pituitary hormone, called luteinizing hormone (LH), also reaches the ovary via the bloodstream to cause ovulation and form the corpus luteum which can then secrete progesterone.

When fertilization occurs the body has to take firm action to prevent another ovum being released and the next menstrual period occurring. The fertilized ovum embeds within the endometrium seven days after ovulation. This is accomplished by the chorionic villi that surround the fertilized ovum and have the ability to erode maternal tissue. The chorionic villi produce a hormone known as chorionic gonadotrophin which reaches the ovary by way of the maternal bloodstream forcing it to produce more progesterone which, in turn, will suppress the pituitary gland secretion of follicle stimulating hormone. The net result is that the corpus luteum continues to increase in size, thus increasing the amount of progesterone secreted, while the suppression of the production of follicle stimulating hormone means that no more follicles ripen in the ovaries.

If fertilization does not occur the corpus luteum begins to shrivel on about the 26th day of the cycle. The consequent fall in progesterone as well as in oestrogen level results in menstruation. If, however, fertilization has occurred, then the production of chorionic gonadotrophin from the chorionic villi results in a dramatic increase in secretion of progesterone from the ovarian corpus luteum which rapidly enlarges. The enormous increase in progesterone production together with its prolonged secretion beyond the 26th day of the menstrual cycle means that menstruation does not occur. The endometrium within the uterus remains intact and the newly implanted pregnancy is allowed to continue growing. Progesterone not only creates the secretory changes in the lining of the uterus, which are essential for the nutrition of the new pregnancy, but it also causes softening and relaxation of the uterine muscle as well as other involuntary muscle throughout the body, especially in the intestine, the bladder and blood vessels. It does not affect the heart itself. Relaxation of the muscle in the walls of many of the blood vessels occasionally results in a fall in blood pressure, especially when a pregnant woman is standing, and this predisposes her to fainting attacks. Relaxation of the muscular wall of the intestine predisposes to constipation, which together with relaxation of the muscular wall of the blood vessels round the anal canal may result in the formation of haemorrhoids or piles. Slackening and relaxation of the muscle wall of the bladder and of the muscle in the wall of the ureters that connect the kidneys to the bladder predispose the pregnant woman to infections in the urinary tract. Progesterone is also responsible for the increase in the size of the breasts during early pregnancy, as well as the nausea which affects most women.

The ovary of the new-born female infant contains all the ova which she is likely to need during her life (together with many more besides). These are formed while the female baby is still in the uterus, and can be damaged during their development. While X-rays will not damage the baby itself, it is known that they can affect or damage the genetic pattern of the chromosomes within the developing ova of the baby. Pregnant women are therefore X-rayed as little as possible. Intensive X-ray investigations are not advisable because of the possibility that the child may develop leukaemia or that future generations may be adversely affected.

Ovulation

Ovulation is a name given to the actual production of an egg by the ovary. The ovaries of the new-born female contain approximately one million ova, which is many more than she will require during her reproductive life. During each menstrual cycle about 250 ova commence to develop, but usually only one is destined to be properly ripened and shed in the middle of the cycle. A developing ovum lies within a small cyst known as a Graafian follicle which gradually enlarges and migrates towards the surface of the ovary. When it is fully ripe it bulges as a dome-shaped protuberance from the surface of the ovary, measuring almost half an inch in diameter. The actual rupture of the follicle seems to be a natural conclusion to the gradual enlargement of the cyst-like swelling. The follicular fluid contained within the cyst is spilt into the abdominal cavity carrying the tiny delicate ovum into the fimbriated end of the Fallopian tube. The fimbria help to collect and guide the fluid and the ovum into the tube where fertilization takes place. The muscular wall of the Fallopian tube contracts and relaxes rhythmically so that fluid is drawn into it. The minute cells lining the inner surface contain specialized hair-like structures known as cilia which wave in unison and help to move fluid along.

The life of the unfertilized ovum lasts approximately 12 hours and if it has not been impregnated during this time it dies. Once dead it becomes fragmented and is absorbed by the cells lining the Fallopian tube.

Most women menstruate every 28 days and the standard menstrual cycle is, therefore, said to last for 28 days. The first day of the menstrual period is usually counted as day 1. By this calculation a 5-day menstrual period lasts from day 1 to day 5 of the menstrual cycle. Ovulation usually occurs on the 14th day of a 28-day menstrual cycle, but ovulation is always geared to the next menstrual period and not to the menstrual period that has passed, and in fact always occurs about 14 days before the next menstrual period is due. Variations in this timing are not uncommon, but even so the range is usually between the 12th and the 16th day before the next menstrual period. Since the unfertilized ovum can only survive for about 12 hours, fertilization can only occur on the 14th day of a 28-day menstrual cycle. Sperms, however, can live in the female genital tract for 48 or even 72 hours. A woman who is ovulating on day 14 of a 28-day menstrual cycle should, therefore, have intercourse between day 11 and day 14 if she is to become pregnant. It has been calculated, and it seems reasonably certain, that sperms travel from the cervix to the outer end of the Fallopian tube in less than one hour.

So called spurious or irregular ovulation may occur at any time during the menstrual cycle, but is rare. Even allowing for some variation from the usual it can be calculated from the above that fertilization is less likely if intercourse takes place during the first 8 days or during the last 10 days of a menstrual cycle, or conversely that pregnancy is possible if intercourse takes place between day 8 and day 18 of a 28-day cycle. This is the principle underlying the so-called 'safe period', or a rhythm method of contraception (see Chapter 43).

Any alteration of the menstrual cycle from the standard 28 days will, of course, also alter the safe period. Accurate calculation of the safe period during irregular menstrual cycles can be very complicated or indeed impossible. In a woman who has a 24-day menstrual cycle ovulation still occurs 14 days before the next period, that is on the 10th day of the cycle, and similarly a woman who has a 5-week (35-day) cycle ovulates on day 21 of that cycle.

Normal ovulation does not usually give rise to any symptoms, but minor discomfort does make some women aware that they have ovulated. Ovulation pain, known as 'Mittelschmerz', may be felt in one side of the lower abdomen. This is probably caused by the rupturing of the Graafian follicle and may last for five minutes or for up to six hours and may vary in intensity from a very mild ache to quite a severe pain. Most women ovulate from each ovary alternately, but there are no hard and fast rules. The right ovary may ovulate for two, three or even six months in succession and then be followed for a similar length of time by the left ovary. Some women experience pain from only one ovary so that they are aware of ovulation in one side only on alternate months or for two or three consecutive months.

There is an increase in the secretion from the cervical glands at ovulation which may cause a colourless vaginal discharge that lasts for only one or two days and is not associated with any soreness or irritation. Some women also bleed from the uterus at the time of ovulation. This may take the form of a slight stain or it may become quite a pronounced blood loss which lasts for up to 48 hours, or even longer. This bleeding is more socially inconvenient than dangerous. Always seek medical advice if irregular bleeding occurs or if bleeding occurs between menstrual periods

Never assume that it is caused by ovulation unless it occurs exactly fourteen days before the next period and is small in quantity, but even so discuss this with your doctor in order to exclude any other possible cause.

The cells which line the Graafian follicle change after ovulation has occurred to form a structure known as the corpus luteum. The cells enlarge and assume first a pink, then a yellow colour. The function of the cells of the corpus luteum is the secretion of the hormone progesterone. A pregnancy is entirely dependent upon the corpus luteum during its early stages, but after fourteen weeks it becomes self-supporting and is capable of producing sufficient hormone from its own placenta to maintain a satisfactory environment for its survival within the uterus.

It is not known by what mechanism the ovaries decide which is going to function next. If one ovary is damaged, destroyed or removed the other ovary grows slightly larger and ovulates each month. Two ovaries are to a certain extent a luxury as well as an insurance. A woman can function perfectly well with only one ovary, since from this ovary she manufactures sufficient hormones and ova to remain just as fertile as if she had two.

The menstrual cycle

The onset of menstruation or the time of the first menstrual period is usually accepted as being the date at which puberty occurs. This, however, is not strictly true. Puberty represents very extensive changes that occur throughout the whole body, and the process is really the changing from a child into a woman. The completion of this process may take as long as ten years and at some stage during these ten years menstruation begins.

The menarche is the technical term for the date of onset of the first period. This varies in different races and in different parts of the world, but generally occurs earlier in hotter climates than it does in temperate zones. Nevertheless, the age of the menarche is gradually becoming younger and in Great Britain today it usually occurs between the ages of twelve and fourteen, although it is not uncommon at ten or even nine.

The first changes of puberty may be recognized as early as six or seven years and result from the initial secretions of oestrogen from the maturing ovaries. The earliest features that may be noticed are subtle changes in body contour together with very early development of the breasts. These so-called secondary sexual characteristics continue gradually and slowly until the fully mature woman is developed. This is usually at the age of eighteen whereas in the male development may continue for some time longer.

The whole development of the mature female is a very gradual and carefully planned process. The secondary sexual characteristics such as the development of the breasts, the distribution of fat over the body, the growth and distribution of hair, proceed in a very carefully organized and logical manner. Development of the sexual organs, namely the vulva, the clitoris, the vagina, the uterus and the Fallopian tubes and maturation of the ovaries proceed at the same time, and it is during this time that the first menstrual period begins.

The onset of menstruation is usually unexpected, but may be accompanied by premonitory signs and symptoms. The establishing of a normal regular menstrual cycle may take months or even years, and while a large proportion of girls do in fact have a normal menstrual rhythm from the start, it is not abnormal if it takes several years to establish a regular cycle. Irregular bleeding at this time does not require any treatment, but prolonged or excessive menstrual loss should be considered abnormal and medical advice sought.

The normal menstrual cycle is represented by bleeding which occurs from the uterus every 28 days. In order to understand the menstrual cycle, however, it is necessary to understand some of the factors that control menstruation. There are three basic cycles involved.

1 The pituitary cycle

The pituitary controls the menstrual cycle by secreting follicle stimulating hormone which provokes the formation of many follicles within each ovary. The developing follicles secrete oestrogen and continue to develop in competition until finally one follicle alone reaches maturity (occasionally more in the case of a multiple pregnancy) on the 14th day of the cycle. As soon as this happens the other competing follicles atrophy so that only one ovum is normally released during each menstrual cycle. The pituitary gland secretes luteinizing hormone which causes ovulation and stimulates formation of a corpus luteum from the ruptured follicle. This continues for the next 12 days until the 26th day of the menstrual cycle, when, in the absence of pregnancy, the production of luteinizing hormone ceases and the corpus luteum degenerates. This is followed on the 28th day by the onset of menstruation and thereafter the whole cycle begins again with the secretion of the follicle stimulating hormone.

2 The ovarian cycle

Under the stimulus of follicle stimulating hormone from the pituitary glands, follicles commence to ripen in both ovaries. These are tiny cysts, each one of which is capable of producing an ovum ready for fertilization. Only one follicle, however, generally reaches maturity and it does so on the 14th day of the cycle. At the beginning of the menstrual cycle perhaps one hundred or more follicles in each ovary commence to ripen. They produce and secrete oestrogen increasingly as they ripen, and the production reaches its peak at the time of ovulation. The follicle which has been selected for final ripening matures very rapidly and distends the surface of the ovary as a cystic swelling almost half an inch in diameter. On the 14th day it ruptures and discharges the fully mature ovum into the outer end of the Fallopian tube. The follicular fluid which contains a large amount of oestrogen is absorbed. The other competing follicles atrophy and degenerate. It is not known why generally only one follicle is selected when many commence to mature. Some of the so-called 'fertility drugs' contain a follicle stimulating hormone and if this is administered either to a woman who is unduly sensitive or in extra large doses, then more than one follicle may ripen or alternatively one follicle may ripen from each ovary, and it is easy to understand how multiple pregnancies can result.

Just before ovulation the pituitary gland secretes luteinizing hormone, which causes ovulation and the formation of the corpus luteum from the newly ruptured follicle. The corpus luteum secretes progesterone. If fertilization does not occur the corpus luteum begins to degenerate on the 26th day of the menstrual cycle with the resulting fall in progesterone production and subsequent menstruation.

Thus the ovarian cycle results first in the production of oestrogen, then in ovulation and finally in the production of both oestrogen and progesterone which fall immediately prior to menstruation.

3 The uterine cycle

The menstrual cycle normally lasts for 28 days, although regular variations between 21 and 35 days or even longer are considered normal. The first day of the menstrual period is the first day of the menstrual cycle. Bleeding occurs from the uterus as a result of a breakdown and degeneration of the thick and luxuriant lining of the cavity of the uterus. This breakdown is a direct result of the fall in levels of oestrogen and progesterone on the 26th day of the preceding menstrual cycle. If fertilization has not occurred it is necessary for the body to produce another ovum for fertilization. The lining of the uterus that has been hopefully prepared for a pregnancy during the previous month is shed in order that a new lining can be prepared to be ready to receive a fertilized ovum should pregnancy occur during the next month. The superficial layers of the lining of the endometrium disintegrate accompanied by a certain amount of bleeding. The disintegration and shedding of the endometrium takes about three days and thereafter the amount of blood lost during the period gradually diminishes as the endometrium heals.

Following the end of the period the action of oestrogen provokes the regeneration of the endometrium in what is known as the proliferative phase. This results in the rapid growth of a thick and normal lining to the uterine cavity. When ovulation has occurred and the secretion of progesterone begins, the endometrium undergoes what is known as secretory change. This change, directly under the influence of progesterone, is vital for the nutrition of a newly fertilized ovum. The secretory change

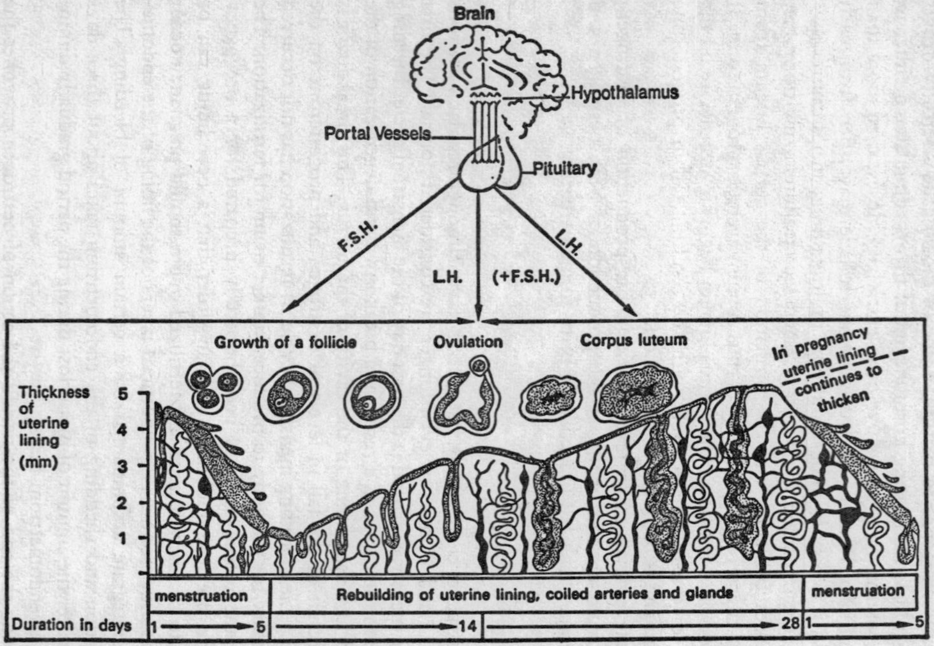

Fig 6 The menstrual cycle

commences on the 15th day and continues until the 26th day of the cycle. The glands in the endometrium enlarge and secrete material for the nutrition of the new ovum.

Most women rapidly establish what is known as a normal menstrual pattern in which not only is their menstrual cycle regulated but also the number of days during which bleeding occurs, together with the pattern of the bleeding. Each woman establishes her own menstrual pattern and while the majority menstruate every 28 days, it is perfectly normal for a woman to menstruate as frequently as every 21 days, or as infrequently as every 3 months. Equally there may be a variation in the duration of bleeding from 2 days to 8 days, as well as a variation in the actual amount of blood lost during a period.

The menopause

The menopause is otherwise known as the change of life or climacteric and occurs most commonly at about the age of 50. When one speaks of the change of life one automatically considers the time or age at which a woman has her last period. Just as puberty spans over a number of years in which the onset of menstruation is only one isolated factor, so the true menopause extends over quite a number of years during which the cessation of menstruation is only one particular and dramatic symptom.

The expectation of life in Roman times was about 24 years but by the fourteenth century it had risen to 43 years. At the beginning of this century it had risen only to 48 so that the problems of the menopause have only become really important during the last seventy years.

At a certain time in every woman's life all the ova which have not been used begin to atrophy and the ovaries themselves gradually cease to function. Menstruation ceases when the cyclic production of the hormones oestrogen and progesterone drops below a critical level.

No one can say for certain at what age the menopause actually begins, because the gradual lowering of hormone levels is so slow that it is initially unnoticed. The majority of women are only aware of the change of life after noting some abnormality of their periods whereas some complain of menopausal symptoms before they notice any alteration.

There are many horrifying stories associated with the change of life. Few, if any, are true. The menopause does present the average woman with some problems, but most doctors agree that the vast majority can be easily overcome with sympathetic advice or a small amount of treatment.

The changes that occur before, during and after the cessation of menstruation are nearly all due to a fall in the level of oestrogen in the body. This begins three or four years before the periods actually stop, so that the earliest symptoms of the change of life can occasionally be recognized for several years while menstruation is still occurring. It should be emphasized that the majority of women can pass through the change of life experiencing very little or nothing in the way of symptoms and without anyone else knowing or appreciating what is happening.

Several small changes may be noticed in the earlier part of the menopause: an increase of premenstrual tension where this has been comparatively mild or even absent; nervousness and irritability; gradual weight gain and some redistribution of the body fat from the arms and legs to the shoulders, buttocks and abdomen; mild indigestion or change of bowel habit, together with several other very minor symptoms.

The actual cessation of the menstrual periods is gradually occurring at an older age (just as the first period is occurring at a younger age) and the average age is now about 48.5 years. This happens normally in one of three ways:

1 The periods stop suddenly without prior warning.
2 They continue with their normal cycle but the amount of loss gradually decreases until there is none.
3 They continue normally but the time between them gradually increases until after a gap of several months no further menstruation occurs.

Any divergence from the list above is abnormal and a doctor's advice should be sought. Bleeding between periods, bleeding after intercourse, prolonged bleeding, heavy bleeding, frequent or irregular periods, or blood-stained vaginal discharge, are not symptoms of the normal menopause. Report them to your doctor without undue delay.

The main symptoms of the menopause, apart from the cessation of menstruation, are sweating and hot flushes. These may come at any time of day or night and may vary from once a week to as often as thirty or forty times a day. They may be very mild or sufficiently severe to cause a great deal of distress and discomfort. The feeling of heat and claustrophobia may force a woman to open windows for fresh air; when the hot flush wears off it is followed by a feeling of coldness and she shuts the window and puts on extra clothing or bedclothes. Although the hot flushes feel as though the face is burning like the setting sun, actual flushing of the face is very rare. It is almost impossible to recognize a hot flush from the facial appearance alone. Hot flushes are usually associated with sweating which is often hardly noticeable but which may sometimes be particularly profuse, especially at night, making a woman change her nightdress several times and occasionally her sheets as well. There is no way of knowing if a woman is going to suffer from hot flushes and sweats during her menopause; nor is there any way of knowing how many sweats and flushes she will have.

Neither the first symptoms of the climacteric nor the menopause itself need affect the daily routine, bodily functions or sex life of a woman. There is a tendency to gain weight, more noticeable because of the redistribution of fat over the body, but this can be resisted by moderate but efficient dieting.

The majority of changes in the body after the menopause are nothing to do with hormone levels themselves but are simple processes of ageing which occur in everybody, male or female. There are, however, some changes which are specifically related to a fall in oestrogen level. The vagina becomes drier and the muscles of the pelvic floor and perineum become rather wasted. These in turn may lead to problems such as vaginal discharge, difficulty or pain with intercourse, frequency of micturition and even vaginal or uterine prolapse. Nearly all these changes can be reversed by giving small doses of oestrogen. This can sometimes be seen in a post-menopausal woman who is suffering from depression as well as some atrophic changes in the vagina. If she is given a small and carefully calculated amount of oestrogen, the depression is relieved and the vaginal changes reversed; all this, together with a return to normal sex life, results in a remarkable improvement in disposition and outlook. Oestrogen must always be prescribed by a doctor and never self-administered.

A great controversy rages concerning the advisability of giving oestrogen before, during and after the menopause. Some say that hormones should not be administered, but there is an argument for the administration of small doses of oestrogen in a cyclic regime which offset the majority of the symptoms of the menopause. If patients who are approaching the menopause are put on a replacement therapy (which contains oestrogen and may also contain progesterone) they are relieved of some of the symptoms they might have developed prior to the cessation of their periods. A woman will know she is entering the menopause because even while taking a low dose of hormone she will occasionally miss periods despite a lack of other symptoms.

The majority of gynaecologists agree that a woman who has no symptoms or abnormal physical signs does not need hormones, but that treatment should be considered if she has symptoms which can be attributed to the menopause or to a postmenopausal drop in hormone levels.

The breasts

The breasts have developed over millions of years, during the evolution of the human race, from sweat glands which have become adapted to the production of milk. At birth the breasts are represented by small nipples which are the same in both sexes. The glandular tissue from which the breasts will later develop is present and this is occasionally illustrated by the phenomenon of 'mastitis neonatorum', in which the oestrogen from the mother causes the breasts of the new-born infant to swell and enlarge to an appreciable extent for one or two days.

Under normal circumstances the breast development does not commence until the ovaries begin to secrete oestrogen at the age of seven, eight or nine. Both the nipple and the breast tissue then gradually develop and growth continues as a slow and regular process until the onset of the first period. At this time, or shortly afterwards, the breasts may enlarge rapidly as a result of the release of large quantities of hormone into the circulation. The initial development of the breasts is entirely dependent on oestrogen. Progesterone, however, is required to develop the particular properties that are necessary for lactation, that is the production of milk. The fully developed breast does not begin to produce milk until after delivery because lactation depends on a hormone called prolactin which is secreted by the pituitary gland only at this time.

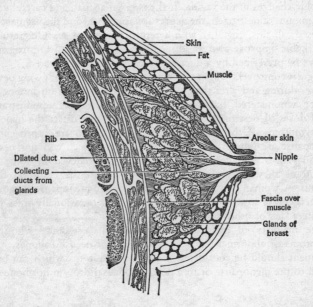

Fig. 7   The breast during lactation

The breasts contain a certain amount of fibrous tissue that divides each into approximately twenty lobes, and each lobe contains the milk-secreting glands. The lobes are a highly complicated arrangement of glandular tissue that gradually forms into a single duct which eventually opens in the nipple. Thus the nipple contains approximately twenty ducts, one from each lobe of the breast. Beneath the nipple each of the ducts widens into a pouch which is used to store milk during lactation. Milk can most easily be produced from the lactating breast by exerting pressure deep under the nipple itself.

Oestrogen is responsible for the development of the breasts themselves and their glandular tissue, and progesterone is necessary to mature the glands, but prolactin must be present to enable them to produce milk.

The breasts do not contain any muscle and it is, therefore, essential that they should have good support during pregnancy, especially if they are full or heavy. If the breast tissue is once allowed to sag or stretch it will never recover and no amount of exercise will restore the former breast contour.

3 The Male Reproductive Organs

The male reproductive organs are designed to fulfil three functions: firstly, the manufacture of sperms in the testicles; secondly, the process of erection and the deposition of the sperms as close to the cervix as possible by the penis; thirdly, the manufacture of male sex hormones by the testicles.

The penis

The penis or phallus is the organ through which the male deposits sperms at the top of the vagina. It consists mainly of erectile tissue and in the flaccid state measures between three and four inches in length and less than one inch in diameter. The urethra is a hollow tube that runs the length of the penis and extends from the bladder to open in an elliptical opening at the tip of the glans of the penis. This tube is not only used for the passage of urine during micturition, but also for sperms during ejaculation. The glans is a particularly sensitive area which, in the uncircumcised male, is normally covered by the foreskin or prepuce. The skin covering the penis is very loosely attached to the deeper structures, thus allowing for swelling during erection and freedom during the act of sexual intercourse.

Under the influence of sexual excitement the erectile tissue of the penis becomes filled and engorged with blood so that the organ becomes distended and rigid. In its erectile state the penis measures more than six inches in length and more than one and a half inches in diameter at its base.

The testicles

The sperms are actually formed within the testicles which are suspended beneath the penis in the scrotum. The testicles serve two functions: firstly spermatogenesis, the production of sperms, and secondly the production of testosterone which is the important male hormone.

The testicles are oval in shape being about one and a half inches long and less than one inch in diameter. They have a very rich blood and nerve supply, and are extremely sensitive to pressure or injury. They are connected to the base of the bladder by a tube, the vas deferens, along which the sperms pass to the seminal vesicles at the base of the bladder where they are stored.

The production of sperms within the testicles is a carefully regulated process that commences fairly early in childhood and continues until old age. Men of 90 can produce perfectly good and viable sperms.

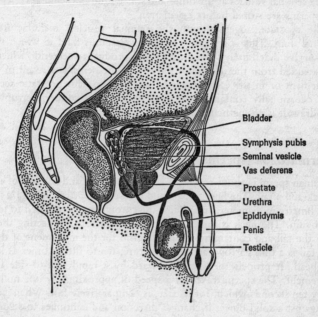

Fig. 8   The male reproductive organs

The scrotum

The scrotum is a bag of loose skin containing the testicles which is suspended from the perineum behind the penis. The testicles are suspended outside the body since they are meant to function at a temperature below that of normal body heat. If they are overheated by hot baths, electric blankets, tight underpants, etc., spermatogenesis stops and over a long period of time this is one of the commoner causes of infertility in the male. The skin of the scrotum is loose and particularly well equipped with sweat glands which enable it to maintain the testicles at the correct temperature by a process of constant evaporation and water loss. The wall of the scrotum also contains the cremaster muscle which contracts if the outside temperature is unduly cold and draws the testicles up towards the body, thus maintaining them at their functioning temperature.

The prostate and seminal vesicles

The prostate is a gland situated at the base of the bladder and also at the base of the penis. The seminal vesicles are attached to the prostate, one on each side. The vas deferens joins the testicle and epididymis at one end to the seminal vesicles at the other and it is within the seminal vesicles that the sperms are stored before ejaculation.

The prostate, together with the seminal vesicles, manufactures the seminal fluid. This is a slightly alkaline gelatinous fluid in which sperms can survive indefinitely. The prostate also produces a secretion which may be extruded from the urethra at the end of the penis as a result of sexual excitement or in the early stages of intercourse. This prostatic secretion may occasionally contain sperms and this is why coitus interruptus, or withdrawal, is an inefficient method of contraception.

Spermatozoa (sperms)

A human sperm is about 1/25th of a millimetre long and consists of a head, a neck and a tail. The head is oval and measures approximately 1/250th of a millimetre in diameter. It contains the chromosomes required to fertilize the ovum. The neck is a short cylindrical structure connecting the head with the tail and containing the mechanism for the movement of the tail. The tail is a thin narrow tapering structure, ten to fifteen times as long as the head. It propels the sperm forward by a rapid side-to-side lashing movement. The sperm travels at a speed of approximately one millimetre every ten seconds which, for its size, is comparatively fast. When it comes up against a solid object it changes direction and continues to swim until it meets a further obstruction.

The storage of sperms

The formation of sperms in the testicles is a continuous process known as spermatogenesis. The life of a sperm may be as long as two or even three months. When it has been produced in the testicle it is transmitted along one of many channels until it reaches the epididymis, where it may remain for several days or even for as long as two weeks according to the degree of sexual activity. The sperms are eventually transferred from the epididymis via the vas deferens to the sac-like seminal vesicles at the base of the bladder where they are stored until ejaculation. The seminal vesicles together with the prostate secrete the seminal fluid.

Ejaculation

Ejaculation occurs at the time of male orgasm. The ejaculation consists of rhythmic muscular contractions throughout the whole of the male genitalia during which the seminal vesicles contract and emit the seminal fluid containing the sperms into the male urethra. Further spasmodic muscular contractions rapidly convey the fluid down the urethra to be ejaculated from the opening at the end of the penis. The average orgasm or ejaculation consists of four to ten of these forceful contractions, and during each one seminal fluid is ejaculated from the penis. The average amount ejaculated is three to five millilitres, each millilitre containing between 50 and 200 million sperms. The total number of sperms in a normal ejaculation may, therefore, vary from 150 million to 1,000 million.

4 Development of the Baby

Ovulation

Ovulation is described on page 47. The human process of ovulation is in no way related to sexual activity. It occurs in the protected virgin just as efficiently and frequently as it does in the married woman.

Conception

Migration of sperms

The migration of the sperms from the vault of the vagina to the outer part of the Fallopian tube, and hence to the ovum, is not satisfactorily understood.

Approximately 400 million sperms are present in each ejaculation and they are initially protected by the semi-gelatinous seminal fluid which liquefies after an interval of 15 or 20 minutes, and the sperms are then exposed to the vaginal acidity. Being very sensitive to acid, those which have not gained access to the cervical canal are rapidly rendered immobile or killed. Many lame, abnormal or damaged sperms are thus automatically destroyed, although they may occasionally fertilize an ovum, resulting in a 'blighted ovum'. Those that reach the cervical canal are protected and nourished by its alkaline mucus. For a few days before ovulation the mucus in the cervical canal is especially prepared for sperms and becomes transparent and less viscous than during the remainder of the menstrual cycle.

If only 10 per cent of the sperms reach the cervical canal a total of approximately 40 million sperms will have gained this favourable haven. The journey of about 23 centimetres from the cervix, up the uterus and along the Fallopian tube takes approximately 45 minutes and between 1,000 and 2,000 sperms reach the outer portion of each Fallopian tube. The cells lining the Fallopian tube secrete an alkaline mucus which is rich in sugar and nourishes the sperms on their journey. They will survive in the outer part of the Fallopian tube for between 48 and 72 hours, lying in wait for the newly forming follicle to discharge its ovum. If ovulation has occurred within 18 hours before the sperms reach the outer end of the Fallopian tube then fertilization occurs immediately the sperms reach the ovum.

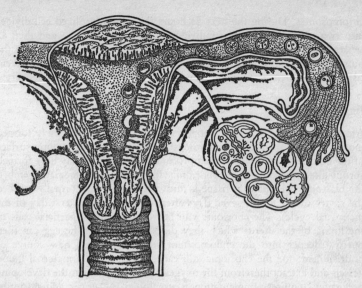

Fig. 9 The journey of the developing ovum along the Fallopian tube from fertilization to implantation in the endometrium

Fertilization

While only one sperm is capable of actually fertilizing an ovum, it is probable that many sperms have to be present in order for fertilization to occur. The ovum is surrounded by a gelatinous material which can be liquefied by hyaluronidase, an enzyme carried by the sperms. No single sperm can carry sufficient hyaluronidase to liquefy enough of the gelatinous material to penetrate the ovum. The hyaluronidase of several sperms is thought to be required for sufficient liquefaction to allow one sperm to penetrate the ovum.

The actual mechanism of penetration of the ovum by the sperm is not known. It is believed that the sperm makes head-on contact with the ovum and gradually penetrates the wall of the ovum by virtue of its hard swimming velocity. In the human the lashing tail does not enter the ovum but is left on the outer side of the capsule. It is also likely that only one sperm actually penetrates the ovum, unlike some animals where several sperms do so although only one is used for fertilization.

During the first few hours after penetration of the ovum by the sperm, the female and the male nuclei, which contain the chromosomes that will endow the offspring with its hereditary characteristics, enlarge and move towards the centre of the ovum where they fuse or coalesce to form a single nucleus. Within a short time the nucleus divides into two equal parts, each part containing an equal portion of maternal and paternal chromosomes. During the next 72 hours the whole fertilized cell divides into two and subsequently subdivides to form 4, 8, 16, 32 and then 64 separate cells, when it is known as a morula. This process continues in the human for 266 days from conception, when the specialization of different tissues is complete and a 3-kg baby has grown and is ready for delivery.

Implantation

After four days a cystic space appears in the centre of the newly formed morula and it is then called a blastocyst. The cells around the outer surface of the blastocyst continue to multiply and by the seventh day have formed sprout-like projections called chorionic villi which will immediately embed the blastocyst in whatever tissue it finds itself in. It has normally reached the cavity of the uterus seven days after fertilization (the 21st day of the menstrual cycle). The chorionic villi burrow into the superficial cells of the lining of the uterus which they digest and erode. The egg can then burrow deeper into the endometrium where it finds a new source of nourishment, for the chorionic villi can gently open the maternal blood vessels and extract therefrom the oxygen and nutrients that the developing pregnancy requires. Implantation is usually in the upper and posterior aspect of the cavity of the uterus. The blastocyst is not visible to the naked eye and a woman will not yet know that she is pregnant, since she has not missed her first menstrual period and even the earliest symptoms of pregnancy do not begin to manifest themselves for several days.

Sex of the child

The determination of sex

All human cells contain 44 chromosomes plus two sex chromosomes, giving a total of 46 in all. The 44 normal chromosomes affect the structure and function of the body and are responsible for all its hereditary character-istics. The normal female cell contains two sex chromosomes, both of which are X chromosomes. These are responsible for all the female charac-teristics and are denoted as XX. The normal male cell contains two sex chromosomes of which one is an X chromosome and one is a Y chromo-some, and they are denoted as XY. The ovum consists of 22 chromosomes plus one sex chromosome which must be an X chromosome. Sperms each contain 22 chromosomes plus one of the sex chromosomes, which may be either an X or a Y chromosome. The human male cell containing 44 chromosomes plus XY divides to form sperms each with 22 chromosomes plus either X or Y. Obviously equal numbers of sperms containing X and Y chromosomes are formed. If the ovum is fertilized by a sperm which contains 22 plus X chromosomes, then the offspring will be 44 plus XX, which is female. If on the other hand the ovum is fertilized by a sperm containing 22 plus Y chromosomes, the offspring will be 44 plus XY, which is male.

The sex of the child is, therefore, entirely a male responsibility and no woman should ever apologize or feel sorry for failing to produce a child of the sex her husband or partner wanted. The mother cannot influence the selection of X or Y containing sperms. An escape clause is possible because some people believe that women have a method of differentiating between 'male' and 'female' sperms, but this has not been proved.

Predestination of sex

There is no scientific evidence that the production of male or female children may be an hereditary phenomenon. It is appreciated that some families produce a long list of males whilst other families produce a large number of female children, but nevertheless statistically each pregnancy stands an equal chance of being male or female and any long run of one sex is entirely fortuitous. It may well be that the present state of our knowledge is incomplete and that eventually some factor will be discovered which does show why some families are predisposed to produce one sex.

One very interesting factor about sex determination is the repeated production of male children by the sub-fertile couple. This is particularly noticeable when the male is the sub-fertile partner and tends to support the old adage that 'anyone can produce a son but it takes a real man to produce a daughter'. The reason for this is not known.

X and Y chromosomal sperms are produced in equal numbers and, despite many popular theories, there is no certain method of separating X from Y and thus deciding the eventual sex of the child. A lot of experimental work has been done on this problem with a certain amount of success in the veterinary world, where the predetermination of sex is of more commercial value than in humans. Experiments have been conducted using human sperms and it has been suggested that passing an electric current through seminal fluid will separate 'male' and 'female' sperms so that the sex can then be selected for artificial insemination, but this is not, at present, a practical proposition.

The various theories regarding what should be done to produce either a male or a female child are not supported by scientific evidence. Theories such as the time in the menstrual cycle, or the time at night at which intercourse should take place, or that a male child is born when ovulation coincides with a particular phase of the moon, are without foundation. There is no realistic way as yet by which sex can be predetermined in the human. Various methods have been used throughout history and it is commonly thought that an acid medium will predispose to male fertilization. While this may be true, there is no medical evidence to support it. For centuries grand ladies in various countries have douched with a variety of acid mixtures from vinegar to lemon juice prior to intercourse, in the hope that this will allow them to conceive a male child. Since the fertilizing sperm must gain access to the cervical canal in order to survive and the mucus in the canal of the cervix is uninfluenced by vaginal douching, the argument for this is not very strong. It is weakened even further when it is appreciated that the normal acidity of the vagina is much greater than that of either dilute vinegar or lemon juice. Similarly, the taking of acid or alkaline diets and medicines will not help.

Many non-medical, and some medical, authorities believe that the 'male' and the 'female' sperms have different characteristics, especially regarding their motility and their ability to survive, and that these properties can be utilized to preselect sex in 80 per cent of people. Some consider that they have ample evidence to prove this.

The theory is as follows: male sperms swim faster but female sperms survive longer in the female genital tract. Ovulation occurs on day 14 of a 28-day cycle (see page 47). If intercourse takes place on day 12, and not on day 13 or 14 of the cycle, then only female sperms will survive to fertilize the egg on day 14. If intercourse takes place on day 14, then the faster swimming male sperms will reach the ovum first. Remember that the egg will survive only for about 18 hours if it is not fertilized.

Prenatal determination of sex

There is no way in which the sex of the unborn child can be accurately determined without some danger to the fetus. The only certain method of finding out the sex of the unborn child is to withdraw some of the fluid surrounding the baby by a process known as amniocentesis. The cells which it contains are stained by a special method and then carefully examined under the microscope. If the XX chromosomes are present they form a characteristic stain within the nucleus of the cell, known as a Barr body, which can be seen when the cells are examined under the microscope. By this method it is possible to determine the sex of a child with 100 per cent accuracy at any stage after about the 12th week of pregnancy. Examination of the baby's cells is used only for definite medical indications because it does present a slight hazard to the unborn baby, as well as to the mother. It is not used unless the advantages of the knowledge obtained outweigh the disadvantages. At the time of writing it is not considered that the satisfaction of curiosity regarding sex is an adequate excuse for performing amniocentesis. The only exception to this is where the infant may be thought to suffer from mongolism or a sex-linked disease such as amyotonia congenita, when abortion may be considered.

X-rays will not determine the sex of a child *in utero* because simple X-rays only outline the bones.

Counting the baby's heart rate in the uterus is probably the simplest (though not very accurate) method of determining sex The normal heart rate is between 120 and 160 beats per minute. A heart rate which is persistently below 140 beats per minute is usually male, whereas one which is persistently above 140 beats per minute is usually female. The fetal heart should be counted before the fetus has been disturbed by examination. This method is, however, only about 70 per cent reliable and the expectant mother is advised against choosing the colour of her layette on the results.

Suspension of an object on the end of a piece of string over a pregnant uterus is believed by many people to give an indication of the sex. When the object moves in a clockwise direction the child is said to be male and if it moves counter-clockwise it is said to be female.

There are many other methods, according to folk lore, of assessing the sex of the infant, including the time at which movement is first felt, the shape of the abdomen, the amount of nausea and sickness and the occurrence of nose bleeds.

There is a certain amount of medical evidence that the female baby produces a greater effect upon its mother than does a male baby and that the carrier of a female child will, therefore, suffer from more nausea and sickness and will 'feel more pregnant' than the carrier of a male child. A woman who may even be unaware of the fact that she is pregnant, except for the absence of her menstrual period, is more often carrying a male child.

Although parents all over the world are always anxious for any indication of the sex of their unborn child, the majority of them would, in retrospect, prefer not to know the answer till the child is actually delivered. It would be rather an anticlimax if the sex of every child were known for months before delivery.

Ultrasonic scanning may be able to define the penis and/or the testicles of a baby *in utero*. The ability of the scan to define these organs depends upon the position of the baby and the duration of the pregnancy. By this method a male infant can be identified with considerable accuracy but obviously there is no means of positive identification of the female infant.

Boy : girl ratio

More male children are delivered than female children. The ratio is 106 boys to every 100 girls. It is considered that the incidence of male pregnancies at conception is even greater than this, a ratio of about 113 male to 100 female, but the preponderance of male babies is reduced because of the higher incidence of miscarriage amongst the male conceptions. The reason for the higher incidence of male conceptions is not known. The ratio of males to females varies slightly with different races and in different geographic areas.

Development of the embryo

Seven days after fertilization the ovum enters the cavity of the uterus where it embeds itself in the endometrium. At this stage the fertilized ovum begins to differentiate into its various parts. A cavity which has formed within the cellular mass gradually enlarges to occupy most of the central space of the developing pregnancy. At the same time a very specialized group of cells (the inner cell mass) commences to grow rapidly and protrude into the cystic space which will eventually become the amniotic cavity, and the inner cell mass will develop into the fetus itself. When the pregnancy embeds itself in the lining of the uterus there is no fetus present—just a mass of cells which will later develop into a baby.

The trophoblast, which surrounds the embryo and is responsible for embedding it in maternal tissue, develops rapidly to form sponge-like projections which erode further into maternal tissue, to obtain the increasing requirements of the rapidly growing pregnancy. The embryo will develop into not only the baby itself but also the umbilical cord, the placenta, the amniotic fluid, and the amniotic and chorionic membranes.

Size of the baby during pregnancy

2nd week (this is the end of the 2nd week, i.e. at the time of fertilization on the 13th or 14th day of a normal 28-day cycle). The pregnancy consists of only one fertilized cell and is invisible to the naked eye.

3rd week. During the 3rd week the fertilized ovum travels along the Fallopian tube and arrives in the cavity of the uterus, where at the end of the 3rd week it embeds in the lining of the uterine cavity. The total pregnancy is still not visible to the naked eye.

4th week. The pregnancy is embedded and grows rapidly during this week so that by the 28th day, or the end of the 4th week, it is just visible to the naked eye. The corpus luteum in the ovary continues to mature and to increase its production of progesterone, so that menstruation is suppressed. Under the influence of progesterone the cells lining the inner surface of the uterus change into the highly secretory and active form which they continue to adopt throughout pregnancy. This is known as the decidua of pregnancy, forming a very thick and vascular lining to the uterus.

5th week. At the end of the 5th week the fertilized pregnancy is approximately 2 mm in length and is visible to the naked eye. The fetus, within the newly formed amniotic sac, is beginning to take shape into its major component parts. The spine is beginning to form and a rudimentary nervous system is just recognizable.

6th week. During the 6th week the formation of the head is rapidly followed by the chest and abdominal cavities. The rudimentary brain is completed and a spinal column as well as a spinal cord is properly formed. The tail of the fetus becomes less noticeable and the limb buds begin to appear at the corners of the body. The heart is forming within the chest cavity and by the end of the 6th week the first simple rudimentary heart and circulation are beginning to function. Heart motion or heart beat may be seen on an ultrasonic scan at this time. Blood vessels are forming in the umbilical cord. The earliest parts of the stomach and intestine are formed within the abdominal cavity.

The face has not yet taken shape, but small depressions are appearing where the eyes and ears will be situated. The mouth and jaw are also beginning to develop.

The length of the fetus is approximately 6 mm.

7th week. By the end of the 7th week the limb buds have grown rapidly and are now clearly distinguishable as arms and legs, at the ends of which clefts are appearing which will later separate into fingers and toes. Blood cells have formed within the circulation and blood vessels now extend into the head and throughout the body. The heart, although still a very simple structure, has started to beat with sufficient force to circulate cells through the blood vessels. The chest is properly formed but the lungs remain as tiny, solid organs one on each side of the mid-line. The intestine is almost completely formed but has not yet assumed its correct position. The liver and kidneys have developed but are small and incapable of functioning. The brain and the spinal cord are growing rapidly and, with the exception of nerves to the limbs and skin, are almost complete. The development of the head is proceeding at great speed and it is gradually assuming its final shape. At this stage, however, it is still bent forward on the chest and rather strange looking lumps are present over the back and base of the head. The depressions which are to become the canals of the ears have deepened and the inner parts of the ears are forming. The eyes themselves are also developing, although the skin over them (which is subsequently to become the eyelids) remains completely intact. The nose is not yet formed but apertures for the nostrils are appearing. Development of the jaws and mouth is continuing.

The length of the fetus is approximately 1.3 cm.

8th week. All the major internal organs are now formed, although in a somewhat rudimentary state, and they enlarge and continue to progress towards assuming their permanent shape and position. The heart is beating strongly now that the circulatory system has been established in the fetus. The lungs have grown considerably but remain solid. This is the main time for growth of the eyes and the inner part of the ear, including the middle ear which is responsible for balance and hearing. There is no external part of the ear at this stage. The head of the fetus is still very large in proportion to the body. The face is now beginning to assume some recognizable characteristics with depressions present where the eyes are destined

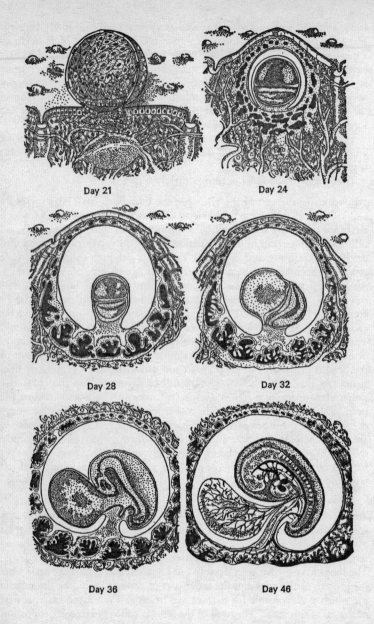

Day 21   Day 24

Day 28   Day 32

Day 36   Day 46

Fig 10   Stages in the growth of the foetus counting from the first day of the last normal period (not to scale)

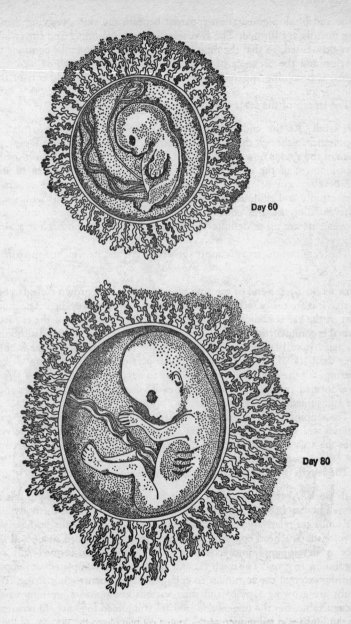

Day 60

Day 80

to be and black pigmentation apparent beneath the skin overlying them. The nostrils are formed. The two sides of both the upper and lower jaw have now fused, so that the mouth is recognizable. The limbs continue to develop and the presence of shoulders and elbows, as well as hips and knees, is becoming apparent. The first, but very tiny, movements of the spine begin.

The length of the fetus is approximately 2.2 cm.

9th week. At the end of the 9th week the fetus has a more mature appearance, although the head is still bent forward on the chest. Development of the eyes is now complete, but the eyelids are still intact over them. Development of the inner ear continues. A nose has now appeared and the development of the mouth proceeds. The limbs continue to grow very rapidly and rudimentary hands and feet are now obvious with some differentiation of the ends of the limb buds into fingers and toes. Movements are more definite but not apparent to the mother for a long time yet.

The length of the fetus is approximately 3 cm and its weight approximately 2 g.

10th week. By the end of the 10th week the eyes have grown considerably in size and are easily recognizable beneath the unformed eyelids. The inner part of the ear is completely formed and the external part of the ear (the pinna) is commencing to grow. The face is more recognizable and although the head is still large as compared with the rest of the body, the bumps over the back of the head and the upper part of the neck are now disappearing. All the internal organs continue to develop. The ankles and wrists have formed and fingers and toes are easily distinguishable, although they are still joined together by webbing.

The umbilical cord is properly formed and blood is circulating along its arteries and vein. The placenta has not yet formed but the chorionic villi over the area of implantation, which will eventually become the placenta, are growing and maturing.

The length of the fetus is 4.5 cm and its weight is approximately 5 g.

11th week. At the end of the 11th week the fetus is easily recognizable as a small human baby, although the head is relatively large for the body and the limbs are relatively short, small and thin because few muscles have yet developed. The head continues to assume its more rounded shape and the face is developing rapidly. The eyes are completely formed and are continuing to grow. The inner ear and middle ear are completely developed and the external ear continues to enlarge and assume its adult shape. The limbs are growing rapidly and their various components are now easily recognizable, but the fingers and toes are still joined together. Movements of the limbs and spine increase.

The ovaries or testicles have formed within the body and the external genitalia are developing but the eventual sex cannot yet be distinguished.

The heart is completely formed and a satisfactory circulation is present for blood is being pumped to all parts of the body as well as through the umbilical cord to that part of the chorion which will eventually become the placenta.

The approximate length of the baby is 5.5 cm (as long as a little finger) and its weight is 10 g.

It is interesting to note that at the end of the 11th week of pregnancy all the essential organs of the fetus are formed and the majority of them are beginning to function. Although eleven weeks may sound a long time, it is only the time span between, for instance, 1 June and 17 August. It is during this time that congenital abnormalities may occur if some factor has been introduced that has the ability to interfere with the formation of a particular organ at a critical stage of its growth, so that its natural and normal development is disturbed. Once an organ has been properly formed it cannot come to any great harm, whatever happens to the mother or the fetus. It is important to realize that major congenital catastrophes can only result from factors which adversely affect the growth and development of the baby before the end of the 11th week. Any factor operating after this time will probably have no adverse effect at all, or, at very worst, will only have a minute effect upon the development of any particular organ.

12th week. The head continues to assume a more rounded form but is still bent forward. The face is now properly formed and eyelids are present. The external ear continues to develop. The internal organs continue their growth and development. Muscular development in the body and in the limbs increases the amount of fetal movement which originally began about the 8th week. The growth of the external genital organs continues.

The approximate length of the baby is 6.5 cm and its weight about 18 g.

13th week. At the end of the 13th week the pregnancy has reached the end of the third calendar month. The uterus is now distended by the pregnancy and measures approximately 10.2 cm in diameter. It can be palpated in the lower abdomen as a very soft, cystic swelling arising out of the pelvis. The amniotic sac which is distending the uterus contains approximately 100 ml of amniotic fluid and the growing fetus is suspended within this fluid. The fetus has plenty of room to move within the amniotic cavity and it only comes in contact with the amnion (and therefore the wall of the uterus) if it happens to bounce against it. The head is now rounded and, as the neck is fully formed, it moves freely on the trunk. The face is also formed with the mouth, nose and eyes properly developed. The external ear is also properly developed. The internal organs are fully formed but the lungs, liver, kidney and intestine continue to grow and mature. The external genital organs continue to develop and the sex of the

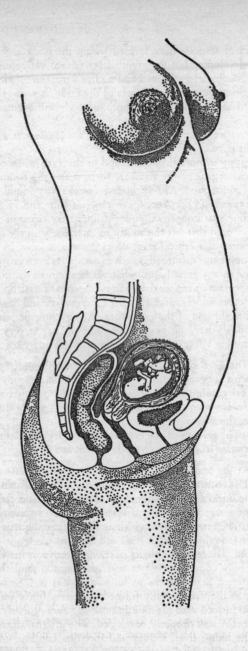

Fig 11   The abdomen at the 12th week of pregnancy

infant is now obvious. Fetal movement increases but is not yet sufficiently vigorous for the mother to be aware of it.

The length of the baby is approximately 7.5 cm and its weight approximately 30 g.

By the end of the 13th week the baby is properly formed. If delivered it could not survive because although all the organs are present they have not yet matured sufficiently to perform the duties for which they are designed. Syphilis, viral and rare tropical diseases are the only known infections which can now cross to the fetus and cause it any harm. There are several specific drugs which, if taken in normal doses from this stage of pregnancy, may cause abnormal growth of a particular organ, but there is no drug which can cause gross congenital abnormality unless it is taken in such large doses as to jeopardize the mother's life.

The remainder of the pregnancy is designed not only to allow the fetus to grow to a size at which it is capable of independent survival, but also to give all the vital organs in the body sufficient time to mature and develop their highly complex processes which are essential for independent survival. It can be appreciated, therefore, that while the weight of the baby may be important, it is upon its degree of maturity that the survival of the fetus really depends.

16th week. By the end of the 16th week the limbs are properly formed and all the joints are moving. Vigorous movements continue but are rarely felt by the mother. The fingers and toes are normal and fingernails and toenails are present. The head is still relatively large for the size of the body but fairly rapid growth continues to enlarge the body. Primary sex characteristics continue to develop and the sex of the infant is now obvious to the untrained observer.

A fine downy hair, lanugo, forms over the whole fetus including the face. The eyebrows and eyelashes start to grow.

The approximate length of the baby is 16 cm and its weight about 135 g.

20th week. The baby is now growing rapidly in length and in weight. Hair appears on the head. Muscle is rapidly increasing in the limbs and very active movements can easily be observed and felt by the mother. The fetus has a relatively large amount of liquor amnii (amniotic fluid) in which it can move and rotate with ease.

The length of the infant is approximately 25.5 cm and its weight about 340 g.

24th week. The fetus continues to grow and its vital organs are now sufficiently mature for it to survive for a short time if delivered prematurely. It is unlikely to maintain independent life for any length of time, however, as the lungs are inadequately matured. It does, however, now have a chance of survival if it is treated by experts in an intensive-care premature-baby unit. The arms and legs have a normal amount of muscle,

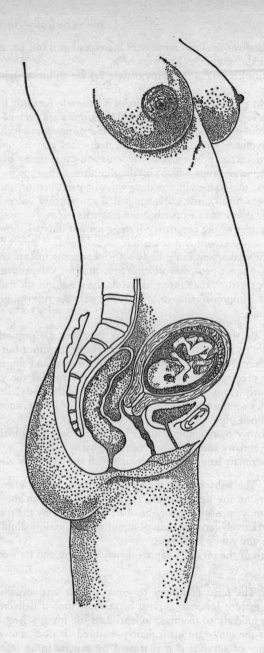

Fig. 12   The abdomen at the 16th week of pregnancy

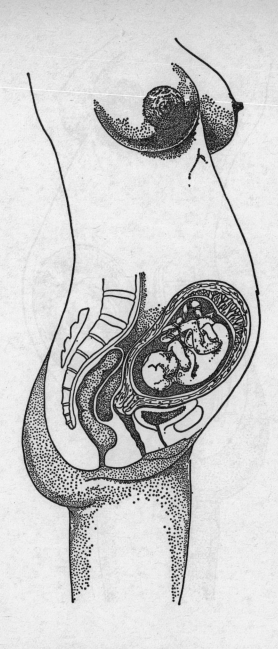

Fig 13 The abdomen at the 20th week of pregnancy

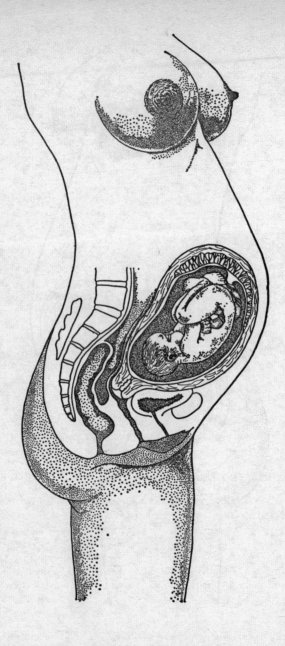

Fig 14   The abdomen at the 24th week of pregnancy

although the baby remains rather thin because deposits of subcutaneous fat have not yet been laid down.

The approximate length of a child born at this stage is 33 cm and its weight 570 g.

28th week. At 28 weeks the fetus is viable, which means that, according to legal definition, it is capable of a separate and independent existence and if prematurely born it must be registered. The definition of viability and the date of viability during pregnancy were laid down approximately one hundred years ago and nothing has happened in the intervening years which has altered the baby's chance of independent survival before the end of 28 weeks of pregnancy. Some babies delivered before the 28th week of pregnancy do survive with very highly specialized expert medical and nursing care and attention but they are few. The chances of survival at 28 weeks are up to 75 per cent in the very best premature-baby intensive-care nurseries, providing of course that the child has no congenital abnormality and its very delicate organs have not suffered any damage or injury at birth.

Before the 28th week the termination of pregnancy is abortion. This may be legally performed if the provisions of the Abortion Act 1967 are complied with (see Chapter 44). After the 28th week of pregnancy a woman is said to go into premature labour and it is not a legal offence to induce premature labour in any circumstance even at 28 weeks and one day, even though it may be known that the baby's chances of survival are virtually nil.

The fetus is now covered with vernix, which is a greasy, adherent, cheese-like material over the whole of the baby's skin, protecting it from becoming waterlogged by its continual immersion in the liquor amnii. The baby's body has grown more than the head has grown during the past few weeks so that the head is now only slightly out of proportion to the size of the body.

The length of the baby is 37 cm and the weight is 900 g.

32nd week. The child is now perfectly formed and its head is in proportion with its body. A large amount of vernix is present over the whole body. If the baby is delivered the eyes will open spontaneously, especially if the baby is inverted (that is facing downwards, not head downwards) and the chances of survival are up to 95 per cent in the best premature nurseries.

The amount of subcutaneous fat that has been deposited is increasing, but the child is still relatively thin. Its length is approximately 40.5 cm and its weight 1.6 kg. It will usually be lying with its head towards the mother's pelvis.

36th week. At this stage the baby is almost fully mature and stands more than a 95 per cent chance of survival if delivered. The main reason why babies fail to survive if they are delivered at this stage is because the lungs

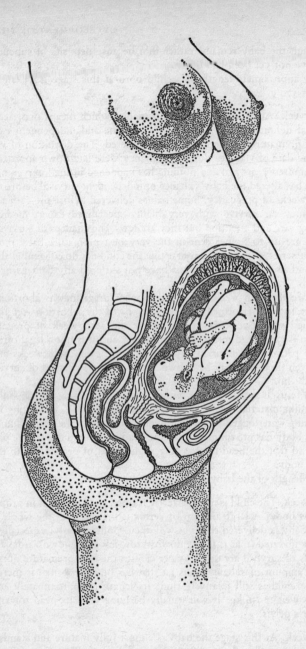

Fig. 15　The abdomen at the 28th week of pregnancy

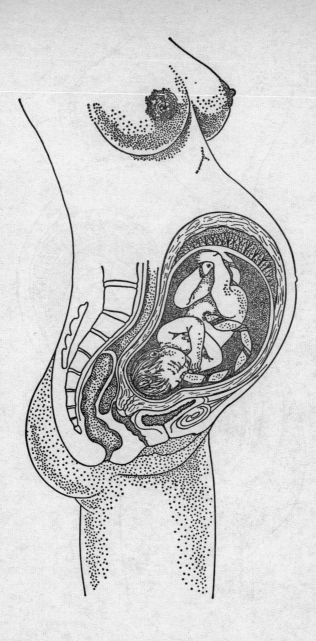

Fig. 16 The abdomen at the 32nd week of pregnancy

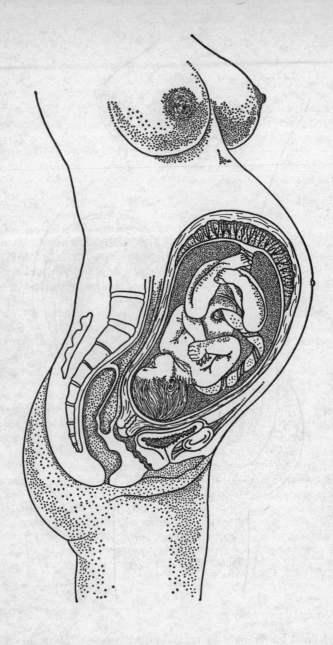

Fig 17   The abdomen at the 34th to the 36th week of pregnancy

may be insufficiently developed. A great deal of subcutaneous fat has been laid down. A large quantity of vernix is still covering the baby and small amounts may be present in the amniotic fluid. The baby should have assumed its permanent position as a cephalic or head presentation, and in approximately 50 per cent of women having their first baby it is at this stage that the head will descend into the pelvis. If the head does not descend or engage at the 36th week there is no need for concern. Women having their second or subsequent baby will notice that the head does not engage until the 40th week, or very frequently until the onset of labour. In a male infant the testicles have descended into the scrotum.

The length of the baby is approximately 46 cm and its weight 2.5 kg.

40th week. The average pregnancy is supposed to last 280 days, or 40 weeks, from the first day of the last normal menstrual period (or 266 days from conception) but it must be remembered that this is an average, not a rule. Some women will have normal pregnancies of shorter duration, whilst others will have normal pregnancies of longer duration, and similarly, some babies will mature and be ready for delivery before the 40th week whilst others will be slow to mature and will not be ready until after the 40th week. The time of delivery is discussed on page 113, and has nothing to do with the baby's subsequent physical or intellectual ability. The mature baby is properly developed and has a large quantity of subcutaneous fat which has been deposited over the previous ten weeks and which gives its limbs and body a rounded appearance. The lanugo has disappeared, or almost disappeared, from the body but may still be present over the shoulders, arms and legs and occasionally on the forehead. The hair on the head varies in length from 2 to 4 cm. The body is covered entirely with vernix except for the mouth and on the eyes. The vernix is particularly thick on the skin creases of the groin and the elbow, as well as round the neck, under the armpits and behind the knees. The sclera, or white part of the eye, is fairly white in colour and the iris is blue. Babies are always born with blue eyes, although occasionally the colour may change within a few minutes of delivery. The nails are properly developed and protrude to the end of the finger but not beyond. They are very soft and will not damage the skin by scratching during the first 24 hours of life.

The baby increases in weight by approximately 7 per cent per week from the 36th to the 40th week, that is about 1 per cent, or 28 g a day. The approximate length of the baby at term is 50 cm and its weight approximately 3.4 kg.

When is a baby fully formed?

The baby is fully formed by the end of the 12th week of pregnancy and from then onwards it only grows and matures. The process of maturing, however, is certainly as important as the process of growth. At 12 weeks a baby has all the appropriate organs but they are not yet sufficiently well developed to function satisfactorily or independently.

At the 28th week of pregnancy a baby is stated to have the ability to undertake a separate existence and the term 'viable' is used. Each day, however, that the child can remain *in utero* beyond the 28th week increases the chance of survival, because it becomes more mature each day. Its heart is more capable of controlling the altered circulation after birth; the brain is developing so that it is more able to control the fundamental functions of the body; the lungs are developing and are more able to exchange oxygen; the liver with all its complex metabolic processes is also developing and maturing with each day that passes. It is not, therefore, the size of the baby that is the most important factor, but its maturity, and it is upon this that its eventual survival depends. In other words, a baby who is 38 weeks mature stands a much better chance of surviving than a baby who is 34 weeks mature. And similarly a baby who is 34 weeks mature has a much better chance of surviving than a baby who is 30 weeks mature.

Some babies, for instance those of diabetic mothers, may be unduly large but this does not increase their chance of survival. A baby weighing 2.5 kg who is 38 weeks mature stands a better chance of survival than a baby who is 34 weeks mature and weighs 3.6 kg. In the latter instance the vital organs of the baby, while not being completely mature, still have to provide all the oxygen and vital functions for a 3.6 kg baby, whereas in the former instance the better developed organs have only to supply the needs of a 2.5 kg baby.

Development of the placenta

The chorionic villi, or sponge-like protrusions, which surround the newly embedded embryo rapidly increase in both number and size. At about the 6th week of pregnancy blood vessels are formed within the fetus, and by the 8th week within the chorionic villi, thus enabling them to transport materials more readily to the developing fetus. As the embryo enlarges it gradually fills and then commences to distend the cavity of the uterus and by the 12th week of pregnancy the active growth of the pregnancy itself is beginning to exert pressure on the walls of the uterus and cause its further growth and distension. It is at this stage that the chorionic villi at the site of the original implantation develop with immense speed to form the placenta (or afterbirth), while the chorionic villi over the remainder of the embryo gradually shrivel and die. After the 14th week a proper placenta is formed and takes over the functions of basic nourishment and hormone production.

The newly formed placenta gradually enters larger maternal blood vessels, but the chorionic villi penetrate only as far as the middle layers of the cells lining the inner surface of the uterus. They do not penetrate the muscle of the uterus, nor do they penetrate the major blood vessels which are supplying the uterus.

The action of the chorionic villi upon the maternal tissues results in the creation of a lake or pool which fills with maternal blood and is surrounded on its outer side by the cells lining the inner side of the uterus, and on the fetal side by the placenta itself, and into which are suspended the individual villi or finger-like processes of the placenta. Blood arrives at the placenta from the fetus by means of the umbilical arteries; it circulates through the placenta and through the chorionic villi and returns to the fetus by way of the umbilical vein.

The placenta is responsible for the selective transfer to the fetus of oxygen and other necessary substances as well as removal from the fetus of its waste products. Everything that is required for the growth and maturation of the fetus must pass the placenta, so the placenta is responsible for the passage of not only oxygen, but also carbohydrate, fatty acids, protein, complicated amino acids, vitamins and essential elements such as calcium. Excretion products from the fetus are absorbed into the maternal circulation and some of these, such as carbon dioxide, are exhaled by the mother from her lungs, whilst others such as urea are excreted by her kidneys.

The placenta reaches maturity at approximately the 34th week of pregnancy. After this it slowly undergoes very mild ageing or degenerative changes.

At term the placenta, or afterbirth, weighs approximately 570 g or about one-sixth of the baby's weight, and is a flattened disc-like mass measuring approximately 18 cm in diameter and 3.2 cm in thickness.

The umbilical cord is usually attached to the centre of the fetal surface of the placenta, which has a shiny bluish colour on which can be seen the blood vessels which supply the placenta. The maternal, or deeper, surface of the placenta is usually divided into twelve to fifteen lobules or segments and is a dull red or brownish colour.

The maternal and fetal circulations are entirely independent. The fetal blood circulates from the fetus into the placenta and returns again to the baby. The maternal circulation arrives at the uterus by means of the uterine artery and leaves it via the uterine veins. This blood forms the pool, or lake, of blood into which the lobes of the placenta are immersed. At no stage, with the exception of a few cells as described below, do the circulations or cells from the circulations of the mother and fetus mix. Materials are transmitted rapidly across the barrier formed by the placenta either from the fetus to the mother or from the mother to the fetus. This barrier is sometimes only one cell thick.

Bleeding occurring during pregnancy, either early or later, comes from

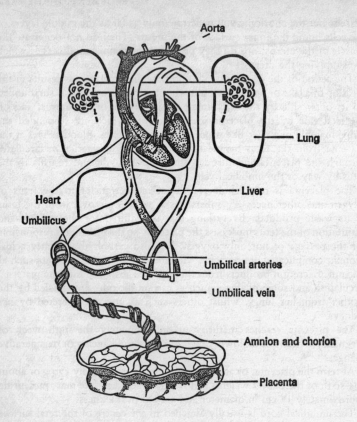

Fig. 18 The placenta and the fetal circulation

the pool of maternal blood lying immediately beneath the placenta. The blood is always maternal blood and never blood from the fetal circulation, since it is impossible for blood to escape from the fetal circulation.

Small finger-like processes of the placenta may occasionally break off and be washed away with the maternal blood into the mother's circulation. This may occasionally include a few of the circulating red cells from the fetus. The intrusion of these fetal cells into the maternal circulation occurs intermittently throughout the whole of pregnancy, and careful examination of the mother's blood will occasionally demonstrate cells either from the placenta itself or from the fetal circulation. At the time of delivery quite a large number of both placental cells and circulating fetal blood cells escape into the maternal circulation and it is the marked leakage of cells at this particular time that is responsible for Rhesus sensitization.

Hormones produced by the placenta

The placenta produces a large number of hormones, one of the most important being progesterone. It begins to produce progesterone after about the 10th week of pregnancy and, by the end of the 14th week, should be manufacturing sufficient to ensure the survival of the entire pregnancy and so replace the progesterone previously made by the corpus luteum.

The placenta makes a large number of placental proteins, of which human placental lactogen (HPL) is one of the most important, and oestrogens (excreted as oestriol). These hormones may be used later in pregnancy as an indicator of placental activity and function.

Abnormalities of the placenta

These are described under the headings of Abortion, Blighted ovum, Hydatidiform mole, Bleeding in pregnancy, Death in utero, Post-maturity, Pre-eclampsia and Postpartum haemorrhage.

The membranes

The membranes consist of two very thin structures called the amnion and the chorion. The membranes form the lining of the inner aspect of the uterus during pregnancy and they are responsible for forming the bag within which the water or amniotic fluid is contained. The most important duty of the membranes is to maintain and keep the amniotic fluid within the cavity of the uterus, because without the amniotic fluid a pregnancy cannot continue. If the membranes rupture the waters break and the amniotic fluid will drain away, which is a characteristic occurrence either at the onset of labour or at some stage during the process of labour.

The membranes are also known as the caul. David Copperfield was supposed to have been born in a complete caul, which used to be considered a good omen and an indication that the person would never drown at sea. Even today some people have a fear that a child may suffer adversely as a result of being born with the membranes unruptured. It is almost impossible for this to happen, but should it occur there is certainly no harm done to the baby since the membranes can be easily broken and removed from the baby's face and mouth.

The amniotic fluid

Throughout its whole development and growth the baby is surrounded by the amniotic fluid, otherwise known as the liquor amnii or just simply liquor. It is contained by the amniotic membrane within the amniotic cavity, and is formed very early in the development of the human embryo. The amniotic fluid gradually changes its constituents as pregnancy progresses.

In early pregnancy the size of the amniotic cavity is larger than is required by the small fetus, therefore affording the growing fetus complete freedom to move and develop.

At about the 16th week of pregnancy the baby has complete freedom to move, turn and rotate but can now be palpated by the skilled examiner through the wall of the uterus. This freedom continues until about the 30th week of pregnancy, when the baby has a tendency to become fixed in a longitudinal position within the uterine cavity. In some pregnancies, however, there is still sufficient fluid even at 34 weeks to allow the baby to rotate or turn quite freely.

Approximately 1 litre of amniotic fluid is present at the 36th week of pregnancy, after which the amount of fluid gradually diminishes until the expected date of delivery is reached, when the amount present is usually just under 1 litre. If delivery does not occur at the 40th week the quantity of amniotic fluid is reduced more rapidly, so that by the 42nd week 100 or 200 ml may be all that is remaining.

Functions of amniotic fluid

1 Amniotic fluid provides a liquid environment in which the fetus can develop and exercise in absolute freedom.
2 It causes enlargement of the amniotic cavity and, therefore, of the uterus, so that the developing fetus is not distorted by pressure from the wall of the uterus.
3 It provides an environment of constant temperature.
4 Its constituents vary as pregnancy advances and as the requirements of the fetus change.
5 It provides a means of excretion of substances from the fetus, especially urine.
6 The fetus also swallows liquor. It is not known how much nutritional benefit this may have for the fetus, but it enables it to develop its mouth, as well as its swallowing and breathing mechanisms.
7 The amniotic fluid functions as a shock absorber which is most efficient in preventing damage to the fetus as a result of a blow or undue pressure. If undue force is brought to bear upon any particular part of the uterus then the placenta may suffer damage, or may even be separated, but it is virtually impossible to damage the fetus itself as a result of direct or indirect injury.

Many women fear that their baby will be damaged by a fall or a direct blow upon the uterus or abdomen during pregnancy. If a pregnant woman does suffer from direct injury, or if she falls down on her abdomen, she is unlikely to have caused injury to her pregnancy but she should consult her doctor if she develops pain or if she is unduly concerned. Falling down stairs, tripping over the edge of a carpet or pavement, and motor-car accidents are the three most common causes of abdominal injury during pregnancy. Contrary to some of the ancient legends, injury to the abdomen will not cause deformity or congenital abnormalities of the fetus. Obviously pregnancy does not prevent maternal bones being broken or other injuries occurring, but direct injury to the baby itself is very unlikely.

Origin of amniotic fluid

The method of formation, disposal and the control of amniotic fluid are not really understood. It is probably formed from the cells which line the amniotic membrane and during the second half of pregnancy the fetus urinates into the amniotic fluid. Some of the amniotic fluid is probably absorbed either into the umbilical cord or into the cells lining the amniotic membranes, and during the second half of pregnancy the fetus swallows some amniotic fluid. The amniotic fluid is formed by tissues of fetal origin and not of maternal origin. It is secreted and absorbed continuously.

Leakage of amniotic fluid

When the membranes rupture during labour amniotic fluid leaks out of the uterus and down the vagina. Rupture of the membranes before the onset of labour is inevitably followed by labour either prematurely or at term. In certain instances leakage of amniotic fluid precedes miscarriage. When the membranes rupture there is a sudden rush, or gush, of liquor which is unmistakable. Should this happen the pregnant woman must go to bed immediately and notify her doctor or midwife, or telephone the hospital.

Sudden rupture of the membranes with the loss of a large amount of liquor is always obvious, but there may occasionally be a small leakage of liquor which is much more difficult to diagnose. Some pregnant women occasionally leak small quantities of urine during the second half of pregnancy and this is easily confused with amniotic fluid. Bath water does not normally enter the vagina, but sometimes during pregnancy a small quantity of water may do so and escape shortly after bathing. If a small rupture has occurred in the membranes it will result in a small but continuous leakage of amniotic fluid from the vagina. If she has any doubt about the origin of the water the patient should put on a sanitary towel, go to bed and, if the leakage continues, notify her doctor or telephone the hospital. If the leakage of amniotic fluid has occurred prematurely she will be admitted to hospital where it may be possible to prevent the onset of premature labour by rest and the administration of drugs.

Amount of amniotic fluid

The quantity of amniotic fluid varies during a pregnancy, as stated above, but it also varies from person to person and from pregnancy to pregnancy. Within reasonable limits the amount has no effect upon the fetus or upon its growth and development. In some pregnancies there is a small amount of amniotic fluid, which may not be of any significance, or may sometimes be associated with conditions in which the baby does not get sufficient nutrition in the uterus and grows poorly (intrauterine growth retardation). Certain kidney abnormalities are also associated with decreased liquor. It does mean, however, that the baby has less room in which to turn and it is important that he should assume his correct position—cephalic (head) presentation—at about the 30th or 32nd week of pregnancy.

If an excessive quantity of amniotic fluid is present it is called polyhydramnios.

The umbilical cord

The umbilical cord extends from the umbilicus of the fetus to the surface of the placenta. It carries the fetal blood from the fetus to the placenta via the two umbilical arteries, and the returning blood via the single umbilical vein.

The blood vessels in the umbilical cord have a very thin muscular wall and are easily damaged. They are surrounded by a jelly-like substance known as Wharton's jelly and are coiled in a spiral fashion. The umbilical cord is approximately 50 cm in length and in a fully mature pregnancy is about the thickness of the index finger. It is surrounded by a very thin, delicate, skin-like membrane.

On rare occasions the umbilical cord becomes tied into a true knot which may be pulled tight either by the fetus within the uterus, or at the time of delivery. A true knot which is loosely tied does not affect the circulation of blood, but if it becomes tightly pulled then the blood flow will be obstructed and the fetus will die rapidly from lack of oxygen. This type of knot in the cord is rare, but is an unpreventable cause of death. In early pregnancy the baby can move freely within the uterus and undoubtedly turns over and over many times. It is extraordinary that true knots do not form in the cord more frequently.

The umbilical cord may become wrapped around an arm or a leg, or it may become twisted around the neck of the baby. Instances have been recorded in which the umbilical cord has been coiled as many as six or seven times around a baby's neck and the child still survived unharmed. Nevertheless, this does present a hazard to the baby, mainly during labour. The placenta is usually attached to the top or the fundus of the uterus and as the baby descends during the second stage of labour so the cord which is twisted round the neck tends to be pulled tighter with each descending movement. The cord is usually sufficiently long to allow this to happen without any effect on its circulation, but if it is rather short then the circulation will gradually be occluded as the head of the baby descends and the cord is tightened round the neck. Happily this catastrophe is extremely rare, but unfortunately it is impossible to diagnose before delivery or before sudden and dramatic fetal distress has occurred during the second stage of labour.

Fetal movements

Fetal movements are essential for a baby to mature properly, because he will only develop those muscles that he can use and exercise to the fullest extent while in the uterus. Her baby's movements also remind the mother that he is still present, alive and kicking.

For a further description of fetal movements see Chapter 11.

The fetal heart

The fetal heart begins to develop during the 6th week of pregnancy and the fetal circulation is established by the end of the 7th week. The fetal heart can be seen beating on an ultrasonic scan at the end of the 6th week and can be heard with the use of Doptone apparatus as early as the 12th week of pregnancy, although it is sometimes difficult to detect until the end of the 14th week. It can be heard with an ordinary stethoscope at about the 24th week of pregnancy. The times at which the fetal heart can be seen and heard are used as valuable milestones to judge the progress of a pregnancy.

There are certain qualities of a baby's heart beat such as volume, tone and rhythm as well as a normal rate which any skilled observer will recognize. It is most unusual for the tone and rhythm to vary greatly during pregnancy. A baby's heart beats relatively quickly while he is in the uterus. The speed varies from 120 to 160 beats per minute and sounds very fast when you hear it for the first time. Small variations in this speed will occur when the baby moves or following palpation of the abdomen, but before the onset of labour it is unusual for the rate to vary outside the normal range.

Weight of the baby

The average weight of full-term new-born infants in England is 3.2 to 3.4 kg. Any baby whose weight at birth is below 2.5 kg is stated to be premature or small for dates. Babies more than 4.5 kg are usually considered to be overweight at birth; they nearly always develop perfectly normally, but, as in the case of a premature baby, frequently require extra care and attention during the first few days of life.

It is strange how some women wish to dramatize their personal experiences during delivery. Everyone is familiar with the manner in which women will recount their own blood-curdling experience during childbirth to a newly pregnant acquaintance. Such exaggerations also apply to babies' birthweights, so that it is extraordinary how many children delivered fifty years ago are supposed to have weighed over 4.5, 5 or even 5.4 kg. There is some evidence to suggest that the average weight of the normal healthy baby has slightly increased over the past fifty years, but this increase is only from 3.26 kg in 1920 to 3.35 kg in 1970.

Factors affecting birthweight

Most babies weigh between 3.12 kg and 3.84 kg. It is impossible to predetermine the weight of a baby by any known influences that can be exerted upon a woman during pregnancy. A multitude of different factors affect the birthweight of a baby, only a few of which can be controlled. If a normal pregnant patient asks 'What can I do to have a small baby?', or 'What can I do to have a large baby?', the simple answer is that there is very little anyone can do to influence the rate of growth of the baby in the uterus. Heavier women tend to have heavier babies, and lighter women tend to have lighter babies. It is also true that women who gain excess weight during pregnancy tend to have babies who are slightly heavier than those of women who gain a normal amount of weight.

Age. The majority of women will deliver their heaviest child when they are about 35 years of age. On a rough working average the baby born to a woman of 35 will be approximately 170 g heavier than the baby born to a girl of 17.

Number of children. In subsequent pregnancies babies tend to become slightly longer and heavier. A woman who has had several children will find that her last is slightly heavier than her first.

Sex. Boys are usually heavier than their sisters and, all other factors being equal, male babies weigh approximately 113 to 170 g more than female babies. This difference is purely an average and does not, of course, apply to all new-born infants.

Race. Babies of German parentage are usually heavier (3.52 kg) than those of British parentage (3.40 kg). These in turn are usually heavier than American Negro babies (3.22 kg) while the average birthweight of the Japanese baby is even less (2.95 kg).

Economic factors. The average weight of babies delivered to women of the upper social classes is higher than the average weight of those delivered to women in the lower social classes. This is partly because premature labour is more common in the lower social classes resulting in the delivery of small infants which reduces the overall average birthweight. Quite apart from prematurity, however, the weight of infants born at term to women who are in the lower socio-economic groups is on average 0.3 kg less than those born to women in the higher socio-economic groups. There are many factors which influence the birthweight of babies in these two particular groups. The affluent patient has more time for rest and leisure and may have a more complete diet. She generally pays more detailed attention to her pregnancy and follows more meticulously the advice and instruction she is given. She is thus less likely to smoke or suffer from anaemia, pre-eclampsia and other factors that adversely influence the outcome of a pregnancy.

Maternal disease. In the past maternal disease was thought to have a large influence on the birthweight of the baby. Today there are only two serious maternal diseases which exert a major influence upon fetal weight.

Diabetes, or a condition known as gestational diabetes (a state of very early diabetes in which the urine may contain sugar for the first time during pregnancy and which can only be diagnosed by special blood tests), may result in a large baby and it is for this reason that the mothers of all babies who weigh 4.5 kg or more at birth should have a special test performed to exclude diabetes or gestational diabetes.

Raised blood pressure and renal disease (chronic nephritis) may in some instances result in the formation of a small placenta, which in turn results in a small baby. Such a small baby, having been delivered, will of course develop quite normally, as will the large diabetic baby.

Parental size. The old and long-standing aphorism that women produce babies to suit themselves is still true. A small woman will usually produce a smaller baby than a tall woman. Similarly, a short woman married to a tall man will usually produce a small baby suitable to her own particular stature. The majority of women, however, produce an average size baby. If a woman's first baby is large, then her subsequent children are likely to be large also. Similarly, if a woman's first baby is small then her subsequent children are likely to be of similar size.

Maternal weight. Within reasonable limits maternal weight does not appear to affect the birthweight of the baby. A large woman is, however, more likely to produce a large baby and a small woman to produce a small baby. Obesity, however, does not have any effect upon birthweight.

Diet. It is difficult to influence the birthweight of a baby by diet during pregnancy. The baby is a parasite and behaves as one. It will extract from the maternal circulation its exact and complete requirements regardless of the mother's condition. Many women in a state of severe malnutrition give birth to perfectly healthy, normal babies who show no deficiency whatever. This is particularly applicable to the intake of iron and of calcium. A woman may become very severely anaemic due to iron depletion, but her new-born child will have perfectly normal bones at birth, whereas his mother's bones have become softened and even bent because of the calcium taken from her by her child. A woman who is having a normal and reasonable diet cannot affect the birthweight of her baby either by increasing her calorie intake or by going on a strict reducing diet.

Heredity. Many obstetricians ask about a pregnant woman's own birthweight because there is some evidence to show that large babies or small babies do occasionally run in families. People's ideas of their own particular birthweight are, however, notoriously inaccurate.

Smoking. The baby of a woman who smokes more than ten cigarettes a day is likely to be lighter than normally expected. Smoking thirty cigarettes a day may reduce the baby's weight by as much as 10 per cent and almost certainly causes mental and physical retardation in later childhood. It is generally considered that smoking has an adverse effect on the blood supply to the uterus and reduces the oxygen supply to the baby. Women must not smoke during pregnancy; quite apart from the general ill health which may be caused by smoking, they must realize the possible harm they may do to their unborn child if they continue smoking after the 16th week.

5 Early Pregnancy

Symptoms

Certain characteristic symptoms occur very early in pregnancy and most women go to their doctor for confirmation of pregnancy as soon as they are aware of them.

Absence of menstrual period (amenorrhoea)

Failure of the period to come at the usual time is generally the first sign of pregnancy. A missed menstrual period in any woman of child-bearing age who is having sexual intercourse should be presumed to be due to pregnancy until proved otherwise. Once the menstrual periods have established a normal rhythm, pregnancy is the commonest cause for their delay or absence. Stress, strain, psychological upset, severe systemic diseases such as anaemia, diabetes, and tuberculosis, or change of climate, change of occupation or sudden shock may all be the reason for the absence of a menstrual period. Some women do not have any periods while they are using the contraceptive pill.

Partially suppressed periods

Occasionally in early pregnancy the level of progesterone produced by the corpus luteum is inadequate to suppress completely the menstrual period. In this circumstance a small amount of uterine bleeding may occur which the woman naturally interprets as a normal period. The amount of loss, however, is usually less than normal and occurs for a shorter duration than usual. It is very seldom accompanied by any pain. Partially suppressed periods confuse not only the diagnosis of pregnancy but also the date of fertilization and, therefore, the expected date of delivery. Women who have partially suppressed periods during the early part of their pregnancy usually only do so for the first one or perhaps two, the second one being shorter than the first. On very rare occasions a woman will 'menstruate' throughout the duration of her pregnancy and it is not unknown for periods to occur for the first four, five or even six months. The presence of such partially suppressed periods does not appear to affect the fetus adversely, but 'bleeding in early pregnancy', although recognized as a partially suppressed period, must be considered as a threatened abortion and treated by bed rest. Obviously such a condition will not arise until the time of the second suppressed period because the woman will only then consider a diagnosis of pregnancy and appreciate in retrospect that the first period was not entirely normal.

Frequently women will feel most of the premonitory symptoms of menstruation and be sure that a period is about to appear. Symptoms of impending menstruation vary greatly from person to person and they frequently include a variable degree of engorgement and tenderness in the breasts, lower abdominal discomfort, a feeling or sensation of tension together with many other ill-defined and minor phenomena. These rather vague premenstrual symptoms do not prejudice a pregnancy in any way. They frequently continue for a day or two after the expected date of the period.

Nausea

Nausea or a sensation of feeling sick is very common in the first three months of pregnancy and is frequently the first symptom noticed by women. The nausea tends to be more severe in the early morning although it can occur at any time of the day. It follows an individual pattern not only in each person but also in each pregnancy. Some women experience nausea in the morning alone, others in the evening. The more unfortunate may suffer for most of the day. It is frequently, although not necessarily, followed by vomiting, when it is known as 'early morning sickness'. Nausea is accompanied by a sensation of fullness in the upper abdomen which may become so severe that women will actually make themselves vomit in order to relieve this pressure.

The exact cause of the nausea is not known but it is probably associated with a high hormone level especially that of progesterone. It may be provoked by sickly smells and especially the smell of cooking fat, and can be considerably alleviated by avoiding these and any other factors which tend to precipitate it. It is also relieved by raising the blood sugar level which can be easily accomplished by taking small frequent meals. These should not contain large quantities of sugar because a high concentration of sugar in the stomach will itself increase the amount of nausea. A drink of tea or milk together with a piece of dry toast is usually sufficient.

Nausea can be controlled to a certain extent by the doctor's or midwife's reassurance. It is a phenomenon of normal pregnancy and, generally speaking, a lot of nausea means a better and more secure pregnancy. This does not mean that a woman who does not suffer nausea does not have a good or a stable pregnancy. The symptom can usually be controlled by careful attention to diet, but for those who find it too severe there are some anti-histamines which can safely be taken in early pregnancy to control the nausea or at least improve the symptom even if they do not completely eliminate it.

Nausea usually diminishes in severity after about the 10th week of pregnancy and decreases quite dramatically from the 13th week, disappearing completely by the end of the 14th week. It is unusual for it to continue into the 15th week but if it does do so it does not indicate abnormality.

Vomiting

Vomiting in early pregnancy is usually associated with severe nausea, but this is not an unbroken rule. The vomiting, or 'morning sickness', generally occurs in the early morning relieving a fairly severe degree of nausea. Actual vomiting often happens rather suddenly without the disagreeable symptoms that precede it in the non-pregnant person. Vomiting itself can be most unpleasant especially in the early morning because there is no food in the stomach and only a small quantity of mucus is brought up. It may occur at any time later in the day and will usually be worse if a woman is subjected to stress, strain or worry.

Excessive vomiting known as hyperemesis gravidarum occasionally occurs and the woman is usually treated in hospital (see Chapter 18). The vomiting itself does not harm the woman nor does the exertion harm the uterus or the fetus. It is not true that an excessive amount of vomiting is associated with any abnormality of either the pregnant woman or her baby, except in very rare instances. Excessive vomiting, however, should always be carefully investigated and any woman who is being sick more frequently than three or four times a day should consult her doctor or midwife.

Early morning sickness can be controlled by a very careful diet regime first thing in the morning. The woman should rest quietly on waking and not leap out of bed to start her housework. One of the easiest and best methods of controlling the sickness is to have a small drink of some bland fluid such as sweetened tea containing a small amount of milk and a dry biscuit or some dry toast. Butter and other fats are better avoided especially in the early morning. For the rest of the day her diet should consist of small and frequent meals again avoiding fat and excessive intake of concentrated sugar. Powerful anti-emetics are to be avoided but some antihistamine drugs, such as Avomine, will help to control vomiting and may even eliminate this unpleasant symptom. The intensity of the vomiting may vary from day to day but it usually starts to decrease spontaneously about the 10th week of pregnancy and is usually gone completely by the end of the 14th week.

Micturition

Sometimes one of the earliest signs of pregnancy is an increase in the frequency of micturition. The majority of women pass urine between two and six times each day and do not have to get up to empty their bladder at night. It is not unusual in the early months of pregnancy for a pregnant woman to have to pass urine every two hours during the day and for her to get up at least twice during the night. This is not abnormal so long as there is no pain or discomfort and is due to pressure from the enlarging uterus, which is still within the pelvis, on the bladder. Frequency of micturition tends to become less marked during the fourth month but may again become more severe towards the end of pregnancy, especially after the baby's head has engaged in the pelvis.

Constipation

Constipation is an early symptom of pregnancy but is not sufficiently definite to assist in its diagnosis. The action of the hormone progesterone relaxes the muscle of the intestine reducing its movement and causing varying degrees of constipation which, unless treated, will probably continue throughout the whole pregnancy.

Taste

Alterations in taste may be among the earliest of pregnancy symptoms. Some women will recognize a strange taste in their mouth even before they miss their first period. Such a taste is characteristic to each individual and is usually described as metallic.

Shortly after the first missed period the majority of pregnant women start to 'go off' certain things. A dislike of cigarettes or tobacco smoke is probably the most commonly noticed of these early changes and may be followed shortly afterwards by a dislike of other things that are normally very much appreciated such as alcohol, especially spirits and red wine, coffee, fat and occasionally meat itself.

It is very difficult to differentiate between smell and taste and a pregnant woman often has a different appreciation for different smells and perfumes and usually an intense dislike of the smell of cooking fat.

Skin changes

Changes in the skin are not very common in early pregnancy but in some people they do occur relatively early and occasionally they are noticeable. Dry skin tends to become drier quite early in pregnancy. Some women develop spots on the face, especially around the mouth, such as they had many years before, especially preceding a period, and from which they have not suffered recently. These spots may disappear quite quickly and the complexion returns to normal. On rare occasions, however, they may persist for several weeks or even months.

Breast changes

Together with the missing of a period the breast changes are usually the most convincing evidence of early pregnancy. The premenstrual fullness of the breasts continues when the period does not appear and within a matter of days the symptoms become even more marked. The breasts feel full, slightly tender and more sensitive than usual, especially in the region of the aerola (the pink area around the nipple) and the nipple. There may also be a sensation of tingling. The breasts enlarge quite slowly but definitely so that by the end of the sixth week after the last menstrual period there is a very appreciable change in their size. The small tail of breast tissue that lies almost inside the front of the armpit may become particularly swollen and tender. There is also an increase in the superficial veins over the breasts, and at about the same time tiny nodules called Montgomery's tubercles appear on the areola. Six or twelve of these small raised bumps will be found on each breast. The nipple also enlarges and becomes more prominent.

Quickening

Feeling fetal movements is not really a sign of early pregnancy since the baby's movements are not normally felt in a woman having her first baby until between the 18th and 20th week of pregnancy or in a subsequent pregnancy between the 16th and 18th week. It only too often happens, however, that for some reason or other this is the first symptom recognized by a pregnant woman. The movements themselves are difficult to recognize at first, being very similar to the sensation of wind moving around inside the abdomen, and have often been likened to a butterfly fluttering. (See Chapter 11.)

Diagnosis

Pregnancy tests

The diagnosis of early pregnancy is most easily and satisfactorily accomplished by performing a pregnancy test on the urine of the pregnant woman.

Many people want to know how a pregnancy test works. It is really very simple, but in order to understand it completely you will have to read the section that explains the production of chorionic gonadotrophin. This is a hormone produced by the new pregnancy even before it embeds in the lining of the uterus on the 21st day of the menstrual cycle. Its production increases day by day so that by the 28th day there is sufficient to suppress the next menstrual period, and by the 35th day there is so much that it can be detected in the urine by means of special tests.

Chorionic gonadotrophin is found in its most concentrated form in the first specimen of urine passed in the early morning since nothing has been drunk for six to eight hours.

The former tests for pregnancy involved injecting the urine into animals. The chorionic gonadotrophin caused characteristic changes in the ovaries or in other parts of the genital tract of the various animals. These changes in the laboratory animals indicated the presence of a high concentration of chorionic gonadotrophin in the injected urine and therefore meant that the urine came from a pregnant woman. These tests used to take anything from twenty-four hours to seven days according to the different type of animal used.

The purely laboratory tests of today use an immunological technique. A specific antibody has been developed to chorionic gonadotrophin which makes it easily detectable in a test tube or on a simple microscope slide. These modern tests for pregnancy are as accurate as the use of laboratory animals, if not more so; they are much quicker, much more simple, much kinder and, of course, cheaper. The tests take anything from about two minutes to two hours depending on the particular type of test being used.

A positive result indicates pregnancy in over 99 per cent of instances. A negative test, however, does not necessarily mean that a pregnancy is not present because the test may have been performed too early in the pregnancy or for some particular reason the level of chorionic gonadotrophin may not yet have become sufficiently high for the test to become positive. If all the signs and symptoms of pregnancy are otherwise present the test should be repeated after a further seven days.

A special fraction of human chorionic gonadotrophin known as the 'ß-subunit' can be detected in the blood of a pregnant woman as early as the 21st day of the cycle or 7 days after fertilization and 7 days before her next period is due.

X-rays

X-rays are no longer used merely for the diagnosis of early pregnancy, having been superseded by electronic methods of looking at or listening to the fetal heart, although there are some special circumstances where an X-ray in later pregnancy may be necessary. Until recently X-rays were used for the diagnosis of pregnancy but even in the best hands it was not possible to confirm a pregnancy by X-ray until after the 14th week which is the earliest time at which the bones of the fetus can be discerned.

Ultrasound

An extension of the simple ultrasonic device used for listening to the baby's heart is the ultrasonic scanner which uses high frequency sound waves above those the human ear can detect. It may be used, without harm to mother or baby, to diagnose a pregnancy as early as six weeks from the last period. In addition, ultrasonic scans are used extensively in later pregnancy to study the growth of the baby, diagnose twins and find out to which part of the uterus the placenta has become attached.

The fetal heart

The fetal heart can normally be heard by the stethoscope at about the 24th week of pregnancy. The more modern method of listening to the baby's heart is by means of ultrasonics, using the Doptone or the Sonicaid apparatus which can detect the fetal heart at the 14th week of pregnancy and frequently as early as the 12th week. Ultrasound has replaced the use of X-rays as a means of determining the presence of a fetus in the uterus in early pregnancy, and furthermore it does not carry the disadvantages of X-rays. Ultrasonic scans will demonstrate movement of the fetal heart as early as the end of the 6th week of pregnancy.

Clinical examination

The diagnosis of pregnancy before the 8th week by simple clinical examination alone is extremely difficult. The most certain method of establishing an early diagnosis is by means of a pregnancy test which will be positive about 12 days after the first day of the missed period.

Most doctors get a pretty shrewd idea that a pregnancy is present from the history given by the patient. If all the usual symptoms of early pregnancy are present then it is fairly good presumptive evidence that the woman is pregnant. Most women, however, want a definitive answer which it is impossible to give based on the symptoms alone. Examination of the patient herself may show the characteristic breast changes. Vaginal or internal examination will not show any significant changes until about 6 weeks after the first day of the last period. These changes when they do appear will include a bluish or violet discoloration of the vagina, a softening of the cervix, a slight enlargement and softening of the uterus together with a palpable pulsation of the uterine artery which cannot be detected in the non-pregnant state. All these physical signs are rather uncertain and if a definite answer is required then the pregnancy will usually have to be confirmed by performing a pregnancy test upon the urine. A special blood test (page 100) in very early pregnancy or ultrasonic scan at 6 weeks will also confirm pregnancy.

6 Changes in the Body during Pregnancy

The uterus

Growth

Everyone knows that the uterus grows during pregnancy but what most women do not know is the size of their uterus before they show any obvious signs of early pregnancy. They also wish to know whether the size of their uterus is normal for the duration of their pregnancy. One of the first things to realize is that the clinical diagnosis of very early pregnancy is almost impossible by ordinary routine examination and it is for this reason that pregnancy tests were designed and are performed. The earliest detectable changes in the uterus do not occur until approximately 6 weeks after the first day of the last menstrual period when the uterus becomes softer as well as larger. Its very softness makes it so difficult to palpate that it is frequently impossible to determine its exact size; indeed the uterus may become so soft at about the 8th or 10th week of pregnancy that it may be extremely difficult to feel it at all.

Before the onset of pregnancy the uterus varies in size from person to person, but on average measures approximately 7 cm in length, 5 cm in width and over 2.5 cm in thickness, while at full term it can measure as much as 38 cm in length, 25.5 cm in width and 20 cm from front to back. The weight of the uterus itself increases throughout pregnancy approximately twenty times from a pre-pregnant weight of 40 g to almost 800 g immediately after delivery.

The enlargement of the wall of the uterus during pregnancy is entirely due to the enlargement of the muscle. This is accomplished by an increase in size of the existing muscle fibres, not the creation of new muscle fibres, so that despite the enormous increase in the size during pregnancy the actual thickness of the wall of the uterus at full term is almost exactly the same as it was before pregnancy began.

It is very difficult to appreciate absolute size when it is given as a simple measure. To compare the sizes of the normal uterus in the early stages of pregnancy we can consider that if it begins as a tangerine orange, then at 6 weeks it will be the size of a normal apple. At 8 weeks it will be the size of an average orange and at 10 weeks the size of a Jaffa orange. At 12 weeks the uterus will be as large as a grapefruit and at 14 weeks approximately the size of a small melon.

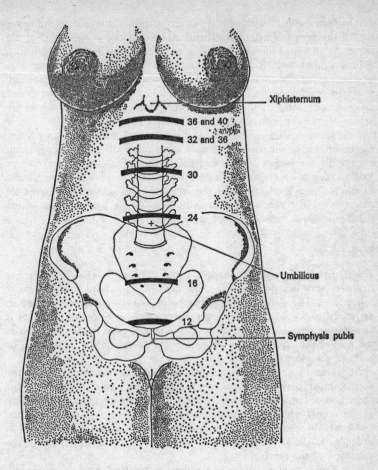

Fig. 19 The height of the uterus at different stages during pregnancy (in weeks)

The uterus is normally mobile and is free to move within the pelvis not only when the bowel and bladder fill and empty, but also during intercourse or even when walking. In the 12th week of pregnancy the uterus becomes too large to remain hidden in the pelvis. It is at this stage that it can be felt in the lower abdomen rising out of the pelvis, or even earlier if the bladder or rectum are unduly full.

From the 12th week of pregnancy the uterus enlarges at a regular rate to reach the umbilicus at about the 22nd week (see fig. 19). At about the 16th week it is half-way between the symphysis pubis and the umbilicus. At the 30th week the uterus will be half-way from the umbilicus to the xiphisternum, which is the small piece of cartilage attached to the lower end of the breast-bone, to which the ribs are joined in the front of the chest. At 36 weeks the uterus reaches the xiphisternum in the mid-line.

In a woman who is having her first baby, a phenomenon known as 'lightening' may occur at or about the 36th week of pregnancy. Lightening is caused when the baby's head descends into the cavity of the pelvis and this is accompanied by lowering or dropping in the level of the top of the uterus—hence the term or phrase 'lightening'. The baby continues to grow and the uterus enlarges further so that by the 40th week of pregnancy the top or fundus of the uterus will have again returned to the xiphisternum even while the baby's head is engaged in the pelvis. In the multiparous woman (that is a woman who is having a second or subsequent baby), the fundus of the uterus reaches the xiphisternum at the 36th week of pregnancy and remains there until the head of the baby engages in the pelvis, usually at term or the onset of labour.

Structure

The structure of the uterus changes during pregnancy. The changes are at first very slow and poorly defined but later they are more rapid and easily discernible. The body of the uterus becomes very soft and rounded in early pregnancy but as it enlarges and moves up into the abdomen it resumes its pear-like shape. Most of the new muscle fibres that form in the wall of the uterus during pregnancy are present in the upper part, or body of the uterus.

At about the 30th week of pregnancy, the repeated contractions of the uterus, most of which occur in the upper part, gradually lead to the formation of the lower uterine segment. This is the lower part of the body of the uterus which gets thinner during the last 10 weeks of pregnancy and gradually enlarges in order to accommodate the baby's head and in order to facilitate the subsequent mechanism of labour, especially the dilatation of the cervix.

The cervix, which before pregnancy is firm and hard, very rapidly becomes soft as well as larger but does so very slowly throughout pregnancy. The canal of the cervix remains filled by a tenacious plug of thick mucous material which occludes it and prevents any infection ascending from the vagina into the uterus.

The blood supply

The blood supply to the uterus, as indeed to all the pelvic organs, increases very rapidly and dramatically during early pregnancy. Some of the earliest physical signs upon which pregnancy can be diagnosed are in fact the result of the rapid increase in blood supply The cervix not only starts to become soft but first of all it assumes a blue or purple colour. In the non-pregnant woman the arteries that supply the uterus cannot normally be felt when vaginal examination is performed, but their pulsation can be easily recognized as early as the 6th week of pregnancy. The blood supply to the enlarging uterus increases rapidly as pregnancy advances, so that at full term it is approximately 25 per cent of the total body circulation.

Uterine contractions

Contractions of the uterus occur throughout life but become especially well marked and important during pregnancy, when they are known as Braxton Hicks' contractions. They are extremely important both for the growth of the uterus and for the satisfactory circulation of blood through the uterine vessels. A Braxton Hicks' contraction occurs approximately every 20 minutes throughout pregnancy and is usually felt as a painless but nevertheless quite definite hardening of the wall of the uterus itself which lasts for about 20 seconds.

The Fallopian tubes

The Fallopian tubes change very little during pregnancy, although they do increase slightly in size, and their blood supply, like the blood supply to all the pelvic organs, is also increased. The vital role of the Fallopian tubes during the first seven days of pregnancy in transporting the newly fertilized ovum to the uterus is described in Chapter 2. Having undertaken this vital function they take no further part in the pregnancy.

The ovaries

The ovaries are responsible for the production of the ova and once an ovum has been fertilized the Fallopian tubes transport it to the cavity of the uterus.

Following ovulation the corpus luteum develops in the ovary and is responsible for the production of progesterone. The corpus luteum continues to enlarge for the first 12 weeks of pregnancy and if it is damaged or removed during this time the level of progesterone in the body will fall suddenly resulting in the disintegration of the decidua lining the pregnant uterus. This will result in both death of the ovum and shedding of the lining of the uterus together with the ovum.

As soon as the placenta is properly formed at about the 12th or 14th week of pregnancy, it begins to produce hormones of which progesterone is the first. By the end of the 14th week it is producing enough progesterone to make the pregnancy self-supporting, so removal or destruction of the corpus luteum will not usually affect the pregnancy. The corpus luteum gradually shrinks after the end of the 14th week and although It may be recognized even up to the end of pregnancy it ceases to exert any significant influence on the pregnancy itself.

The corpus luteum may occasionally cause pain or tenderness in the side of the pelvis during early pregnancy. The exact reason for this is not known and no treatment is required because the pain always subsides spontaneously.

The ovaries themselves enlarge during pregnancy and may occasionally develop small cysts. These are normal changes and a few months after the end of pregnancy the cysts disappear and both the ovaries return to their normal size and shape.

The vagina

Some of the earliest noticeable changes in pregnancy occur in the vagina. The blood supply is increased, a certain amount of congestion occurs and, as the circulation slows down, the colour changes from the normal pale pink to a darker, suffused pink or even pale blue or lilac. This becomes more marked as pregnancy advances, so that at term both the vagina and the cervix may be purple.

Vaginal secretions begin to increase early in pregnancy causing a certain amount of mucoid discharge. The quantity of discharge varies from woman to woman throughout pregnancy, but a certain amount is considered normal. If it becomes offensive, profuse, causes any pain, soreness or irritation, it has probably become infected and should be mentioned at the next antenatal clinic, so that appropriate treatment may be given.

The bladder

An increase in the rate or frequency of micturition is often one of the earliest symptoms of pregnancy and may continue until delivery. This is because the uterus is still within the pelvis for the first three months and presses on the bladder. So long as there is no pain or discomfort when passing water frequency should be accepted as normal in early pregnancy.

The blood

The amount of blood normally present in a woman of average height and weight is approximately 5 litres. Very extensive changes take place in the blood during pregnancy caused initially by the rise in hormone levels which results in a gradual increase of the amount of blood circulating throughout the body. After mid-pregnancy the uterus needs about 25 per cent of the circulating blood. The breasts and other organs that increase in size also require an increased blood supply. These demands can be met either by depriving other organs of their normal blood supply or by increasing the total amount of blood available within the body. It is the latter alternative that the body adopts and from the 10th to the 34th week of pregnancy the amount of blood circulating throughout the body gradually increases by as much as 30 per cent or even 40 per cent. The circulating volume thereafter remains relatively constant until very close to term, when it may fail slightly. As soon as the hormone levels fall after delivery the blood volume rapidly returns to normal.

The rapid increase in the amount of blood circulating in the body during pregnancy is mainly accomplished by an increase in the serum or plasma. Unless this increase is also accompanied by a similar rise in red cells, these will be diluted in the blood resulting in anaemia.

The pregnant woman needs a great deal of iron and nutrition. The baby takes iron from his mother to form his own blood and, in addition, her own bone marrow needs it to manufacture a larger number of red cells for the increasing volume of blood that her body demands. It is obvious, therefore, that anaemia can very easily develop and one of the major principles of antenatal care is its prevention by giving the mother plenty of iron and vitamins and frequently checking her blood. If all pregnant women attended the antenatal clinic early in pregnancy and took their full complement of iron and vitamins, anaemia during pregnancy would be comparatively rare.

The blood pressure

Important changes may occur in the blood pressure very early during pregnancy. One of the major actions of the hormone progesterone is to cause relaxation of the involuntary muscle of the blood vessels as well as of the uterus, the bladder and intestine. Relaxation of the muscular wall of the blood vessels causes some delay in the circulation through some of the tissues (it is this slowing down in circulation of blood supply to the vagina that is responsible for its change in colour in early pregnancy). The slowing in the circulation causes a fall in blood pressure which is very common in early pregnancy. This may lead to a sensation of light-headedness or even fainting, especially after prolonged standing in one position (as in a bus queue). You should be aware of this tendency to faint in early pregnancy and therefore avoid standing in one position. If this is unavoidable, you should move your weight from one foot to the other to help the circulation through the legs. If you feel light-headed or feel as though you are going to faint, an actual fainting attack can be averted by taking a few rapid very deep breaths.

The fall in blood pressure in early pregnancy is usually only small in amount and is perfectly normal. It is frequently associated with a certain amount of tiredness or lack of energy and lassitude, and this may be interpreted as one of nature's ways of ensuring that you rest and do not indulge in too much exercise during this vital stage of pregnancy.

After about the 14th week of pregnancy the tendency to light-headedness or fainting disappears because the blood pressure rapidly returns to normal as the body increases the amount of blood within its circulation. It will remain at or about the same level until the onset of labour. Your blood pressure will be checked at every antenatal clinic because any abnormal rise may be one of the first signs of pre-eclampsia and the associated complications can be prevented if diagnosed early.

The heart

The work of the heart is considerably increased during pregnancy. The increase in work load is small at the onset of pregnancy but it may increase by as much as 40 per cent at about the 28th week. It is small wonder, therefore, that many women feel tired and lethargic towards the end of pregnancy and this is one reason why there should not be too large a weight gain. Cosmetic reasons apart, the more weight gained, the more work the heart has to do.

The heart itself behaves in quite an astonishing way during pregnancy. If you feel your own pulse when you are 36, 38 or even 40 weeks pregnant, it will feel exactly the same as it did before you became pregnant. While resting, the rate is about 80 beats per minute and you will detect little change from the 70 beats per minute of the normal non-pregnant pulse. The heart enlarges during pregnancy and is so adaptable that it can increase its amount of work by at least 40 per cent with only a slight increase in rate and no change in rhythm. The increase in heart rate of 10 beats per minute represents 14,000 beats per day! It manages to accomplish all this even though it is gradually being pushed further up into the chest by the enlarging uterus. The increased load on the heart during pregnancy is another vital reason why anaemia, as well as excessive weight gain, should be avoided.

The heart returns to its normal shape, size and position within three or four days of confinement.

The lungs

The lungs change very little during pregnancy but they do have to work at a considerable disadvantage during the last four months. The enlarging uterus pushes up against the diaphragm and gradually squeezes them into a smaller and smaller area within the chest. The reaction of the chest is to spread the ribs out sideways in order to provide the lungs with more room.

A certain amount of automatic compensation occurs within the lungs so that even at the 40th week of pregnancy you will be able to breathe quite easily and normally. You will notice, however, that you do occasionally take big, deep or sighing breaths. Sometimes normal non-pregnant people do this, but you may notice yourself doing it more frequently and this is absolutely normal. If you have a twin pregnancy, or if for some other reason your uterus is unduly large, then you may find that breathing can become difficult towards the end of pregnancy. This may be especially noticeable when you sit down, and the lower you sit the more noticeable will it be. It is for this reason that you will be more comfortable in a comparatively high chair which also has a relatively straight back, for the further down or the further forward you slump, the more difficult does it become for your chest to move and your lungs to expand satisfactorily. You may also need extra pillows in bed to ensure maximum comfort at night.

The lungs return to normal almost immediately after delivery.

The nervous system

No fundamental changes occur in the central nervous system during pregnancy although certain emotional changes, and even variations in personality, are evident very soon after conception and continue to a greater or lesser degree until about six months after delivery.

Several physical changes in the body do, however, have some effect on the nervous system, causing tiredness, lassitude or occasional feelings of faintness (sometimes actual fainting) during the first 14 weeks of pregnancy.

Headaches, not generally considered a feature of pregnancy, are suffered more frequently by some women when they are pregnant. The reason for this is not known.

Backache is usually the result of bad posture or weight gain in association with the softening of the ligaments in the spine. It has nothing to do with the central nervous system although patients who have previously suffered from a slipped disc should be especially careful during pregnancy.

As pregnancy advances into its last 8 or 10 weeks, the baby's head may bounce on nerves in the brim of the pelvis resulting in shooting pains down either the front or the back of the legs. These are usually transient, although occasionally causing considerable discomfort, and nearly always disappear when the baby moves its head, and certainly go after delivery.

The skeleton

The main changes that occur in the skeleton during pregnancy take place in the pelvis. The pelvic bones themselves do not alter, but the ligaments, especially in the region of the sacro-iliac joints at the back and the symphysis pubis in front, soften and become more elastic. The bones can therefore move quite appreciably during pregnancy to increase the capacity of the pelvis, and especially in labour to facilitate the passage of the baby.

Most of the ligaments in the body soften during pregnancy and are more liable to be stretched. It is most important that the ligaments in the back and in the feet should not be overstretched. Correct posture goes a long way towards preventing this, and shoes giving proper support to the feet should be worn throughout pregnancy.

During the last two months of pregnancy the ribs may be increasingly pushed upwards and outwards by the pressure of the uterus. This is more often on the right side, and may lead to pain and discomfort known as costal margin pain which disappears after delivery.

The skin

Pigmentation

An increase in pigmentation of the skin occurs during pregnancy (see Chapter 12). It is generally accepted that this is greater in women with dark hair than in women with fair hair, and red-heads have very little or no extra skin pigmentation during pregnancy. As well as the specific pigmentation which may occur on the breasts and on the abdomen, moles and freckles tend to both darken and increase in size. Excess or extra hair does not form during pregnancy but it often happens that previously very fair and unnoticed hair on arms and legs, and occasionally even on the abdomen and back, becomes darker and is then noticed for the first time. The colour of the hair will return to normal after delivery although some women do complain that the hair on so-called 'hairy warts' does not always return to its former colour.

Irritation

Generalized irritation of the skin frequently associated with dryness is not uncommon during pregnancy. The cause of this is unknown but it may be due to a shortage of one of the members of the vitamin B group, and so it is wise to make sure that an adequate amount of vitamin B is taken. Otherwise there is very little that can be done for this condition besides treating the underlying dryness, which may be causing the irritation, with oil or creams.

Local areas of irritation can result from any skin disease or, for instance, from such simple things as varicose veins which can occasionally cause a most annoying itching and irritation of the overlying skin. Vulval irritation may be caused by vaginal discharge and, if so, the discharge itself should be treated. Irritation around the anus may be the result of piles or of sweating and overweight. Cleanliness and hygiene will do much to alleviate these complaints.

Stretch marks

Beneath the surface of the skin there are elastic fibres which, under normal circumstances, allow the skin to stretch and contract to maintain its normal flexibility and pliability. If these elastic fibres are overstretched so that they rupture, the skin over them will be unduly stretched and a 'stretch mark' will appear. Stretch marks appear with alarming suddenness (literally overnight) and they are brightish red in colour. Once they have begun they may extend or adjacent marks may appear.

During pregnancy stretch marks may occur on the abdomen. They may also appear on the breasts in early pregnancy, when they are usually associated with sudden breast enlargement resulting from the rapid rise in hormone levels. Their appearance is not associated with any generalized increase in weight, although overweight women are more likely to develop them. The red discoloration continues throughout pregnancy but eventually fades leaving silvery, rather thin scars which will never entirely disappear.

Stretch marks may occur at puberty on the buttocks and also on the breasts, especially if a girl is overweight.

Dry skin

The skin certainly seems to change during pregnancy but the reason for these alterations is not known. Women who have a greasy skin usually find it becomes more greasy and those with a normally dry skin find it becomes drier. Little can be done for those whose skin becomes more greasy other than ensuring that too much weight is not gained and keeping skin creases and folds scrupulously clean.

Increased dryness of the skin will do no harm although it may cause a mild itching or irritation. Dry skin, of course, tends to wrinkle and therefore meticulous care should be taken of the skin during the entire pregnancy. This is best accomplished by rubbing a small amount of oil or baby lotion gently over the affected parts once or twice a day. A little bath oil or baby oil in the bath gives the whole body a thin, but nevertheless adequate, coating of oil which will help prevent dryness and alleviate irritation.

Scrubbing, hard water, harsh soaps, strong detergents and face powder all tend to dry the skin and should be used with caution on skin with this tendency. Particular attention must be paid to the skin on the face, by using satisfactory make-up and applying a liberal amount of a good moisturizing cream at night.

The breasts

Changes in the breasts are probably the earliest symptoms of pregnancy. Most women are aware of some fullness in the breasts immediately preceding the menstrual period which normally disappears as soon as the period commences. With the onset of pregnancy, however, it continues and gradually becomes more obvious. By the 6th week of pregnancy, that is, two weeks after the first missed period, the breasts will show very definite enlargement. They will be firm and there will be a certain amount of tenderness throughout the whole of the breast tissue. There is at this time an increase in both the size and the number of the veins on the surface of the breasts and these are easily visible. Even before these obvious changes, sensations of tingling may occur, and some women complain of an increase in the sensitivity of not only the nipple but the whole breast as well. Occasionally, there may be actual pain in the breast itself, caused by the rapid enlargement in the breast tissue.

Millions of years ago the breast was developed from an ordinary gland in the skin and as the human race has evolved the breast has differentiated into an organ capable of producing enough milk to feed a baby. The nipple itself is surrounded by an area of pink, rather tender and delicate skin which is known as the areola. Six to fifteen smaller vestigial glands are situated in the areola and are not normally visible or palpable in the non-pregnant woman. They do, however, respond to pregnancy in exactly the same way as the breast itself. At about the 6th week they become obvious as small, raised, pink nodules approximately 3 mm in diameter, known as Montgomery's tubercles. They are not usually tender but may occasionally become so, and their presence is one of the most reliable early signs of a first pregnancy. They are less reliable as a diagnostic sign in subsequent pregnancies because they do not shrink completely after delivery.

7 Duration of Pregnancy

Normal pregnancy

The period of gestation is 266 days from the date of conception. This is simply an average. The duration of pregnancy, on the other hand, is calculated as being 280 days from the first day of the last normal regular menstrual period which is the same as ten lunar months, or forty weeks. It has always been stated that pregnancy lasts for nine months. This is not exactly true because pregnancy usually lasts for nine calendar months and seven days. Because of the confusion that arises when people try to interpret forty weeks as being nine months, it is usual for doctors and midwives to discuss the duration of pregnancy in weeks and never in months. The same principle has been followed throughout this book.

Calculation of the expected date of delivery is always from the first day of the last period and is extremely simple. If three calendar months are subtracted from the first day of the last period and seven days then added the date arrived at will be 280 days from the first day of the last period. In other words, if the first day of the last period is on 6 June, the subtraction of three months goes back 6 May, 6 April, 6 March and then seven days added brings the expected date of delivery to 13 March. Similarly, if the first day of the last period is 20 February, taking off three months 20 January, 20 December, 20 November and adding seven days is 27 November, which is the expected date of delivery.

The expected date of delivery is an average over a large number of patients. There is no guarantee that any woman will deliver on the 280th day after the first day of her last period, and in fact her chances of doing so are approximately 5 per cent. The chances of delivering on any day in the two weeks before or in the two weeks after that date are approximately 85 per cent.

If the normal menstrual cycle is less than 28 days then the expected date of confinement will be a few days earlier, whereas if the normal menstrual cycle is longer than 28 days the expected date of confinement will be later. This is because ovulation occurs early in a short menstrual cycle and late in a long menstrual cycle. The expected date of delivery will, therefore, be seven days earlier if the normal menstrual cycle is 21 days and will be seven days later if the normal cycle is 35 days, or even fourteen days later if the average normal menstrual cycle is 42 days.

It is important to emphasize that the expected date of confinement is *an expected day* and is only worked out as an average. Women become somewhat impatient towards the end of pregnancy and look forward with eager anticipation to the expected date of their confinement. They are often greatly disappointed when the expected day arrives and passes and there are still no signs of labour, especially when they repeatedly receive anxious enquiries from well-meaning friends. Women should not set their hearts on delivery by a certain date, but should set their sights on delivery within either two weeks before or two weeks after the expected date so that they avoid this intense disappointment.

It is interesting that age, height, size, colour, race or climate does not exert any influence upon the duration of pregnancy. Multiple pregnancies do on average deliver earlier than single pregnancies, and the actual average duration of a twin pregnancy is 37 weeks.

Calculating the date of delivery

See table on pages 116 and 117.

Accessory methods of calculating the date of delivery

Numerous precautions are taken throughout pregnancy to check that the expected date of delivery has been correctly estimated. At the first examination the size of the uterus is assessed to ensure that this agrees with the date of the last period. The fetal heart may be heard by an ultrasonic detector as early as the 12th week of pregnancy. Fetal movements are felt by the pregnant woman between the 18th and 20th week in her first pregnancy, and between the 16th and 18th week in subsequent pregnancies. The fetal heart can be heard with an ordinary stethoscope at the 24th week of pregnancy. Throughout pregnancy the size of the uterus is carefully assessed, noted and compared with the expected date of delivery. The growth of the pregnant uterus is described in Chapter 6.

These and many other small factors all contribute towards confirming the correct date of delivery. An X-ray examination is unlikely to help and should be avoided.

An ultrasonic scan can be performed if there is any real doubt about the maturity of the fetus (see Chapter 22). An ultrasonic scan will usually be performed at or about the 16th week of pregnancy and will give an accurate date of delivery to within 7 days. An earlier scan will be even more accurate but is not usually performed unless there is a good indication.

Amniocentesis in the last 8 weeks of pregnancy will indicate the maturity of the baby. The cells in the amniotic fluid are stained to show the exact duration of pregnancy. This method is not used unless there is some anxiety about the condition of the baby or ultrasonic scans were not performed earlier in the pregnancy.

Prolonged pregnancy

Prolonged pregnancy is one which continues more than 14 days past the expected date of confinement. The labour and the baby are then considered postmature.

Occasionally prolonged pregnancy becomes a legal issue when paternity is disputed, and the longest pregnancy accepted in the British courts of law has been over 340 days. Many pregnancies of over 320 days are recorded but really long pregnancies are usually of normal duration, having been conceived after some months of non-pregnant amenorrhoea.

The reason for the onset of labour is not known, but in order to try and understand how and why postmaturity affects the baby, it is best to consider the placenta and the baby together. The placenta, or afterbirth, reaches maturity at about the 32nd or 34th week of pregnancy, and from this date onwards it gradually becomes less efficient. At the same time the demands on the placenta are increasing because each day the growing baby requires more and more oxygen, and its needs also become more complicated with the baby's continued maturation and development. At the 32nd week of pregnancy there is an enormous reserve in the placenta, but as the placenta ages and the baby grows the reserve is slowly reduced. At 40 weeks the baby has grown to its fullest extent and the placenta still contains sufficient reserve to withstand the trials of labour.

Postmaturity

From the 40th week onwards the baby seems to realize that it is on a losing wicket. It is doubtful if it increases in size and it certainly begins to reduce some of its requirements. The fat which it has stored beneath its skin is gradually used and although the baby's brain, liver, lungs and heart continue to mature and its bones continue to get harder, it may in fact actually lose weight. By the 42nd week the baby will have very little fat beneath its skin and by the 43rd week probably none at all, so that if delivered the baby will look thin, rather scraggy, dry and rather wrinkled. The fingernails will be long. Desquamation, or peeling, of the superficial layers of the skin will be obvious over the hands and feet and, within a day or two of birth, over the skin creases of the knees, elbows, wrists and groins. These postmature changes in the baby are designed to conserve its resources and not place undue demands upon the continuously ageing placenta. Once it is delivered the child will rapidly replace its subcutaneous fat and within a few days will look like any normal baby.

Opinions are divided on the possible dangers of postmaturity. Most obstetricians would agree that patients with pre-eclampsia should not be allowed to go past their expected date. It may also be inadvisable to allow women over the age of 35 who are expecting their first child to go much beyond their expected date. Most obstetricians, however, would agree that

Calculating the date of delivery

The line of heavy black figures gives the date of the first day of the last menstrual period. Immediately underneath this date, and in lighter type, is a second date 280 days later. This is the expected date of delivery.

January	1	2	3	4	5	6	7	8	9	10	11	12	13	14	15	16
October	8	9	10	11	12	13	14	15	16	17	18	19	20	21	22	23

February	1	2	3	4	5	6	7	8	9	10	11	12	13	14	15	16
November	8	9	10	11	12	13	14	15	16	17	18	19	20	21	22	23

March	1	2	3	4	5	6	7	8	9	10	11	12	13	14	15	16
December	6	7	8	9	10	11	12	13	14	15	16	17	18	19	20	21

April	1	2	3	4	5	6	7	8	9	10	11	12	13	14	15	16
January	6	7	8	9	10	11	12	13	14	15	16	17	18	19	20	21

May	1	2	3	4	5	6	7	8	9	10	11	12	13	14	15	16
February	5	6	7	8	9	10	11	12	13	14	15	16	17	18	19	20

June	1	2	3	4	5	6	7	8	9	10	11	12	13	14	15	16
March	8	9	10	11	12	13	14	15	16	17	18	19	20	21	22	23

July	1	2	3	4	5	6	7	8	9	10	11	12	13	14	15	16
April	7	8	9	10	11	12	13	14	15	16	17	18	19	20	21	22

August	1	2	3	4	5	6	7	8	9	10	11	12	13	14	15	16
May	8	9	10	11	12	13	14	15	16	17	18	19	20	21	22	23

September	1	2	3	4	5	6	7	8	9	10	11	12	13	14	15	16
June	8	9	10	11	12	13	14	15	16	17	18	19	20	21	22	23

October	1	2	3	4	5	6	7	8	9	10	11	12	13	14	15	16
July	8	9	10	11	12	13	14	15	16	17	18	19	20	21	22	23

November	1	2	3	4	5	6	7	8	9	10	11	12	13	14	15	16
August	8	9	10	11	12	13	14	15	16	17	18	19	20	21	22	23

December	1	2	3	4	5	6	7	8	9	10	11	12	13	14	15	16
September	7	8	9	10	11	12	13	14	15	16	17	18	19	20	21	22

| 17 | 18 | 19 | 20 | 21 | 22 | 23 | 24 | 25 | 26 | 27 | 28 | 29 | 30 | 31 | January |
| 24 | 25 | 26 | 27 | 28 | 29 | 30 | 31 | 1 | 2 | 3 | 4 | 5 | 6 | 7 | November |

| 17 | 18 | 19 | 20 | 21 | 22 | 23 | 24 | 25 | 26 | 27 | 28 | | | | February |
| 24 | 25 | 26 | 27 | 28 | 29 | 30 | 1 | 2 | 3 | 4 | 5 | | | | December |

| 17 | 18 | 19 | 20 | 21 | 22 | 23 | 24 | 25 | 26 | 27 | 28 | 29 | 30 | 31 | March |
| 22 | 23 | 24 | 25 | 26 | 27 | 28 | 29 | 30 | 31 | 1 | 2 | 3 | 4 | 5 | January |

| 17 | 18 | 19 | 20 | 21 | 22 | 23 | 24 | 25 | 26 | 27 | 28 | 29 | 30 | | April |
| 22 | 23 | 24 | 25 | 26 | 27 | 28 | 29 | 30 | 31 | 1 | 2 | 3 | 4 | | February |

| 17 | 18 | 19 | 20 | 21 | 22 | 23 | 24 | 25 | 26 | 27 | 28 | 29 | 30 | 31 | May |
| 21 | 22 | 23 | 24 | 25 | 26 | 27 | 28 | 1 | 2 | 3 | 4 | 5 | 6 | 7 | March |

| 17 | 18 | 19 | 20 | 21 | 22 | 23 | 24 | 25 | 26 | 27 | 28 | 29 | 30 | | June |
| 24 | 25 | 26 | 27 | 28 | 29 | 30 | 31 | 1 | 2 | 3 | 4 | 5 | 6 | | April |

| 17 | 18 | 19 | 20 | 21 | 22 | 23 | 24 | 25 | 26 | 27 | 28 | 29 | 30 | 31 | July |
| 23 | 24 | 25 | 26 | 27 | 28 | 29 | 30 | 1 | 2 | 3 | 4 | 5 | 6 | 7 | May |

| 17 | 18 | 19 | 20 | 21 | 22 | 23 | 24 | 25 | 26 | 27 | 28 | 29 | 30 | 31 | August |
| 24 | 25 | 26 | 27 | 28 | 29 | 30 | 31 | 1 | 2 | 3 | 4 | 5 | 6 | 7 | June |

| 17 | 18 | 19 | 20 | 21 | 22 | 23 | 24 | 25 | 26 | 27 | 28 | 29 | 30 | | September |
| 24 | 25 | 26 | 27 | 28 | 29 | 30 | 1 | 2 | 3 | 4 | 5 | 6 | 7 | | July |

| 17 | 18 | 19 | 20 | 21 | 22 | 23 | 24 | 25 | 26 | 27 | 28 | 29 | 30 | 31 | October |
| 24 | 25 | 26 | 27 | 28 | 29 | 30 | 31 | 1 | 2 | 3 | 4 | 5 | 6 | 7 | August |

| 17 | 18 | 19 | 20 | 21 | 22 | 23 | 24 | 25 | 26 | 27 | 28 | 29 | 30 | | November |
| 24 | 25 | 26 | 27 | 28 | 29 | 30 | 31 | 1 | 2 | 3 | 4 | 5 | 6 | | September |

| 17 | 18 | 19 | 20 | 21 | 22 | 23 | 24 | 25 | 26 | 27 | 28 | 29 | 30 | 31 | December |
| 23 | 24 | 25 | 26 | 27 | 28 | 29 | 30 | 1 | 2 | 3 | 4 | 5 | 6 | 7 | October |

providing everything else is normal there is no harm in allowing a normal pregnancy to run into the second week past the expected date. It is when the 42nd week is reached that clearly some division of opinion arises. Some obstetricians consider that most patients should be induced when they reach the 42nd week of pregnancy, while others consider that there is little or no indication to perform induction of labour before the 43rd or even the 44th week. It is emphasized that each individual pregnancy is treated on its merits and no hard and fast rule can be laid down.

Milestones of pregnancy

This is a short summary of some of the main symptoms and signs that occur during pregnancy and enable a woman, and her doctor and midwife, to confirm the duration of pregnancy and also the expected date of arrival of her baby. Each point is discussed at greater length elsewhere.

Amenorrhoea. The absence of a menstrual period is the first and the most classic sign of the onset of pregnancy. Occasionally a so-called 'partially suppressed period' may occur in which the menstrual loss is very much shorter and very much less than normal.

Breast changes. The onset of breast changes varies in its timing, but many women notice changes as soon as they miss their first period. These may be very slight initially but they gradually become more noticeable.

Nausea may commence at any stage during the first three months of pregnancy but frequently begins one or two weeks after the first period has been missed. In fact actual nausea may be fairly late in its onset and may be preceded by lack of appetite, a lack of interest in food, or even an active dislike of other things such as smoking or alcohol. Nausea need not necessarily occur in the morning. It can occur at any time during the day or evening.

Frequency of micturition. Increase in frequency of micturition is a common early symptom of pregnancy, usually beginning about the 6th week. An excessive desire to pass urine may occur during the day or at night.

Uterine size. The uterus is enlarged into the abdomen by the 12th week of pregnancy and is easily palpable. From this time on the size of the uterus will follow a characteristic pattern and will enlarge steadily and proportionately as the pregnancy progresses. It normally reaches up to the margin of the rib cage in the mid-line at the 36th week.

Relief of nausea. The nausea, sickness, tiredness and other trying symptoms of early pregnancy usually disappear spontaneously by the end of the 14th week. This is a most characteristic date.

Pigmentation of the breasts, together with the formation of the linea nigra (the black line down the centre of the abdomen) and darkening of moles and freckles, will commence shortly after the end of the 14th week.

Ultrasonic scan Pregnancy can be diagnosed and dated accurately during the 6th week of pregnancy.

Fetal heart. The fetal heart can usually be heard by Doptone apparatus between the 12th and 14th week and by a stethoscope at about the 24th week of pregnancy.

Fetal movements. There is no hard and fast rule about the first sensations of fetal movements, but generally movements of a first baby are felt between the 18th and 20th week, and between the 16th and 18th week in a subsequent pregnancy.

Lightening. In a first pregnancy the baby's head drops down into the pelvis at about the 36th week. This results in considerable relief from pressure in the upper abdomen and is known as lightening. When it occurs it is quite characteristic.

Clinical examination. Frequent clinical examinations throughout pregnancy, carefully noting the size of the uterus and the size of the baby, together with all the above factors, confirm the duration of pregnancy and the expected date of delivery.

8 Phantom Pregnancy

A phantom, or false, pregnancy, which is otherwise known as a pseudo-cyesis, is a condition in which a non-pregnant woman has all the symptoms of pregnancy and firmly believes that she is pregnant.

A woman who is suffering from a pseudocyesis will visit her doctor or the antenatal clinic complaining of all the symptoms and minor discomforts of early pregnancy, including absence of her periods, breast enlargement and breast changes, nausea and vomiting, increase of weight and abdominal distension. The clinical diagnosis of early pregnancy is extremely difficult, especially if such a person has a slightly enlarged uterus or is overweight, and it may be virtually impossible to confirm or deny the presence of a pregnancy by clinical examination alone. Since it is not the normal practice to perform pregnancy tests upon everybody who attends an antenatal clinic, she will probably be accepted as being pregnant and booked for confinement. The symptoms of pregnancy will continue and as the woman gains more weight she will become increasingly convinced about the presence of her pregnancy, although the fact that she is suffering from pseudocyesis may gradually become apparent to her.

True pseudocyesis is extremely rare and it must not be confused with a woman who, having missed one, or perhaps two periods, has no symptoms of pregnancy but visits her doctor to find out why she has missed them, and to ascertain whether or not she is pregnant. The very small group of women who suffer from pseudocyesis are convinced about their pregnancy. It is a condition that occurs mainly in women in their late thirties or early forties who desperately want a child and have been trying to become pregnant for many years. It can also occur in younger women—especially when relatives and friends are having babies or asking and joking about the girl's ability to become pregnant. Women who suffer from false pregnancies are normally emotionally quite stable but may become very unstable over the question of pregnancy.

Pseudocyesis also occurs in some women who have lost a pregnancy or a baby. It may be an emotional reaction, but, in this case, there is increasing scientific evidence to indicate that a temporary hormone imbalance is the cause of all their symptoms.

The diagnosis of pseudocyesis is extremely difficult, especially at the beginning of a false pregnancy. The uterus will remain normal in size and successive pregnancy tests, if performed, will be negative. As the false pregnancy proceeds a marked increase in weight may occur, together with abdominal and breast enlargement, but the uterus will not enlarge nor will the breasts show active signs of pregnancy. None of the other physical signs of pregnancy will develop and all tests for pregnancy will be negative.

A woman who is suffering from true pseudocyesis will insist that she is pregnant despite the assurance that she is not. The problem requires very careful and sympathetic consideration with kindly explanation to the patient as to the reasons why she is not pregnant, together with appropriate proof that a pregnancy does not exist.

Severe emotional disturbance may follow the realization that she is suffering from a false pregnancy and the woman's husband should also be acquainted with all the facts and treated with complete confidence, because his help is invaluable.

9 Antenatal Care

Antenatal care aims at maintaining the good health of the mother during pregnancy which will enable her to produce a healthy, normal infant and remain so herself. It is greatly concerned with health education during pregnancy to ensure the maximum preparation of each individual for her labour and role of motherhood. One of its outstanding features is the early detection of any condition which might adversely affect the health of the mother or her baby.

The history of antenatal care

Antenatal care is a comparatively new approach to childbirth and has only developed since the beginning of this century. Before 1900 women had no supervision during pregnancy and were seen for the first time by a doctor or midwife when labour had become established so that complicating factors were never discovered until late in labour The results were disastrous. Women died in childbirth and their babies were often fortunate to survive.

The serious study of pregnant women began in 1901 in Edinburgh and has been developed throughout many countries. Advances in the care of pregnant women are still continuing and today in this country it is difficult to realize the situation of the past. Today women have nothing to fear from pregnancy and labour, the outcome of which is a happy event in any family unit.

Very few aspects of medicine have changed so dramatically and radically as the care of the pregnant woman over the past fifty years. The introduction of antibiotics and the consequent control of infection have affected all branches of medicine, not least of all women during and immediately after childbirth. However, the complete antenatal care as we now know it is an entirely new concept not even dreamed of fifty years ago. It has moved most of the responsibility for the pregnancy from the pregnant woman herself to her professional adviser, be that doctor or midwife. The maternity services, as represented by the doctor and midwife, have cheerfully and gladly accepted the responsibility of looking after the pregnant woman. The history of antenatal care is one which will stand repeated examination

Fifty years ago antenatal clinics as we now know them did not exist

The pregnant woman either wrote to or went to see her doctor, midwife or hospital in order to book a place for her confinement. When she had done this she returned home and awaited the onset of labour, or some complication which might befall her during her pregnancy. If the pregnancy proceeded normally and labour duly arrived, the doctor or midwife was summoned at a time determined by the pregnant woman and her husband, or other members of the family brought in to give appropriate advice.

Complete antenatal care is the ideal type of preventive medicine for which doctors have been searching for many generations. Complications can be recognized sufficiently early to be corrected. Tests and other investigations can be performed to detect those patients in whom a complication might arise so that treatment can be given to prevent its occurrence. Even for those who are destined to have a perfectly normal pregnancy, labour and delivery, helpful guidance, reassurance and instruction will help to make their pregnancy a pleasure rather than a duty.

The importance of antenatal care cannot be overemphasized nor can the benefits that good antenatal care bestows upon the pregnant woman be overstressed.

Statistical evidence in the Perinatal Mortality Survey shows that the earlier a pregnant woman presents herself to her professional adviser for her first antenatal visit the higher is the chance that she will have a perfectly normal pregnancy and healthy baby. Also, the longer she defers her first visit, the greater are the chances of her having some complication of pregnancy or a dead baby. It is astonishing, with these facts in mind, that only about 5 per cent of women attended for their first antenatal visit during the first 8 weeks of pregnancy, and that almost 50 per cent of women failed to attend until after the 16th week of pregnancy. The same report also shows that the chance of a woman producing a live, healthy, normal infant is directly related to the number of antenatal visits she makes with a reasonable limit.

For many years obstetricians and midwives have been accused by their patients, often quite rightly, that they keep them 'in the dark' and tell them nothing, and that pregnant women have to obey a long list of rules and regulations without knowing why. When antenatal clinics were new, doctors and midwives were themselves searching for the reasons why some pregnant women developed complications, and why some babies died. It was not until after the Second World War that the answers to some of the problems gradually became apparent, but meanwhile the accent was, and still is, on reassuring the pregnant woman who is intensely receptive to suggestion She needs assurance that her pregnancy is going well, and it is extremely difficult and often impossible for the doctor to say to her 'Because such and such has happened I am afraid the chances of your baby dying are automatically doubled.'

As professional advisers have learned the answers to their patients' questions they have still thought it inadvisable to answer these questions directly because of the worry this might cause the patient herself. Imagine the reaction of a patient who first attends the antenatal clinic at the 30th week of pregnancy on being told that she should have attended the clinic at the 8th week of pregnancy and, on enquiring why, is then told that by this neglect the chances of her child surviving are considerably reduced.

During the past ten to fifteen years women have become more inquisitive concerning the process of labour and their delivery and their seeking for information is to be encouraged. Even so, some women are frequently screened from some of the true or more unpleasant facts if these might disturb them.

Many pregnant women today want to know more about the process of pregnancy and what they can do to ensure its success. Their questions should be answered honestly and sympathetically and they in turn must accept the honesty of the answers they are given. If they enter into a phase of grey depression when they are told that a certain risk is present and do not accept that the risk is not a finality, doctors will refuse to disclose information to their patients.

The majority of doctors and midwives recognize that only knowledge can eliminate fear and depression. They are now attempting to remove the mystique which has always surrounded pregnancy and labour so that pregnant women and their husbands will understand not only the physiology and anatomy, but also the signs and symptoms of complications as well as the methods of dealing with them and their prevention. The effort to replace ignorance with knowledge and understanding is gaining momentum from the combined efforts of midwives and doctors as well as from women themselves.

The vast majority of maternity units under the National Health Service in Great Britain have a course of classes for patients who are attending the antenatal clinic of the hospital. Similar antenatal classes are run by many local authorities for women who are having their babies at home. The majority of these courses include lectures and discussions on pregnancy, labour, delivery, the care of the new-born baby, clothes required during pregnancy and for the new-born infant, as well as visits to the wards and delivery room, instruction and practice in the use of gas and oxygen machines and other simple equipment that may be required during labour. Relaxation classes are usually run parallel with the courses of instruction. A dietician is available to give advice on diet during pregnancy and a social worker to offer advice and help to those who need it. The majority of units also encourage husbands to attend one or more of these discussions or lectures.

The whole concept of this type of antenatal care and instruction is to offer helpful information and to create trust, confidence and understanding between the patient and the people who are going to look after her Fear and misunderstanding are replaced by knowledge and a confident appreciation of the reasons behind the meticulous care that is taken of a woman during pregnancy.

Many changes through the years have been responsible for the progress in obstetric practice. Their effect has been cumulative since no single factor could have changed pregnancy from the days of ignorance, disease, damage and death, to the present haven of knowledge, safety, happiness and health of the mother and her child. It must however be clearly understood by everyone that the maternity services are severely understaffed and are working under very great strain. No allowance has been made by the government for the increasing demands that women, quite correctly, place on the maternity services.

Obstetricians, doctors who specialize in midwifery, have had an immense amount of training.

Midwives have advanced training and they too are experts in the care of women in normal pregnancy, labour and the puerperium. The midwives and obstetricians cooperate to achieve maximum benefits for all under their care.

Anaesthesia. Improvements in the methods of anaesthesia during labour have been an important factor in the evolution of the maternity service.

Paediatricians are trained to care for babies and, with the cooperation that exists between obstetricians and paediatricians, the survival rate of all babies, especially that of the small premature baby, has improved.

General practitioners have been trained in modern methods of maternity care and are encouraged to help in the antenatal supervision of their patients who are to be delivered in hospital. They seek help and advice from specialist obstetricians concerning those patients whom they are looking after at home or in a General Practitioner Maternity Unit. All the facilities of the health service are at their disposal.

Blood transfusion is now safe and this development has done much to ensure the safety, and indeed the lives, of many women. The early diagnosis and virtual elimination of anaemia has had a profound influence upon pregnancy and its management.

Bacteriological advances have done much to eliminate infection during and after delivery and this, combined with the discovery and widespread use of antibiotics, has probably saved more lives than any other recent discovery.

Ultrasound and other techniques have improved and are invaluable aids to obstetricians.

Health visitors, dieticians, social workers, laboratory technicians and physiotherapists are all concerned with pregnancy. These people are highly trained specialists who augment the work of the obstetrician.

Many safe drugs, in addition to antibiotics, are now available for the treatment of abnormalities in pregnancy, labour and the puerperium, as well as for the treatment of the baby.

The hospital maternity units form a centre of cooperative effort, seldom seen in hospital medicine, that is designed especially for the care and welfare of the pregnant woman. Both simple and complicated equipment have been designed to make maternity care more efficient.

The pregnant woman herself, however, is the most important factor in the management of pregnancy. She must learn to look after her unborn baby during the nine months of her pregnancy with the same amount of care that she will take of him after he is born, and to do this she must know all about her pregnancy.

The first visit to the antenatal clinic

The first visit to an antenatal clinic can be quite an ordeal, particularly if it is the first time a woman has set foot inside a hospital. All fears are groundless. Pregnant women are just about the only fit and well people who ever attend as patients in a hospital or go to the doctor. Most know and trust their doctor; he or she is one of the best friends they could possibly have—perhaps not yet, but he will be, especially if he is going to look after them. Perhaps he is married, perhaps he has children; he is human and, like his patients, has loves and hates, fears and friendships, likes and dislikes. He is an ordinary human being who happens to have been trained to practise medicine and look after people.

The general practitioner, the community midwife and the doctors and midwives who work in the hospital are all particularly and specifically trained to take care of women during their pregnancies. They understand the fears and apprehensions, as well as the joys and excitement, that beset a woman at the beginning of her first, or indeed at the beginning of any, pregnancy. As pregnancy progresses the woman gets to know the people who are looking after her, so that after the baby has arrived she wonders how she ever managed without them. They become friends and advisers because they know that in this way they have a happier and more cooperative patient to look after. Obstetrics and midwifery are vocations which doctors and midwives follow because they enjoy their roles. They are intensely dedicated professions. There is no need for any woman to approach her first antenatal visit with fear and trepidation. She will find it most interesting, especially if she knows what to expect.

The antenatal history

In every pregnancy it is essential to acquire as much information as possible about each new patient at the earliest opportunity. This is usually obtained at a quiet, unhurried interview between the obstetrician or the midwife and the patient. The details of the history that are required may seem superfluous and, in order to try and classify them in a more easily understandable fashion, we will consider them under separate headings.

Social history. This is one of the most important considerations concerning any pregnancy. You will be asked your full name, age, date of birth and country of origin. How long have you been married? How long have you been trying to get pregnant? What contraceptive, if any, have you used? What work did you do before you married (or are you doing now)? What is your husband's or partner's occupation? Details may also be required about your housing accommodation, especially if you hope to have your baby at home or return home shortly after your delivery in hospital.

Family history. Is there any family history of twin pregnancy, diabetes or any type or form of congenital abnormality?

Medical history. Have you yourself suffered from any particular medical conditions, especially any disease of the heart, lungs or of the kidneys? What infectious diseases have you had, with special reference to rubella (German measles)? Do you smoke? If so, how much? What is your alcohol intake?

Surgical history. Have you had any operations, broken bones, serious accidents or blood transfusions?

Menstrual history. The doctor will want to know the age at which your periods began, your normal menstrual cycle together with the number of days your periods usually last, and the date of the onset of your last normal, regular period.

Obstetric history. If you are not pregnant for the first time, perhaps the most important part of the history is to record information about your previous pregnancies. This will include particulars of any miscarriages as well as dates of deliveries together with the weights of the babies and details of your labours.

The present pregnancy. Finally you will be asked for details of your present pregnancy, and these will probably include a request to know your weight at the beginning of the pregnancy and a list of the symptoms that you may have had since you first realized you were pregnant.

Once doctors or midwives have all this information, they have a pretty good picture of you, but what is perhaps more important is that they also have an idea of what you expect from them

Examination

Assessment of the woman's health at this stage is, of course, most important and after the interview in which the details of your history have been taken, you will undress for examination.

Height. This is important because it gives a rough estimate as to the size of the bony pelvis for childbearing. In Britain women over 5 ft in height nearly always have pelvic bones of adequate size (as do women who take average sized shoes) and, indeed, those who are less than 5 ft tall often have an adequate pelvis.

Weight. One aspect of antenatal care is weight control in pregnancy. You will be weighed early in pregnancy and then at each visit to the antenatal clinic, to calculate weight gain. It is essential to allow only up to 28 lb weight gain during the whole pregnancy. Diet in pregnancy is most important. You may be asked if you normally diet to keep your figure.

Urine is tested at the first and at every subsequent antenatal visit. At the first visit a special specimen, called a mid-stream specimen, is sometimes obtained after washing the external parts of the vulva to ensure that there is no contamination and that the urine is especially 'clean'. You will be told how to collect this specimen at the time. This is sent to the laboratory for particular examinations to exclude any abnormalities such as unsuspected infection. A small amount of the specimen is tested in the clinic for protein and sugar which, if present, are significant in your antenatal care. You may be requested to bring a clean specimen of urine in a clean container to the antenatal clinic at each subsequent visit. The second specimen of the day is preferable to the first.

Blood pressure. Your blood pressure will be taken and recorded at your first visit and at every subsequent antenatal visit. The blood pressure recording at the first visit is most important because only variations from this level are really significant. A rise in blood pressure is one of the less welcome signs of pregnancy and often indicates the possibility of a complication. One of the commonest abnormal conditions in pregnancy is pre-eclampsia (see Chapter 18) and it is only by careful assessment of the blood pressure that this condition can be detected sufficiently early to be treated successfully.

The breasts are examined for signs of pregnancy and evidence of their activity. Their condition and the state and condition of the nipples are noted, especially if you wish to breast-feed your baby. They are also examined by a midwife who gives appropriate advice on their care during pregnancy (see Chapter 15).

A general medical examination is carried out either by your general practitioner or by a doctor at the antenatal clinic to assess mental as well as physical health. It is surprising how much can, in fact, be noted purely by observation.

Head and neck. The state of your hair, the colour of your eyes, the condition of your teeth, any evidence of pallor or anaemia, any indication of enlarged veins in the neck or swollen thyroid can be noted by a doctor without touching you.

Chest. The heart and lungs are examined by stethoscope although this may be purely a formality in a young healthy woman who has never suffered from any disease.

Abdomen. The abdomen is examined at the first and at every subsequent visit to the antenatal clinic. At the first visit the uterus is usually quite small and all the other organs can be palpated to assess their normality. The size of the uterus is noted and compared with the estimated date of delivery. If you are more than 16 weeks pregnant you may be asked if and when you have felt fetal movements. The exact date at which you first feel the baby move may be rather difficult to define but you should make a note in your diary as soon as you are certain that you have felt it and tell the clinic this date at your next visit. If you are more than 12 weeks pregnant the size and duration of the pregnancy may be confirmed by listening to the baby's heart with electronic equipment such as a Doptone or Sonicaid.

Limbs. Your pulse will be taken and any swelling of the fingers which might be making rings unduly tight is noted. The condition of the finger-nails may indicate any possible anaemia and reveals much about character and how hard a person works. They are very revealing. The legs are examined for evidence of varicose veins or swelling of the feet or ankles.

Vaginal examination during pregnancy

A vaginal, internal or pelvic, examination is usually performed at the first visit to the doctor or to the antenatal clinic:

1 To confirm the presence of the pregnancy.
2 To confirm that the size of the uterus is in agreement with the suggested duration of the pregnancy.
3 To ensure that the pregnancy is normal.
4 To exclude the presence of any tumours or other abnormalities in the pelvis.
5 To diagnose any infections in the vagina or cervix.
6 To diagnose the presence of an ulcer or erosion on the cervix.
7 To take a routine cervical smear to exclude disease or cancer of the cervix.
8 To assess the size of the cavity of the pelvis.

9 To assess the size of the outlet to the pelvis.

A vaginal examination may be performed at other times during pregnancy but generally it need not be repeated until the 36th week when it is performed:

1 To confirm the presentation of the baby.
2 To assess the condition of the cervix.
3 To confirm the size of the bony pelvis.

The assessment of the bony pelvis is easier at the 36th week than in the earlier stages of pregnancy. This assessment is particularly important in a woman having her first baby, especially if the head is not by then engaged within the pelvis. If the head is engaged at the 36th week a vaginal examination may not be performed since the cavity of the pelvis must be adequate for the head and the pelvic outlet had been assessed at the beginning of pregnancy.

Blood tests

Blood tests are of vital importance during pregnancy. Blood will nearly always be taken at the first antenatal visit to either the clinic or doctor, and at intervals throughout pregnancy to ensure that it is proceeding normally.

A haemoglobin estimation. This is an estimation of the quality and the density of the red cells in the blood. It is expressed either in grams (g) or simply as a percentage; 14.7 g is equivalent to 100 per cent. The normal haemoglobin level in the non-pregnant woman is approximately 13 g or 90 per cent. During pregnancy it falls, but should never be less than 12 g or 80 per cent. If it does fall below this figure the woman is said to be anaemic.

Blood grouping. People belong to one of four major blood groups—A, B, AB or O. This knowledge is important not only in case a blood transfusion is necessary at a later stage but because in very rare instances incompatibilities between the mother and her baby may arise when they have different major blood groups.

Rhesus factor. It is important to know if the woman is Rhesus negative or positive (see Chapter 20). If a woman is *Rhesus negative* a test for Rhesus antibodies is performed.

A Wassermann reaction. This is a routine screening test for the presence of syphilis. Some patients become very indignant when they realize that a test is being performed for syphilis but it is of the utmost importance. Syphilis is a disease which can be transmitted to the unborn child after the 20th week of pregnancy. Adequate treatment before the 20th week of pregnancy will prevent its transmission to the fetus. If a woman is unaware that she has the disease and is not treated her child can be severely and unnecessarily affected. In most units the Wassermann reaction has been replaced by other, similar, blood tests.

Other blood tests

Most hospitals routinely test patients' blood for alpha fetoprotein (AFP) at about the 16th week of pregnancy. This is high when the baby has spina bifida. Routine testing for German measles (rubella) and other viruses may be performed. These include cytomegalovirus and hepatitis B virus.

Subsequent tests

Blood is taken for haemoglobin at intervals throughout the pregnancy to ensure against anaemia, and more complicated tests may be required to assess the well-being of the fetus (see Chapter 22).

The dietician

At the first visit to the antenatal clinic the dietician should be available to give details about diet in pregnancy. Early pregnancy is the time to discuss diet and weight control as it is easier to be strict about forbidden foods from the very beginning.

The medical social worker

The medical social worker is available to see women who have social problems.

Iron and vitamins

Iron and vitamin tablets are given routinely to most pregnant women. The iron pills come in various sizes and contain different preparations of iron. The vitamin pills similarly contain varying amounts of different vitamins. Generally speaking all these iron and vitamin pills are adequate and satisfactory.

Iron is essential to prevent anaemia which was, until a few years ago, so common in pregnancy that it was considered normal. It is now comparatively rare and your haemoglobin level should stay well above 11 g (75 per cent) throughout the whole pregnancy. A more recent addition to the range of vitamins administered is folic acid which is now given routinely to prevent a particular type of anaemia which occurs during pregnancy, known as megaloblastic anaemia, and which, without this treatment, affects 5 to 7 per cent of pregnant women in Great Britain.

Iron and vitamin tablets are not usually supplied until after the end of the 14th week of pregnancy for two reasons. Firstly, although they are all quite safe, there is an inherent dislike of giving any tablets to any woman during the first 12 weeks of her pregnancy. Secondly, iron tablets can cause disturbance of the intestine and lead to either constipation or diarrhoea, occasionally to nausea and in some circumstances to actual vomiting, and therefore are not given until the nausea which most women experience to a greater or lesser degree during the early part of pregnancy has passed. If iron tablets do cause discomfort, constipation, diarrhoea or nausea, this should be mentioned at the next visit to your doctor or the clinic. People's reactions to different iron preparations vary considerably and any upsetting symptoms will probably disappear completely with another type of iron tablet. Some people who are extremely intolerant of all iron tablets may have to be given iron injections.

There are no side effects from vitamin pills or folic acid tablets.

Subsequent visits to the antenatal clinic

Subsequent visits that you make to either the doctor or the antenatal clinic follow a standard routine unless for some reason the doctor wishes to see you earlier.

Visits are usually every four weeks until the 28th week of pregnancy. Thereafter they are every two weeks until the 36th week and then every week until delivery. At each visit to the clinic you will be weighed, your urine tested, your blood pressure taken and recorded and your abdomen and ankles inspected. Unless there is some specific reason for another internal examination, it is not again performed until the 36th week. Blood samples are taken at intervals and more frequently if there is evidence of anaemia.

Ultrasound scan will usually be performed at the 16th week. This will not only confirm the duration of pregnancy but will also help to exclude abnormalities such as spina bifida, and it will also, of course, diagnose a twin pregnancy. Even if ultrasound examination has been done earlier in the pregnancy it is normal practice to repeat it at the 16th week. Subsequent ultrasound scans may be undertaken for a variety of reasons which are discussed in Chapter 22.

As pregnancy progresses the normal milestones are carefully recorded and slowly but gradually a complete picture of the pregnancy emerges Any variation from normal in the woman, her uterus or her baby is carefully noted and corrective measures are taken. Your cooperation and understanding are, of course, essential, for without them proper care during pregnancy is impossible.

If you have questions that you would like to ask the doctor or the midwife when you visit the antenatal clinic, make a note of these on a piece of paper and take it with you. Most antenatal clinics are rather busy and there is not a great deal of time for answering irrelevant queries. In practice, however, there is always time and you can ask your questions quickly and simply from a list.

The whole art of looking after and taking care of a pregnancy is the preventive medicine that takes place in the antenatal clinic. (For instance, see pre-eclampsia, Chapter 18; anaemia, Chapter 21; monitoring, Chapter 22; twins, Chapter 30.)

From about the 28th week until the end of pregnancy a doctor or midwife can feel the baby as it lies within the uterus and can also define quite accurately the position in which the baby is lying even to the extent of feeling its hands and feet. A baby normally sits on its bottom with its head at the top of the uterus until about the 30th or 32nd week of pregnancy, when for some unknown reason it turns head downwards. It can thus prepare the pelvis and the lower part of the uterus for its subsequent delivery which occurs head first. If the baby does not turn round spontaneously by the 33rd or 34th week of pregnancy the doctor may do an external version. By gently palpating the baby through the anterior wall of the abdomen and the uterus, the baby is turned so that its head instead of its bottom is lying over the brim of the pelvis. A skilled doctor can do this without the mother realizing that the baby is being turned or even moved. In 96 per cent of pregnancies the baby's head is presenting which means that the baby has turned round spontaneously. It is important for the obstetrician to know which part of the baby is presenting at the brim of the pelvis because in the 4 per cent where the breech is presenting, either external version must be performed or adequate plans made for the breech delivery.

Even when the head is known to be presenting, it is most important that its exact position should also be known.

During a first pregnancy lightening normally occurs at about the 36th week. This is the result of the baby's head descending into the actual cavity of the pelvis, which is known as engaging. In subsequent pregnancies the head does not usually engage until the expected date of confinement or the onset of labour.

Engagement of the head in the pelvis does not mean that labour is imminent. It does mean that the size of the pelvis is adequate for the baby's head and that everything is progressing satisfactorily. The date of delivery cannot be predicted from the date of engagement. At the antenatal visit you will be given a 'cooperation card' on which your doctor will write the results of all tests, and at each visit details of your health and the baby's growth.

10 Preparing for the Baby

Hospital or home?

The argument on the rather difficult subject of whether a mother should have her baby in hospital or at home has continued ever since maternity hospitals were first instituted well over sixty years ago. Hospital delivery provides the essential medical and nursing care, as well as the facilities to deal with any eventuality. Domiciliary, or home, confinement provides social advantages and is convenient for the mother who has a young family. Gradually, however, more and more women are having their babies in hospital: at present more than 98 per cent are delivered in a maternity unit.

This increase is due to several factors. Since complications in labour and in the new-born baby may arise suddenly and fatally, most obstetricians prefer to look after their patients in hospital, where there are all the facilities and ancillary services which they may require. Most women prefer hospital delivery because they know this, and also because they are assured adequate rest afterwards.

Yet those in favour of a return to home confinements often quote the Dutch experience where a 50 per cent rate of home deliveries is combined with a low perinatal mortality rate. There are, however, many differences between Holland and Britain. Dutch women are very carefully assessed for a home birth. They belong to a more homogeneous population than ours. The Dutch midwife has a long training experience and is helped in the home by a 'maternity aid nurse'. Perhaps most importantly, all women are within thirty minutes of a hospital should an emergency arise.

It is known that the worst results for mother and baby occur in patients who must be transferred as an emergency during labour. A large survey in Liverpool in 1982, of over 1,000 pregnant women, found that only 28 per cent were suitable for a home delivery. Of these low-risk pregnancies, nearly one-third developed antenatal complications (e.g. high blood pressure, haemorrhage) or problems in labour and immediately after delivery (e.g. fetal distress, retained placenta, haemorrhage). Nearly 7 per cent of the babies needed specialized paediatric care.

Although a choice is still available to those who are medically acceptable for a home confinement, ideally the doctor and community midwife should deliver the woman in a maternity unit rather than her home. The mother can then be transferred back to her own home as soon as her general condition and that of the new-born infant are considered satisfactory. This is planned early discharge and combines the safety of hospital confinement with the mother's swift return to her home.

Hospital confinement

During the last few years the increased number of hospital confinements reflects a new social trend in Britain and with the average duration of stay in hospital of 5 to 8 days and planned early discharge from hospital it is now possible to provide hospital care for all mothers. Hospital is undoubtedly the best and safest place for a baby to be born and should be encouraged by all in the obstetric field.

Nevertheless, women are still allowed a choice between a home or a hospital confinement and this is sometimes critical to the future well-being of the mother and her baby.

Maternal mortality and illness, together with perinatal mortality and illness, have declined phenomenally during the past three decades but even lower rates could be achieved if all mothers were admitted to hospital for their confinement. Hospitals are geared for all obstetric emergencies that may arise and provide an impressive list of facilities, as well as the basic ward, delivery and nursery units. They include antenatal clinics, postnatal clinics, infant welfare clinics and special dental, infertility, tuberculosis, cardiac, diabetic, venereal disease and family planning clinics. The expert staff include obstetricians, physicians, paediatricians, anaesthetists, radiologists, bacteriologists, midwives and nurses specially trained in the care of premature and sick babies.

When a woman is having her first baby and any after her third, it is essential that the confinement should take place in hospital. Only those women having their second or third baby and whose pregnancies are absolutely normal are acceptable for home confinement. Furthermore, any woman under 5 ft in height, under the age of 19 or over the age of 35 should be delivered in hospital. If there has been a serious complication in any previous delivery or if there is any serious anaemia at the beginning of pregnancy, or at any other time during pregnancy, then she should have her baby in hospital. Any woman who develops a rise in blood pressure or has a multiple pregnancy can only safely be delivered in hospital. Medical reasons, or any illness such as diabetes, kidney disease or heart disease, are also absolute indications for hospital confinement where the necessary facilities are easily available should they be required.

A great advantage of having her baby in hospital is that the mother is freed from a mass of worries and responsibilities. If she is at home it is easy for whoever is running the house to bother her with minor domestic problems. There may be a continuous stream of visitors who want to see the baby and it is almost impossible for the new mother to have peace and quiet. Rest and sleep are essential for any woman after labour if she is to recover rapidly from her delivery and enjoy caring for her new baby.

The mother going into hospital will not need as much equipment as she would at home. Most hospitals provide a list of the articles that a mother needs to bring into hospital and she should pack these in a special case towards the end of pregnancy. The list usually includes: soap and flannel, brush and comb, toothbrush and toothpaste, paper handkerchiefs in preference to linen ones, a sanitary belt or disposable paper panties, safety pins, nightdresses, a bed-jacket, dressing gown, slippers and two brassieres. A set of baby clothes will be required when the baby goes home, but while in hospital these are provided.

The midwife

A nurse must study for three years to qualify as a State Registered Nurse after which she can specialize in certain fields. The midwife is a specialist in maternal and child health and after her state registration she must work and study for a further year after which she must pass another examination before being allowed to practise as a midwife. A midwife may also train in a special two-year scheme. The midwives who staff maternity wards have had years of sound experience. During your time in hospital most of the help and advice regarding your baby will come from the midwife whose sole purpose is to guide you and to give you confidence in handling your baby in preparation for your return home.

In a maternity ward a woman has to adjust to a certain routine which may be very disconcerting at first, but it sets a pattern for each individual mother and baby which can be continued when they go home. This is an important fact to remember and it will help a woman organize her daily life when she no longer has the order of the hospital. There are usually no rigid rules about visiting times in maternity wards; they should not interfere with ward routine, the feeding of babies or mothers' resting time, but otherwise any visiting restrictions are gradually being removed.

Home confinement

The one advantage of having a baby at home is that the other children feel they share in the event and will welcome the new baby right from the start. If you want to have your baby at home all the following conditions should be fulfilled at the time of booking:

1 As far as can be ascertained your general physical condition is excellent and you are 5 ft or more in height.
2 You are pregnant for the second or third time and the previous pregnancies, labours and the puerperiums have all been normal.

3 You are under 35 and over 19 years of age.
4 No Rhesus antibodies are present in your blood.
5 Your home conditions are suitable.
6 There is adequate help at home.

The facilities available for patients having a domiciliary confinement are: doctors, consultations with an obstetrician, mobile obstetric emergency unit, maternity packs with sterile supplies and home help. Community midwives are provided by the local health authority under the National Health Service and the necessary arrangements can be made with your own family doctor after he has confirmed your pregnancy.

The standard of home conditions must be high before delivery at home can even be considered. There must be a suitable bedroom where the mother can be delivered in privacy. The doctor and midwife who are going to conduct the delivery will see the room beforehand so that any suggestions about particular changes in furniture can be attended to. The ideal room should be bright and quiet, conveniently near the bathroom and certainly on the same floor. Heating must be provided day and night in cold weather to prevent the baby getting cold. The mother's bed must be accessible from both sides and well situated with regard to light. A cot for the baby, a comfortable chair and a table are necessary. A wash-basin with running water is a luxury which is much appreciated, but bowls, jugs and lots of hot water will do just as well. A really good light is vital. Flooring should be easily washable. If the carpet cannot be moved it should be covered for protection. A large plastic or polythene sheet must be placed over the mattress.

Requirements for a home confinement

A suitable room with furniture as above, two large basins—one for the mother, one for the midwife—one bed-pan, one bucket for soiled dressings, one 2 pint jug for water, plastic sheet to cover the mattress, a nail-brush, one or two hot water bottles with covers, and newspapers.

Personal belongings: two nightdresses, one dressing gown, one pair of slippers, toilet articles, one bath towel, one face towel and face cloth, two brassieres, sanitary belt, sanitary pads (maternity quality).

For the baby's immediate needs: a soft towel to wrap the baby in when born, a baby bath, soft bath towel, soap, soft petroleum jelly, mother's bathing apron, safety pins, cot, low chair for feeding as well as all his clothes, sheets and blankets. Your midwife will give you a full list.

Factors affecting safe confinement

There are so many modern advances and factors that go towards safe confinement that it is impossible to list them all in detail.

Maternal health. The better a woman's general health, the more easily can she maintain it throughout her pregnancy. This applies not only to the elimination of obvious infection and disease but also to the correction of anaemia and other such conditions.

Antenatal care is responsible for the elimination of anaemia, deficiencies, pre-eclampsia, the control of weight gain and the early diagnosis of complications amongst all other essential factors that lead towards safe confinement.

Midwives. The continued training of skilled midwives whose dedication and devotion to their patients has to be seen and experienced to be believed is probably one of the greatest influences on safe confinement in Great Britain.

Doctors. The increase in the necessary training of both general practitioners and specialists to a better understanding of the problems of pregnant women has gone a long way towards affecting the outcome of pregnancy.

Facilities. While many people may criticize the facilities available in Great Britain, there are not many countries that can match the overall standard of care that is provided during pregnancy nor the specialized and emergency facilities.

Modern advances. While some of the medical advances in pregnancy and delivery are not absolutely recent, the advances in the care of the woman and her baby, such as new drugs, the control of infection, better anaesthesia, the understanding of blood groups, the Rhesus factor, blood transfusion, together with the use of certain modern and specialized techniques and apparatus, all contribute to a safe confinement.

The paediatrician. Enormous advances have been made in recent years in the care and welfare of the infant especially the care of the new-born and premature baby. The credit for this must go to the paediatricians as well as to the nurses who take care of these babies in special units.

Liaison. The increasing liaison between all the various medical, social and administrative departments that have to do with the care of the pregnant woman contributes towards an efficient, and therefore safe, confinement.

Natural childbirth

The term 'natural childbirth' is a phrase that has achieved a great deal of notoriety and confuses many people. It seems to have conjured up an image that the majority of doctors and midwives wish to make childbirth 'unnatural' and that they wish to deny women some of the pleasures and experiences of childbirth. Nothing could be further from the truth. Nobody, least of all doctors and midwives who have devoted several years to learning how to deliver women normally and naturally, would attempt to interfere with any normal or natural delivery unless there was some reason to do so.

It is of the utmost importance that all available help should be given in early pregnancy to enable the woman to accept and understand all the physiological, anatomical, as well as the emotional and psychological, changes that are going to occur throughout pregnancy, delivery and the puerperium. These three phases of reproduction must be kept in their correctly balanced perspective and labour itself must not be chosen as the only, or even the most important, event in the whole process if natural childbirth is to be achieved.

The erroneous conception that 'natural childbirth' refers only to 'normal' delivery is commonly held. However, many doctors believe that natural childbirth starts with a harmonious sex life, resulting in conception at a time of choice, with the full implications of the conception being realized before it occurs. A careful understanding of pregnancy and all its changes is perhaps more important than an understanding of delivery itself, but an understanding of the process of labour is essential if labour is to be conducted with the full cooperation of the doctors and midwives, as well as with pleasure to the mother.

Pregnancy, including childbirth, is often stated to be a natural physiological function which may sometimes present physical discomforts and mental strains, but which, when carried out by a healthy, normal, well balanced person, should be accompanied by an immense sense of achievement and satisfaction. This is undoubtedly true, and the more thoroughly educated the pregnant woman is, the greater will be her confidence and her cooperation with her midwife and doctor during the three vital phases of reproduction. Any physical danger or emotional difficulty that might arise is therefore eliminated.

Classes for antenatal instruction and relaxation are provided by most maternity units attached to hospitals. These may be inadequate for the patient who wishes to have a greater knowledge and insight into her pregnancy and delivery, but there are only a certain number of doctors and midwives available for the whole maternity service and extensive antenatal instruction has not yet become a practical possibility.

This book is meant to be educational. It is meant to help. It is meant to instruct. It is meant to assist you in understanding what your pregnancy is all about. An easy and pleasurable pregnancy and delivery depend upon two main factors. Firstly, that you should really want the child you have conceived and, secondly, that you should not be afraid of producing it, nor of the process of pregnancy or your ability to look after the child after he has arrived. The second of these two is by far the more important factor. A great deal of this book has been spent in describing the normal changes of pregnancy and also the complications that can occur. The description of the complications is not meant to frighten or to disturb, but is mentioned so that you can understand some of the things that can go wrong and appreciate why midwives and doctors do various tests and insist on your attendance at the antenatal clinics.

The whole syndrome of fear, pain and tension has been propounded at length for a number of years. This is a syndrome which becomes a vicious cycle. Fear of the unknown begets tension and tension in its turn begets pain, which then in turn creates further fear. A complete knowledge of what pregnancy and labour are all about is half the battle in overcoming this fear, but the other half is self-confidence: you should have sufficient knowledge to start your pregnancy with some degree of assurance and to begin your labour with complete confidence in your own ability to do what is expected of you, knowing exactly what is happening to you and why various investigations are being done.

The birth rate

There are approximately 9 million women between the ages of 14 and 45 in England, and during 1977 there were 569,000 live births, which represents a birth rate of 11.6 per thousand of the population. The birth rate has been falling in England for several years but has recently stabilized between 11 and 12.

There was a total of 5,400 stillbirths during 1977 which represents 0.94 per cent of all live births.

The maternal mortality during the year 1976 was 0.012 per cent which means that approximately one woman in every 7,720 died in childbirth, but it must be remembered that these figures are for the entire country and therefore include those who had no antenatal care and those who suffered from severe heart and lung disease.

There were 52,000 illegitimate live births during 1977 which represents 9.1 per cent of all live births. One-third of these would be women of under the age of 20 years. (See table below).

Illegitimate births to women under the age of 20 in England (1976)

Age of mother	11	12	13	14	15	16	17	18	19
Number of illegitimate births	1	2	34	201	1100	2594	4590	5319	4793

The total number of abortions during 1976 was 101,900 resulting in the deaths of 6 women, as compared with a total of 68 maternal deaths from childbirth out of the total 555,722 mothers who gave birth to live or stillborn infants in that year.

During 1976, 97.4 per cent of all women had their babies in hospital where the average length of stay for each patient was approximately 7 days.

Mothercraft classes

Women should enjoy having babies because happiness for the parents means an equally happy and well-adjusted son or daughter. This attitude is becoming more important as the pressure of living increases. The mental and physical development of children rests with the individual parent, so that the child's happiness and attitude to life will reflect not only the attitude of the parents but will also decide the sort of community in which he will live and shape his future. Where does happiness like this come from? It starts from the simple acceptance of pregnancy with all its implications; the confidence that the woman builds up in her own ability and her absolute trust in the medical people who will guide her. Pregnancy should be regarded as the time when women are healthier than ever before, despite some of its occasional discomforts, but much will depend on how well they listen to their medical advisers and how efficiently they carry out instructions.

Most maternity units have a course of mothercraft classes, which every pregnant woman should attend. The classes usually comprise:

1 Antenatal care, including hygiene of the pregnant woman, the importance of fresh air and exercise during pregnancy, rest and sleep, relaxation, suitable clothing, the bowels, care of the teeth, bathing, smoking, marital relations and diet during pregnancy.
2 The development and growth of the baby in the uterus.
3 Labour, including the signs of labour and what happens during the first, the second and the third stages of labour. Demonstration of the analgesic machine which is used during labour.
4 Breast-feeding and artificial feeding, which should also include care of the nipples and the latest in maternity wear.
5 Planning the baby's layette, including style and fabrics available.
6 Bathing the baby.
7 A visit to the maternity ward and the labour ward.

The new father

A new baby at home means a big upheaval in a father's life. Women rightly expect their husbands or partners to be loving towards them and to admire

their recent achievement, but it should be remembered that men are sometimes neglected when their partners are pregnant and therefore require just
as much attention as the new arrival. Every woman should make sure that
the new member of the family does not mean that her husband or partner
has less of her love, time and affection. It takes a long time to get used to
having a new baby in the house, particularly if you have to get up during
the night to cope with a crying infant. During the first few weeks the
young mother needs extra sympathy and understanding. By sharing some
of the responsibilities, life will become easier for both partners and the
household will settle quickly and smoothly into the new routine.

Layette

There are no set rules about a baby's layette and the list below is intended
only as a general guide:

- Three vests. Wool is warm and soft.
- Two dozen nappies in Turkish towelling.
- Disposable nappies. More and more mothers use disposable nappies to
  save time and effort. Even if not used all the time they are invaluable
  for travel or when you are particularly busy. Nappy liners, which are
  squares used inside towelling nappies, are also useful. The cost of using
  disposable nappies is not much higher than the total cost of using
  traditional nappies.
- Six pairs of plastic pants, which should not be too tight round the
  baby's thighs.
- Three nightdresses in wool and cotton mixture. Babygros are very useful
  and practical. Flameproof fabric is essential.
- Three cardigans.
- A shawl.
- Booties, helmet and mittens. These are really only needed for winter
  babies.

The above items will see a baby through the first few months and some,
of course, will continue in use longer.

The baby's room

Many items are a matter of taste and the size of your budget.

- The cot. A crib isn't absolutely essential: the baby can go straight into
  a cot. The cot should have the British Standard 'Kitemark' regarding
  safety. Special baby mattresses are firm and covered with waterproof
  material, not loose plastic sheeting as this is a hazard to the baby. No
  pillow is needed in the first year.
- Four cot blankets. The cellular type are warm and light in weight.

- Cot sheets. Buy those of a warm flannelette material.
- Carry-cot. This is a very useful item and the baby can even stay in it at night for the first few weeks.
- Bath. Choose a plastic type, making sure that the stand is absolutely steady.
- Two bath towels. These should be reserved entirely for the baby's use.
- Toilet box. The main things you will need in the baby's box are a baby hairbrush, a supply of large curved safety pins, baby soap, cream, petroleum jelly, talcum powder, cotton wool, swabs and a small bowl for swabs.
- Nappy bin. Useful but not essential. Any pail with a lid will serve.
- Low feeding chair. Ideally the chair will be without arms and will have a padded seat for comfort.

If you can possibly manage to give your baby a room of his own, try and make it as bright and cheerful as possible. Babies love clear, bright colours and there is no reason why one should stick to the traditional pastel shades. Babies like to watch things that move, so it is a good idea to have an inexpensive mobile hanging from the ceiling within his field of vision. All paint should be leadless and this is vitally important for such things as repainted cots which the baby will be chewing and licking later. Linoleum or plastic tiles are the best floor coverings, perhaps with a brightly coloured rug. Curtains should be in light washable material, lined to keep out the light when the baby is to sleep. Safety items such as fireguards and window bars are essential and should be installed well before the baby becomes mobile.

The pram

There is a great choice of prams available today and one must be guided by particular needs and the cost. If restricted for space at home it may be best to buy a collapsible pram, or, for the baby's first months, it may be more convenient to have a carry-cot with a chassis on wheels which folds into a very small space. When buying a pram the following features are important:

1 The pram should be the right weight and height. It should be easy for you to push.
2 It is important to be able to see over the hood when it is up.
3 Safety is vital. Only buy a pram which has the British Standard 'Kite-mark'. The brakes should be secure and easy to adjust.
4 A good, firm mattress.
5 It should have an attachable canopy to provide protection against the sun and a pram net to keep cats off when the baby is outside.

Bathing your baby

It is important to have everything ready before starting to bath your baby each day. The room should be warm and the windows closed. Everything should be within easy reach before you begin. A table or trolley should be arranged with something for holding the soap or a bottle of special baby bath solution, a sponge or flannel, hairbrush, cotton wool swabs, talcum powder, lotion, cream or petroleum jelly and a warm towel. A nappy bin should be ready for the soiled nappies and you should wear a waterproof apron to keep your own clothes dry. A comfortable chair is necessary for you to sit on.

Method of bathing a baby

1 The bath should be half filled with warm water. Test with your elbow for temperature. Have everything within easy reach.
2 Undress the baby, leaving on nappy. Wrap him in a warm towel. Clean face very gently using cotton wool soaked in clean water, and then dry face very gently.
3 Shampoo his head with soap, rinse thoroughly and dry his head. Unwrap the towel and remove his nappy.
4 Soap him all over with your hand and put him into the bath. Hold securely.
5 Rinse the soap off with the water in the bath and let him kick about if he wants to.
6 Lift him out of the bath and lay him face down on the towel on your lap.
7 Dry the baby all over, paying particular attention to the creases around the neck, underarms, knees and bottom.
8 Rub a little cream or petroleum jelly between his legs and on his buttocks.
9 Powder the baby's body lightly to make sure it is properly dry.
10 Dress him.

Bathing should always be a happy time for both mother and baby. The time of day you do it depends on whether it makes him sleepy or not. If it does, do it in the evening; if it seems to wake him up then bath him in the morning. The bathing of the baby should fit into the established routine of the household. Fathers should participate if possible so evening may be more convenient, especially as the room is often warmer and the mother more relaxed.

Changing a baby's napkin

Babies should be as comfortable as possible so the baby's napkin may need to be changed both before and after each feed.

There are two widely accepted methods of putting on a baby's nappy:

1 Lay the nappy out flat, fold it into a triangle and then fold into a smaller triangle. Place the baby on the triangle with the point down between his feet. Fold each of the side points downwards between his legs and tuck them well under him, then bring the central point up between his legs. All three thicknesses can then be held in place with one nappy pin. When pinning have two of your fingers between the baby and the nappy to avoid sticking the pin into him. Always use safety guarded pins.

2 Lay out the nappy and fold it lengthwise to produce three thicknesses. Fold up the lower third at one end so that you have an area of six thicknesses. Lay the baby lengthways on the nappy and fold it up between his legs, securing it at the sides with two safety pins. With boys it is best to have the thickest part in front and with girls at the back.

A good deal of work can be saved if a piece of nappy liner is put inside the nappy as this will avoid soiling of the nappy and make washing so much easier. Disposable nappies are increasingly used and these entirely avoid nappy washing.

Baby's day

This should be flexible; here is a routine type of day·

On waking change him, feed him and put him back in his cot. He will probably go back to sleep again.

10.00 a.m. Bath him or just top and tail him. That means his face, hands and bottom. Feed him, dress him and if the weather is good put him in the garden in the pram.

2.00 p.m. Feed him and change him. If he is wakeful, mother him for a short time.

6.00 p.m. If you have bathed him in the morning, just top and tail him, change him and feed him. It might fit into the daily routine better to bath him in the evening. Put him in his nightclothes and tuck him into his cot. The temperature in the bedroom should not fall below 65°F (18°C) when a baby is very young.

10.00 p.m. Change him and feed him.

During the night the baby will probably wake for a feed for the first few weeks of his life. Feed him, change him, make him comfortable and then put him back into his cot and he will probably go back to sleep.

Breast-feeding

Breast-feeding is discussed in Chapter 37.

Artificial feeding

Artificial feeding is discussed in Chapter 37.

11 Advice to Pregnant Women

Advice

Unsolicited

Unsolicited advice is usually both unwanted and inaccurate.

Everyone has a certain amount of knowledge about pregnancy but it is not until a woman has had a baby that she can talk with any conviction or authority about the signs, symptoms or the finer details of what happens to a pregnant woman. It necessarily follows, therefore, that the majority of girls obtain, or are given, information about pregnancy which is really just a reflection of their mother's experiences of pregnancy. These may have been easy or difficult, good or bad, happy or unhappy, but however they are interpreted they will be transmitted to her children. Pregnancy is no exception to the general principle that a child's ideas are gradually moulded and modified by the things that are read or learned during childhood and adolescence. By the time she is ready to start her first baby, a girl will have a fairly definite idea of what it is all about. She may wish to have more information but the basic ground work has nevertheless been systematically laid down over the preceding years and the careful or thoughtless way in which she has been consciously or unconsciously influenced will show in her approach to her own pregnancy.

The public media

Over the past twenty years or so the public media have responded to the general public's demand for more information about medical science with a number of extremely good programmes on radio and television and a mass of articles in journals and magazines. Radio and television, however, have yet to treat pregnancy as an educational subject. The accent has been more on delivery than on the importance of antenatal care and general basic advice, and written articles can only cover small aspects of pregnancy at any one time. Unfortunately, it is only the relatively small proportion of the population who is either pregnant or who has someone in their immediate family circle who is pregnant that is really interested in a fundamental knowledge of pregnancy.

Solicited

It is because there are so many gaps in the average woman's knowledge concerning pregnancy that she is so vulnerable to unsolicited advice and if such advice worries her there is no comprehensive work to which she can turn to relieve her anxiety. This particular book is a genuine attempt to provide information in an unbiased manner although there will always be differences of opinion upon certain matters and undoubtedly in some places this book is either imperfect or will subsequently be shown to need modification. It is nevertheless intended to be fair and impartial; written in the hope that it may provide some guidance to those who require it and some helpful support to those who may be unduly anxious, particularly those who have heard hair-raising stories of difficulties and problems in pregnancy or delivery.

There are many authoritative books on pregnancy or different aspects of childbirth that give very sound advice and useful information. Antenatal classes, relaxation classes, natural childbirth (National Childbirth Trust) and psychoprophylaxis classes all provide an immense amount of invaluable advice and information. Do not listen to unsolicited and often potentially harmful advice.

Rest

How much rest should you have when you are pregnant? It is impossible to say because it varies with so many personal factors. The ideal is 8 hours in bed at night and 2 hours in bed in the afternoon. This, however, is almost impossible to arrange especially in early pregnancy, because those who are pregnant for the first time are frequently going out to work and those who are pregnant on subsequent occasions have to look after their children. Bearing in mind then that the ideal is 10 hours' rest in every 24 hours, you should get as much rest as you can. Remember that in the early part of pregnancy you may feel unduly tired or lethargic and there is simply no point in trying to fight it. You can either give in to it and rest, in which case you will feel much better, or try to resist it with the inevitable result that you become bad-tempered and even more tired. If you have previously arranged to do things and feel too tired, you should have no hesitation in cancelling your arrangements. This can, however, be very difficult unless your husband or partner appreciates the problem, so it is up to you to see that he knows about your needs.

After the end of the 14th week of pregnancy you will feel much better, much less tired and much more energetic. You should still, however, have an adequate amount of rest.

In the last three months of pregnancy you will need more rest and during the last 6 weeks especially you should rest as frequently as possible with your feet up. When you are pregnant you should always avoid sitting with your knees bent and never with one knee crossed over the other. So long as you are fit and well there is no reason why you should not take a reasonable and normal amount of exercise but remember that you do not have to take exercise in order to become a healthy mother or to have a healthy baby. If you want to go for a walk, go for a walk. If you don't want to, then don't.

Sleep

Tiredness is one of the natural phenomena of pregnancy. This usually commences shortly after the first missed period and is characterized by a definite lassitude and tiredness during the day as well as at night. Ten hours' rest is usually advised throughout the whole of pregnancy. The majority of pregnant women will not be able to sleep for 10 hours, but the important factor is rest rather than sleep. The natural tiredness normally occurring in early pregnancy will usually ensure an adequate amount of sleep and it is frequently more severe in subsequent pregnancies than in the first. It usually begins about the 6th week and continues until about the 14th week during a first pregnancy, but may last until the 20th week during subsequent pregnancies.

A woman can be told how long she should spend in bed or resting during the day but no one can predict, or demand, a certain number of hours of sleep. As pregnancy advances sleep usually becomes lighter. The pregnant woman finds it more difficult to get to sleep and then she tends to wake more easily and, therefore, to sleep for shorter periods. There are various reasons for this. The enlarged abdomen produces generalized discomfort. Fetal movements may disturb her just as she is falling asleep. The increased weight of the advanced pregnancy on the abdomen makes it difficult to find a comfortable position. The irritable bladder may wake her during the night. Congestion in the nose is one of the more annoying side effects of pregnancy which may also disturb sleep.

It does not matter what time you go to bed as long as you are going to stay there for 8 hours. Resting during the afternoon is almost as important as sleep at night and, ideally, the rest should be in bed, but if this is not possible then it should be taken on a couch. It is surprising how much refreshment can be gained from even the shortest sleep.

The secret of sleeping during the afternoon and also at night is that of relaxation. On the principle that physical relaxation results from mental relaxation, conscious relaxation will gradually induce somnolence and then sleep. The cultivation of both physical and mental relaxation is an enormous asset. The majority of people who cannot sleep during the afternoon, or have difficulty in sleeping at night, are mentally overactive, worried or concerned, and of course finally they become worried because they cannot sleep.

If for some reason sleep is difficult discuss this with your doctor. Most doctors agree that sleeping pills should be avoided if possible, but it is better to have a good night's sleep with a mild and safe sleeping pill than to fail to sleep altogether and be a neurotic wreck the next day. Doctors will avoid the administration of sleeping pills in early pregnancy, but many pregnant women have great difficulty in sleeping towards the end of their pregnancy and then sleeping pills are occasionally indicated. These must be prescribed by your doctor and taken according to his instructions. Many sleeping tablets are available which are completely harmless during pregnancy if taken in the prescribed dose, but there are others which should not be taken during pregnancy. Never, therefore, take sleeping pills without first consulting your doctor.

Dreams in pregnancy

Most women dream more when they are pregnant than they are accustomed to. The reason for this is not known but it is probably associated with a change in sleeping pattern which results in lighter sleep and 'waking dreams'. Certainly in the second half of pregnancy sleep may be disturbed not only by fetal movements but also by the difficulty in maintaining a comfortable position in bed or by increased frequency of micturition. All these factors may contribute towards an increased frequency of dreams. There are many old wives' tales suggesting that frightening or disturbing dreams may affect a baby either physically or mentally. This is not true. No importance should be attached to this phenomenon and such dreams certainly have no profound meaning or significance.

Exercise in pregnancy

Most people understand exercise as meaning physical activity over and above their normal daily duties. This is not strictly true. Most women have a home to look after and either a job to do or other children to take care of, and these duties in themselves require a considerable amount of work and exercise. It is difficult to imagine a more vigorous exercise than scrubbing a floor or even polishing a table. There is no reason why a woman progressing through a normal pregnancy should not continue with her normal household duties. If, however, complications arise, then her activities may be restricted by her doctor.

For a pregnant woman who goes out to work, the kind of work must be considered. For instance, there is a world of difference between being a shorthand typist sitting at a desk all day and being a conductress on a double-decker bus running up and down stairs all day. Common sense can decide how long most women should continue with such occupations during pregnancy. The maternity allowance is payable after the 29th week of pregnancy (see Chapter 16), but it is obviously inadvisable for women to continue some energetic occupations until this stage of pregnancy and lighter or more acceptable work must be found for them.

It is stressed throughout this book that pregnancy imposes a certain amount of extra work, both physical and metabolic, upon the body, so that rest is essential. This does not mean that normal duties should not be continued, but extra duties which involve tiredness, fatigue or unnecessary physical exercise should be avoided.

Many women are accustomed to a certain amount of physical exercise or sport such as tennis, golf, cycling, swimming, walking or gymnastics and if they are used to this before the onset of pregnancy there is no reason why they should not continue during the pregnancy provided it progresses normally. They must, however, avoid undue tiredness and exhaustion. They should consult their doctor as to when they should start giving up their particular sport because they must not continue merely as a matter of principle. A woman should not commence such extra physical exercise for the first time during her pregnancy. It cannot be too strongly emphasized that if you go around your normal daily duties you have adequate exercise. Extra exercise is not necessary. The main need during your pregnancy is rest not physical exertion.

Walking

There is really no limit to the amount of walking you may do during pregnancy. Ordinary daily duties involve a good deal of walking and if you feel like going out for a walk to get some extra exercise, there is no reason why you should not do so. You should not, however, go on hiking expeditions. By walking you are both enjoying yourself and helping to keep your body fit, but you are not doing anything specific for the benefit of your pregnancy or your unborn baby. Always stop when you become tired. You must never allow yourself to get exhausted.

Swimming

Swimming does not harm pregnant women. It is a mistake to suggest you should not swim while you are pregnant. Certain precautions, however, must be observed. Women who are not used to physical exercise or who do not swim frequently should avoid going in the water during the early part of pregnancy at the time when they would normally have been having a period, that is at the 4th, 8th and 12th week of pregnancy. This precaution is less important if you do take frequent physical exercise or swim at least once or twice a week, but even then it is important that you should never become overtired. Swimming in very cold water is *not* advisable especially as there is more likelihood of cramp during pregnancy. Diving from heights of 3 ft or less is not harmful to any experienced swimmer but high diving must be avoided by all women throughout their entire pregnancy.

Dancing

Apart from simple, ordinary, common-sense restrictions, dancing can be continued until the onset of labour. The amount of energy and exercise involved depends on the type of dancing and both exercise and energy should be restricted as pregnancy advances. Acrobatic dancing is, of course, forbidden at any stage during pregnancy.

Cycling

No harm will result from riding a bicycle at any stage of pregnancy. However, even in early pregnancy reflexes are not as rapid as usual and any accident may result in a miscarriage. Women who cycle in early pregnancy should be ultra-careful. They should not become overtired and should certainly not take part in rallies or races of any kind. As pregnancy advances a woman's balance becomes affected and this together with the gradually enlarging abdomen makes cycling increasingly difficult. It should be discouraged during the second half of pregnancy for, although it is highly unlikely that a baby will be injured even if there is a direct blow on the abdomen, an accident might predispose to miscarriage or premature labour.

Horse-riding

You should not ride horseback at any time in pregnancy. Not only is the actual exercise undesirable, but there is always the risk of damage or injury resulting from a fall.

Water skiing and snow skiing

Water and snow skiing are not advisable especially for the inexperienced. Even experienced skiers will find that their balance and judgment are disturbed during pregnancy and this increases as pregnancy advances.

Skin-diving

This is also better avoided during pregnancy, mainly because a woman's judgment is impaired and this might adversely affect her reactions, with dangerous results. Underwater diving is rigidly forbidden in the later stages of pregnancy. Underwater swimming using a snorkel is allowed providing the swimmer is familiar with the apparatus.

Fresh air

The British are always going out 'for a breath of fresh air'. What are the advantages of fresh air? Most scientists will agree that there is no particular advantage in breathing outside air especially if the 'fresh air' happens to be the exhaust-ridden atmosphere in a city centre.

The amount of oxygen and other constituents is almost identical inside and outside your house and there cannot really be any scientific advantage in fresh air, but there are several small and unapparent advantages. The exercise in taking a short walk outside certainly does no harm and if you have been sitting around most of the day it certainly does quite a lot of good. The psychological effect of getting out is beneficial, especially getting out into the country for even a few hours, even if you only sit and gaze at the beautiful scenery once you have arrived there.

What about fresh air in the house? Should you open windows? The answer is yes. Artificial heating which dries the atmosphere in most homes is certainly not really beneficial, and without making you cold and uncomfortable a little fresh air is well worth it if only to maintain normal humidity. A window partly open at night is almost essential to avoid the discomfort of nasal congestion with the subsequent mouth breathing. You will find you sleep much better and your nose and mouth will be much more comfortable.

Lifting during pregnancy

Hard physical exercise and the lifting of heavy weights are contra-indicated during pregnancy. It is often said that nothing should be lifted during pregnancy, except that which can be easily lifted with two hands without exerting undue effort. This is mainly meant to refer to furniture and other heavy weights. Even when the lightest objects have to be lifted from the floor it is far better to lift them by squatting down rather than by bending forwards with the knees straight, which adds to the natural strain on the back during pregnancy. Pregnant women should cultivate the principle of picking things up from the floor by squatting down on bent knees so that the buttocks come into contact with the ankles.

For the woman who has a young family there is the ever present problem of lifting the children. No one would ever deny a mother the right to lift her child, but she should learn to pick the child up from a squatting position and also adopt the favourite trick of kneeling down alongside or in front of her child in order to cuddle or console it. Looking after children can be one of the most tiring and tiresome occupations for a pregnant woman, but by careful thought a lot of the hard physical work of handling them can be eliminated.

Travel

The whole question of travel presents a simple yet difficult question. If you have a good, stable, normal pregnancy it will not come to any harm if you have to travel. There is, however, one simple exception to this rule. That is horse-riding.

There are one or two rules which ought to be obeyed. Do not travel over long distances unless it is essential. Travelling by train is usually more comfortable and causes less strain than travelling by car, especially for distances over 100 miles, unless you have a particularly good car and a very competent driver. When travelling by car never miss an opportunity to empty your bladder because another 50 kilometres of motorway with a baby bouncing on a full bladder is not very pleasant. Finally, remember that the emotional instability of pregnancy makes the readjustment to the time change of travelling across time zones, for example from London to New York, much more difficult and can impose quite a considerable strain upon you. If your pregnancy has not been stable, that is, if you have had any bleeding during the early part, or if you have suffered from a previous miscarriage or catastrophe, you should not undertake any journey that is not absolutely essential. If you have bled in early pregnancy, then travel by aircraft even much later is not advisable because though it may not do the baby any harm there is always increased risk that the altitude changes may provoke premature labour.

Even if your pregnancy and past history have been absolutely normal, you should not travel abroad or for any great distance during the last six weeks and you should certainly stay fairly close to home for the last four weeks. It is as well to remember that airlines will not normally accept passengers who are more than 35 weeks pregnant. If your pregnancy has been normal and you happen to be returning from abroad after the 30th week you should get a short note from your doctor, stating your expected date of confinement and the fact that you have his permission to undertake the journey, to show to the airline authorities if necessary.

Travel pills

The majority of pills that are manufactured and prescribed for the control of travel sickness are very similar to those given for nausea and early morning sickness during pregnancy. If you are prone to travel sickness this will obviously become worse if you are already nauseated during the early part of your pregnancy. While the majority of travel pills are quite safe and may be taken in early pregnancy, you should never take them without the permission of your doctor.

Driving

There is no reason why you should not drive during pregnancy and, indeed, you may continue to drive until labour commences providing you obey certain simple regulations.

First, remember that your emotional balance tends to be rather disturbed, especially in early pregnancy, and your judgment is not quite as precise and accurate as when you are not pregnant. You should therefore drive with just that little bit more care and give everybody else just a little bit more room than usual. If you are involved in an accident in late pregnancy there is always a possibility of the steering wheel digging into your abdomen. Unless the accident is serious this is unlikely to harm your baby but even so it is an additional reason for driving with even greater care than usual.

Second, you will tire rather more easily and therefore should not undertake long journeys.

The employment of pregnant women

The maternity allowance is normally payable for 11 weeks before the expected date of confinement, that is at the end of the 29th week of pregnancy. (See Chapter 16.)

Whether you work during pregnancy depends on individual circumstances and no generalization is possible, but certain basic rules can be laid down.

Providing pregnancy is normal there is no reason why a woman should not do reasonable work, on condition that it does not expose her to any risk of accident or undue tiredness. Most women are much happier, especially during their first pregnancy, if they continue with their job than they would be if they sat at home being generally bored. The money is probably important anyway. Women who already have children have a full-time job on their hands coping with the house and the children as well as with the new pregnancy. If there is any question or doubt in your mind you should discuss the whole question of work with your doctor or with the doctor at the hospital.

Even in a normal pregnancy it is not usually recommended to continue working after the end of the 29th week. A lot of women argue, however, that they have a sedentary occupation two minutes' walk from home and might just as well go there and bash at the typewriter as stay at home and scrub the floor. Providing they are happy, have sufficient rest, are not becoming overtired and the pregnancy is normal there is no real reason why younger women should not continue a sedentary job, particularly in their first pregnancy and especially if they do not have far to travel. Each individual must, however, be judged on her merits and a compromise, such as part-time work, may be reached. If there has been any complication during the pregnancy or any abnormal past history, an increased amount of rest is usually prescribed so that employment is not generally possible.

Work is still a difficult problem to which there is no simple answer because each pregnancy is worth a different amount to each woman. For instance, a woman of 27 who is not married may wish to get rid of her pregnancy. If she has been married for only three months she may be quite happy and content to continue working. If she has already had one miscarriage she may consider doing less work or perhaps part-time work. If she has been married for five years and has had three miscarriages she will probably consider giving up work altogether. If she has been married for ten years and has had six previous miscarriages she may well consider not merely stopping work but going to bed and resting in bed for a considerable part of her early pregnancy.

Clothes

Shoes

Your feet are very important!

Care and attention to your feet are most important throughout the whole duration of pregnancy. One of the natural processes of pregnancy is that ligaments soften and therefore tend to stretch. This, of course, takes place in the pelvis where it is one of the major factors that enable normal and spontaneous delivery to occur. These changes are not limited, however, to the pelvic bones and ligaments, but occur elsewhere in the body particularly in the feet. A lot of care and attention must be paid to the feet if their ligaments are not to be stretched beyond return. There are two longitudinal arches and one transverse arch mainly supporting the normal function of the foot, and these must be preserved for its normal functioning and pain-free movement.

A combination of the weight increase of pregnancy and the softening of these ligaments can easily result in flattening of the normal arches of the foot with permanent injury to the foot architecture. This is far more likely to occur in a woman who is ill and tired than in one who is fit and well. Standing for long periods tends to stretch the ligaments and should be avoided if possible. This does not mean that a person should not exercise fully and normally; exercise is good for both the ligaments and the muscles of the foot.

Shoes that give adequate support to the feet are essential. Throughout pregnancy all shoes, including walking shoes and slippers, should have a similar height of heel and should provide the foot with satisfactory support. The habit of wearing 8 cm heels during the day and casual shoes with no heels at all in the evening is to be deplored. Those who always walk barefoot at home may continue to do so but standing without shoes ought to be avoided.

Stockings

Tights or stockings may be worn at the beginning and throughout the duration of pregnancy but stockings must be supported by some type of suspender. Garters are dangerous because they constrict the legs and cause varicose veins below the obstruction. Stockings that are supported by an elastic top have the same effect and should not be worn. Tying a knot in the top of a silk or nylon stocking should not be done under any circumstances, for a woman is much better without any stockings than with stockings supported by a tight knot. There is no harm in wearing short or ankle socks and no harm will come to the pregnant woman who does not wear any stockings at all. There are many advantages in wearing tights throughout pregnancy.

Brassiere

A good support for the breasts is essential throughout pregnancy. Many women notice that the breasts enlarge rapidly at the beginning of pregnancy and again at about the 20th week, thereafter remaining approximately the same size until immediately before delivery. Most pregnant women need to buy a new brassiere at the beginning of pregnancy but should not do so until most of the initial breast enlargement has taken place, which is by about the 10th week. The enlargement in mid-pregnancy is due more to enlargement in the size of the chest than to actual enlargement of the breasts themselves. A suitable brassiere bought at about the 10th week of pregnancy which has the correct bust size and an adjustable back can accommodate the increase of chest size at the 20th week.

A brassiere bought for use in pregnancy must provide satisfactory and adequate support. It should have strong and fairly wide shoulder straps and the back should be wide, giving ample support under the arms with fastenings which allow room for expansion as the rib cage enlarges with the advancing pregnancy. Elastic shoulder straps cannot provide adequate support for the breasts during pregnancy and they are not recommended even if they are 'more comfortable'. The advantage of having a well-made and properly fitted brassiere cannot be emphasized too strongly.

Despite the popular misconception, the breasts do not contain muscle and if they are allowed to sag during pregnancy for lack of adequate support, no amount of exercise after delivery will return them to their former firmness. It is obvious, therefore, that good support is absolutely essential

Whether you wear a brassiere at night as well as during the day is an individual decision, but if your breasts become unduly heavy or have a tendency to become pendulous, wearing a 'sleeping bra' is probably advisable, especially during the second half of pregnancy.

Maternity or nursing brassieres. Owing to the increase in the size of the chest wall after the 20th week of pregnancy, women are advised not to buy maternity brassieres until near the end of pregnancy. Many makes and types of nursing brassiere are available and while some are satisfactory, many do not provide adequate support.

Nursing brassieres fall into three main groups. Those which open in the mid-line in front, those which have a removable panel on each breast, and those which can be undone at the back as an ordinary brassiere. The advantages of front fastenings where the child can be suckled at the breast without undoing the brassiere must be weighed against the less adequate support of such brassieres. Those which have a detachable panel on each breast suffer firstly because of the lack of support given to the breast and secondly because of the comparatively inadequate access to the breast during feeding. After all the child feeds from the breast itself and not from the nipple and the surrounding two inches of breast tissue. One of the arts of breast feeding is the proper handling of the breast during feeding and this is made increasingly difficult if the breast itself is constricted by a brassiere. These disadvantages are weighed against the disadvantage of having to undress almost completely for every feed.

Abdominal support in pregnancy

Advice about abdominal support in pregnancy is contradictory. Women disagree about it when they are not pregnant, so why should agreement suddenly materialize when a woman becomes pregnant?

Let us consider the woman who is pregnant for the first time and does not normally wear any abdominal support. Abdominal enlargement will not be a noticeable feature of pregnancy until the 16th week at the earliest. The first thing she will notice about her abdominal contour is that the waist line disappears especially at the sides. Somewhere between the 16th and the 22nd week abdominal distension will commence. A person such as this invariably has good abdominal muscles and there is no need or indication for her to wear any abdominal support. After the 20th week a certain amount of aching in the lower abdomen may occur especially towards the end of the day. This usually goes after a short rest and if you have never worn any abdominal support you need not start now. Your muscles will respond normally to the pregnancy and providing you do not put on extra weight, they will return to normal after delivery. Here is a guarantee: if you are normal weight before your pregnancy, and use no special support, don't wear one during pregnancy, don't gain more than 22 lb, don't have twins or extra amniotic fluid—then three months after delivery your abdomen will be as good as it ever was. No marks, just as flat, just as strong and just as nice in any bikini.

If the muscular discomfort persists or becomes worse it may be relieved by wearing a lightweight elastic abdominal support. A large or cumbersome maternity belt is not necessary. An elastic support gradually stretches as the pregnancy progresses but should continue to provide sufficient support for the lower abdominal muscles.

The girth of the abdomen will normally reach 100 cm at the expected date of delivery and from the 34th week onwards the duration of pregnancy in weeks will be the same as the girth around the umbilicus in inches. Occasionally an excessive amount of water is formed in the uterus and when this happens abdominal enlargement becomes greater than normal. The girth will also be greater than normal in a twin pregnancy. When the abdomen is larger than usual there are many advantages in providing some support. This is best obtained by a lightweight maternity corset with expanding sides. A U-shaped-front corset does not provide satisfactory support.

Women who normally wear some abdominal support will need to provide themselves with support during their pregnancy. They can use their usual abdominal supports during the first 20 weeks. After this a woman who is not overweight and whose pregnancy is proceeding normally may prefer to continue wearing her normal abdominal support which will gradually stretch as pregnancy advances but still give sufficient support to the anterior abdominal wall. Most women who are overweight will require some special maternity corset. This also applies to the woman having her second or subsequent child who has weak abdominal muscles and in whom the abdomen tends to become pendulous as pregnancy advances. It is essential that such a woman should have adequate abdominal support. This is particularly applicable to the person who has previously been delivered of twins, or who suffered from overdistension of the abdomen during a previous pregnancy or who gained too much weight during her pregnancy. Abdominal support should be put on first thing in the morning and should be kept on throughout the day, not put on late in the day when the abdominal muscles have become tired and have started to ache.

The baby inside the uterus lives in an environment surrounded by water. It is extremely difficult to damage or harm a child in the second half of pregnancy. Some women believe that supporting underwear may damage or deform their child. Tight underwear or clothes will not harm or damage a child or lead to congenital deformities. Even hundreds of years ago when it was the custom to bandage the abdomen so tightly that it was difficult to breathe there was no real evidence that it caused any harm to the unborn infant.

Underwear

Despite many prejudices there is no reason why a woman should not continue to wear the type of underwear she wears in the non-pregnant state. There is no particular disadvantage in any material that is used for underwear. Tight fitting underwear may be uncomfortable and is to be discouraged. This is particularly applicable to tight knickers or pants which may cause discomfort and sweating in the groins and between the legs. People who are grossly overweight will notice that sweating in these areas may be particularly troublesome especially if they use underwear made from nylon or other non-absorbent materials. Cotton panties or disposable briefs have many advantages especially in hot weather or if there is an excess of vaginal discharge.

Teeth

Care of the teeth in pregnancy is of the utmost importance because during pregnancy the teeth are very prone to decay. Any dental disease should be promptly treated.

There are supposed to be two main reasons for dental disease in pregnancy. First, and unlikely, the use of calcium by the baby tends to rob the mother of this vital element and she loses calcium from her bones and teeth. Second, and correct, infection in the gums, or gingivitis, predisposes the teeth to infection and decay.

Most people have a satisfactory diet but it has, nevertheless, always been considered necessary to give the pregnant woman dietary supplements of calcium in order to protect the teeth from decay. It is doubtful whether this does anything to protect the teeth or to reduce the amount of decay once the process has begun, but it may be given to protect her bones from losing calcium as a result of her baby's demands.

The calcium in teeth is so firmly fixed that there is no way of extracting it. A human skeleton buried for 10,000 years will have healthy teeth and yet the bones may crumble. Women in some developing countries suffer from osteomalacia, caused by calcium deficiency resulting from many pregnancies, and while their bones become so soft that they actually bend, their teeth remain healthy. One of the most convenient methods of obtaining calcium is by drinking milk and the inclusion of milk in the diet is probably justified by this alone, but it does nothing to prevent dental decay.

Many local authorities have accepted that fluoride is important to the development of teeth and prevention of caries. However, there is still resistance to the idea that fluoride taken by the mother may help the formation of her baby's teeth. Fluoride tablets are available at most chemists.

The main cause of dental disease is gingivitis or inflammation of the gums which become softer and more vascular in pregnancy and are easily injured by food and coarse tooth brushes. Once injured it is easy for infection to be introduced. During pregnancy this happens around the teeth and destroys the delicate membrane between teeth and gums. When the membrane has been destroyed infection enters beside the tooth: the gums become red and swollen and recede to expose the sensitive part of the tooth which is more prone to decay. Careful dental hygiene in pregnancy is therefore essential if the teeth are to be protected from unnecessary damage.

Care of the teeth

1 Clean the teeth in pregnancy as at any other time—after every meal if possible and always before retiring at night.
2 Use a medium brush, or a softer one if the gums have been bleeding. A medium or soft brush is better than a hard one as it gives more friction for the gums. Two or three brushes should be in use, giving each one time to dry before being used again.
3 No one particular paste or powder is better than another for stimulating the gums without causing irritation. It is, in fact, preferable to change toothpastes from time to time unless your dentist recommends a particular brand.
4 Electric toothbrushes are very good especially for those people who are too lazy to use an ordinary toothbrush for 2 to 3 minutes in the proper way!
5 Some dentists believe that small doses of fluoride taken during pregnancy will protect the baby's teeth from decay in later life. Ask your dentist for his advice.
6 Rinse with a mouthwash if the gums bleed; one part hydrogen peroxide and five parts water is useful as it helps to wash away the debris from between the teeth and helps to cleanse the mouth.
7 The gentle use of dental floss will help to remove food particles from between the teeth.

Hair

Most women notice no difference in their hair throughout pregnancy but some find that dry hair tends to become more dry, and greasy hair more greasy. It is therefore even more important to take particular care of your hair throughout the entire pregnancy and to use an appropriate shampoo for your own particular type of hair.

Before deciding to have a perm always tell your hairdresser that you are pregnant. This is particularly applicable if you have dry hair, because this type of hair always tends to crack and break, especially during the latter half of pregnancy.

On very rare occasions quite a lot of the hair breaks, some of it appearing to come out at the roots to such an extent that there is a very noticeable thinning of the hair itself. The exact reason for this is not known but it seems to be connected with the high progesterone levels in pregnancy. If this should happen to you, be careful not to brush your hair too vigorously and make sure that it is properly washed with a very mild shampoo. Your hair will return to normal after you have been delivered and such thinning of the hair does not usually recur in any subsequent pregnancy.

A lot of women complain that their hair is unmanageable in early pregnancy and if they happen to be feeling particularly tired or nauseated then it makes life even more tedious if extra time has to be spent on making the hair look nice and presentable.

Nails

Just as some women notice that their hair becomes fragile during pregnancy, so others notice that their nails become brittle, crack, break and also split. The cracking and breaking are bad enough, but split nails are very difficult to manage because any bit of dirt that gets into a split is extremely difficult to remove. There is no evidence to prove that nail varnish harms or dries the nails and, although this does seem to be generally accepted, few doctors would advise women against using nail varnish if they wished to do so.

Brittle nails will obviously be more easily damaged by housework and other manual duties. They can be protected to a certain extent by wearing gloves for any chores that might damage them or make them unduly dirty.

An age-old remedy for preventing the nails from cracking during pregnancy is to rub baby oil into the base of the nail at night. If your nails normally have a tendency to crack you should start doing this at the beginning of pregnancy. If your nails have begun to crack you will not notice any benefit until the massaged part of the nail has grown its full length, which takes approximately two months. It is very simple, quick and easy to do, and it can be quite effective.

The bowels

The regulation of the bowels throughout pregnancy is most important and can be accomplished to a great extent by means of careful diet. Perhaps the most important aspect of diet is a satisfactory and adequate water intake Pregnant women should drink at least four pints of fluid each day although they must be careful that the fluid is one which does not have a high calorie content. The best fluid of all is plain water. A good balanced diet is essential and this should contain a larger amount of roughage than normally. Roughage is found in green vegetables, fruit, oatmeal and wholemeal flour. Learn to spare the time to go to the toilet; hurry can destroy good bowel habits.

Taking strong purgatives is neither necessary nor desirable in early pregnancy, and while mild preparations may become necessary later on, even they are better avoided if possible. For people who have never taken medicine to keep the bowels open a small dose of magnesium sulphate or one of the proprietary brands of fruit or health salts will probably be sufficient. If these prove inadequate a slightly stronger purgative such as Milpar may be necessary. Some women find that constipation is a very troublesome problem and may have to take a senna preparation such as tablets or granules of Senokot, though long term use of senna may actually increase constipation.

The ideal should be to open the bowels normally at least once a day, but if one or perhaps two days pass in which the bowels are not open there is no need to take an extra large dose of purgative on the following day. The correct dose of any medicine habitually used to keep the bowels open is that amount which will open the bowels each day and no more.

Sexual intercourse during pregnancy

A great deal of advice has been given and written in books concerning sexual intercourse in pregnancy. There is no reason why normal intercourse should not continue throughout a normal pregnancy until labour begins. It is probably fair to add, however, that the pregnant woman should be treated with a modicum of respect. The breasts may become very tender in pregnancy and pressure can be quite painful so that technique may have to be changed accordingly. The enlarging abdomen will also dictate appropriate changes in technique (the normal position is not ideal in the circumstances).

There are, however, certain exceptions. Any woman who has suffered from a previous miscarriage ought to avoid intercourse for the first 14 weeks of pregnancy, and any woman who has suffered from recurrent miscarriages should avoid intercourse until this has been specifically permitted by the doctor. Any threat to miscarry, or bleeding at any stage in pregnancy, must automatically result in cessation of sexual intercourse until the doctor advises that it may be resumed. This is not only important in early pregnancy, but it is of the utmost importance during the last 10 or 12 weeks.

There is no chance of infection being caused by intercourse. In the past it was often stated that any woman who had intercourse after the 6th week of pregnancy ran the risk of creating infection not only in the uterus but in her baby. This is completely untrue. It is also untrue that sexual intercourse should stop at the 32nd week of pregnancy because of the danger of infection or harm to the baby or of premature labour. However, when a woman *has* had an irritable uterus or even premature labour in the pregnancy, intercourse should stop as seminal fluid is very rich in hormones called prostaglandins which may cause the uterus to contract.

The human female is one of the very few mammals to permit sexual intercourse during pregnancy and it is not surprising that occasionally the libido, or sexual desire, changes. Libido is often reduced in pregnancy, especially during the first 14 weeks, after which it increases till about the 30th week and then declines gradually as the expected date of confinement approaches. You should discuss this with your husband or partner.

Frigidity

Frigidity, or lack of sexual desire, sometimes occurs in pregnancy. If this happens do not worry; your desire will return later. Occasionally loss of libido will continue throughout pregnancy and it is a common symptom after delivery, sometimes lasting for several weeks or even months. When this happens you require gentle understanding until your sexual appetite returns, which it most certainly will, in due course.

Smoking in pregnancy

Most people agree that heavy smoking should be discouraged at any time and this is certainly true during pregnancy. There is ample statistical evidence to show that women who smoke a large number of cigarettes during pregnancy have smaller babies than those who are non-smokers and that smoking after the 16th week probably causes both mental and physical retardation in later childhood. This is possibly the result of an adverse effect exerted by cigarette smoking on the placenta which may reduce the oxygen supply and the nutrition to the fetus in the uterus. The majority of women who smoke soon discover that a dislike of cigarettes is one of the earlier symptoms of pregnancy and is frequently associated with nausea and early morning sickness. They usually stop smoking for at least the first three months and this is certainly to be encouraged; nor should they start again.

Most doctors consider that smoking is positively harmful to the unborn child and they prefer women not to smoke during pregnancy. Smoking is absolutely forbidden in any woman who has or has suffered from kidney disease, raised blood pressure, pre-eclampsia, or any sort of bleeding at any stage during her pregnancy, who has been delivered of a dead baby or whose child has died within the first two weeks of life, because it may jeopardize placental development and function

Alcohol

It is known that large amounts of alcohol taken during pregnancy can be very harmful to the fetus and cause congenital abnormalities. Modern advice is that no alcohol should be taken during pregnancy and some authorities believe that a woman should not consume alcohol for several weeks before pregnancy begins. There is, however, no proof that the odd glass of wine or sherry or beer is harmful.

Bathing

Pregnancy need not alter your previous habits and bathing or taking a shower is not contra-indicated during normal pregnancy. One word of warning, however, is that your baths should not be too hot or too long. There is a tendency to fainting in early pregnancy and if you get up quickly from a long hot bath you can quite easily feel dizzy or faint. Later in pregnancy you may feel clumsy and your balance may be slightly affected by your enlarged abdomen, so you must take the greatest care not to slip when getting into and out of the bath, especially if you use oil in your bath water.

In the old days bathing and swimming were not advised because it was thought that water entered the vagina and carried infection with it. This is not true. It is very unusual for bath water to enter the vagina and even if it does it will do no harm.

The vulva and the surrounding area should be washed as usual during pregnancy and particular care should be taken to wash all soap away and dry yourself adequately.

Douching

Douching is not a particularly British habit. Most authorities agree that it is not advisable during pregnancy because there is always a danger of the pressure forcing some water from the vagina through the cervix and into the uterus where it may jeopardize the continuation of pregnancy and even cause abortion, miscarriage or early labour. While she must never douche with a powerful Higginson's or other form of syringe, there is no objection to a woman using a bidet at any stage during pregnancy unless she has suffered some vaginal bleeding, the bag of waters has ruptured or she is in labour.

Some women who have been douching almost daily for many years insist, very inadvisedly, on continuing during their pregnancy. Antiseptic solutions should never be used even in the non-pregnant state because these solutions may not only injure the vagina but also kill the normal defensive organisms which are naturally present there. Any woman who insists on using a douche during pregnancy must use a very low pressure apparatus with either plain water or water to which a small amount of salt has been added (1 teaspoon to the pint).

The abdomen

The care of the abdomen during pregnancy is very simple and yet very complicated. Various aspects will be found under the headings of exercise, clothing and care of the skin, but perhaps the most important of all is weight gain. The whole secret of preserving your figure and not getting stretch marks is the control of the amount of weight you gain during your pregnancy. This is emphasized repeatedly throughout this book. If you do not gain more than 9 kg in weight throughout your pregnancy then your abdomen will return to normal after you have been delivered; the muscles and the skin will be just as good as they were before you became pregnant (that is providing you have not had twins).

The question of abdominal support is discussed on pages 158–9. The care of the skin of the abdomen should be similar to the care of the skin on the rest of your body. It is quite common for a pregnant woman to massage oil into her abdomen every night before going to bed. This is to be encouraged because it helps keep the skin in good condition and because it also means that these women are anxious to take care of themselves. However, if you put on too much weight, no amount of oil will prevent stretch marks.

The navel, or umbilicus, also needs special care during pregnancy. It should be gently cleaned and dried with cotton wool. At about the 30th week of pregnancy it will commence to flatten and by the end of pregnancy it will almost certainly be completely flat. This is quite normal and it returns to its previous shape within a few days of delivery.

Fetal movements (quickening)

The growing baby begins to move as soon as its muscles have developed. The first muscles form alongside the spine as early as the 8th week of pregnancy, and shortly afterwards the baby is making his earliest primitive movements. Muscles can develop only if they are exercised frequently so that their gradual formation and growth in the arms and legs are associated with an increase in both the amount and the strength of fetal movement. By the 12th week they are sufficiently powerful to be detected by the use of medical apparatus. However, you will not be aware of these movements until the uterus is sufficiently enlarged to allow them to be transmitted from the uterus to the delicate nerve endings in your anterior abdominal wall.

During your first pregnancy you will notice fetal movements somewhere between the 18th and 20th week, but do not be alarmed if movements are not felt until about the 24th week. During subsequent pregnancies movements will usually be felt somewhere between the 16th and 18th week, although some mothers claim that they feel them as early as the 14th week.

The earliest movements are very difficult to identify since they are usually felt as vague flutterings or butterflies in the lower abdomen, which are very similar to the sensation caused by wind rumbling around the intestine. Gradually, day by day, the movements become stronger and more persistent until, even in the first pregnancy, it is obvious that your baby is moving. As he becomes more mature, the character of the movements changes until he produces thumping or kicking movements which become more powerful as pregnancy progresses.

Your baby will not move continuously. The earliest movements may be intermittent and indeed it may be a considerable time before you are aware of the fact that fetal movements are actually occurring. This is partly because of their gentleness, but also because of their intermittent nature.

It is not known if babies go to sleep in the uterus, but they do lie quietly without moving for periods of up to several hours, and nearly always (often at about the 24th week) a baby will lie quiescent for up to 24 hours. This lack of movement does not mean that your baby has come to any harm: he always starts moving again, usually more vigorously than before. Unless a woman has been informed that this may happen it is likely to cause her undue concern.

Babies may develop a rhythmic type of movement in late pregnancy felt as a jerking every few seconds for up to several hours. This is due to hiccoughing and may be present after the birth. It does no harm.

Many women say that the baby is more active as soon as they go to bed at night. This is probably because they are more conscious of movements while resting quietly than when they are up and about with other things to occupy their thoughts.

A child who moves a lot in the uterus is not necessarily destined to be an active or athletic person, nor is a child who moves very little necessarily destined to be slow and lethargic. Similarly, the sex of the child cannot be foretold by the degree of movement within the uterus.

The majority of movements of the mature fetus are gentle because the baby's head is engaged in the pelvis and he does not have such a compara·tively large space in which to move. These can best be described as squirming movements caused by the infant exercising not only his arms and legs but also his spine. He will occasionally kick or squirm in a particular place which becomes tender and painful. When this happens there is no cause for concern; just wait until he moves into a more comfortable position. Most of the dramatic movements of the fetus within the uterus come from the feet; the back and the head have a squirming type of movement. When the head is presenting the feet will be found in the upper part, or at the fundus, of the uterus, so that most of the more violent type of movement will be felt there. After about the 24th week your baby may often produce sudden thumps and kicks after a time of comparative quiet. These can be, and often are, most disconcerting owing to the ease with which they may disturb your train of thought or interrupt a conversation.

The most active fetal movements usually occur between the 30th and 32nd week of pregnancy. Your baby is, by now, very strong and has plenty of room in the uterus in which to move, kick and even punch. It is surprising that comparatively violent movements of a baby are seldom, if ever, painful.

When the head is situated over the brim of the pelvis it rotates and moves and may cause considerable discomfort, especially to the bladder, resulting in frequency of micturition and sometimes difficulty in holding water. When the head is engaged in the pelvis a different type of pelvic discomfort is felt. The baby's head can move even when it is engaged in the pelvis and this movement can result in pressure on nerves causing pain which may radiate down the front or back of the thigh and occasionally through to the back, even causing sciatica-like pain.

Since the fetus has to learn to use all his muscles while in the uterus, it follows that he must use his diaphragm and his respiratory muscles. There is quite a lot of evidence to show that babies do in fact inhale the amniotic fluid as well as swallowing large quantities which are then passed as urine.

Your baby will stay in the same position after the 32nd or 34th week of pregnancy because the head is fixed in the brim of the pelvis. The back remains on one particular side and therefore most of the movement caused by the legs and feet will be felt on the opposite side in about the same place until delivery. Babies do buck and hit the uterus with their buttocks and this is felt on the opposite side to the limbs.

Uterine contractions

All involuntary, or non-controllable, muscle (the heart, intestine, blood vessels, uterus) contracts and relaxes in a rhythmic manner throughout the life of its owner. Contractions and relaxations of the uterine muscle occur from the cradle to the grave although they become more marked during a woman's reproductive life. They may be particularly noticeable on the first day of the menstrual period when they may manifest themselves as the cramp-like pains, called spasmodic dysmenorrhoea, so familiar to many women. The uterine muscle contracts normally at about 20 minute intervals throughout adult female life including pregnancy. During pregnancy, because of the relaxing effect of the hormone progesterone, the contractions are not usually noticeable until about the 20th week after which they may be felt regularly until delivery. They are felt as a tightness which spreads over the entire uterus and are occasionally associated with discomfort but not actual pain. These contractions, called Braxton Hicks' contractions, are a normal phenomenon of normal pregnancy. The uterus can be felt to harden quite noticeably during the contraction which lasts for approximately 30 seconds before passing off as smoothly and as quietly as it began. They are probably of immense value to the fetus because they squeeze out any 'stale' blood in the large veins in the wall of the uterus which then refill with 'fresh' blood after the contraction has passed. As pregnancy advances towards term a woman is much more likely to be conscious of the Braxton Hicks' contractions. However, even as term approaches, although she may sometimes feel slight discomfort, they will not become painful.

Some people consider that the onset of true labour is the conversion of painless Braxton Hicks' contractions into the more forceful uterine contractions of labour, which, when they reach a certain pressure or tension, cause pain. The severity of this pain is directly related to the force of the contraction, which is the tension generated by the muscle.

Braxton Hicks' contractions may be distinguished from true labour by the following characteristics:

1 They may occasionally be uncomfortable but they are not painful.
2 They last for approximately 30 seconds whereas the contractions of true labour are usually longer.
3 They are seldom more frequent than every 15 or 20 minutes, while the contractions of true labour occur with increasing regularity so that they are spaced 15, 10, 5 and eventually 3 minutes apart.
4 True labour contractions become gradually harder and more prolonged as the interval between the contractions gets less.
5 Braxton Hicks' contractions are never associated with a loss of blood whereas true labour contractions are frequently accompanied by the show which so often signals the onset of labour.

Braxton Hicks' contractions occurring at night are often mistaken for the onset of true labour. If you are in any doubt, get out of bed and make yourself a warm drink with two codeine or paracetamol tablets and you will probably settle down and return to sleep. If, in fact, true labour has begun the contractions will continue with renewed vigour and you will either be unable to sleep or will wake again.

Warnings: symptoms of danger

There are ten groups of symptoms which may occur during pregnancy that merit serious attention. They do not indicate that disaster has occurred or is likely to occur, but they should be considered seriously and reported to the doctor or midwife either immediately or as soon as is reasonably possible. The first five listed below should be reported immediately, while the second five may be reported at the earliest convenience, which usually means within 24 hours.

1 **Vaginal bleeding.** When vaginal bleeding occurs in the first 28 weeks of pregnancy it indicates that the pregnancy is unstable and that there is a threat of miscarriage or abortion. If the amount of bleeding is slight, immediate rest in bed is indicated and the doctor can be notified as soon as reasonable, but if the bleeding is heavy or associated with pain you should go to bed at once and notify the doctor immediately. Any vaginal bleeding after the 28th week of pregnancy should be notified immediately to your doctor or the hospital with the exception of the pink, mucous stain which occurs at the onset of labour, and is usually accompanied by uterine contractions of which you will be aware.

2 **Severe continuous abdominal pain.** Onset of severe, incapacitating, continuous abdominal pain should be notified immediately. This type of pain may be associated with some premature separation of the placenta (see p. 266) or with any other acute abdominal emergency, but it is emphasized that this type of pain is continuous and not intermittent and usually occurs in the lower abdomen.

3 **Breaking of the waters, or rupture of the membranes.** When this occurs the onset of labour usually follows fairly quickly. Some types of miscarriage or abortion are preceded by rupture of the membranes and it is the first symptom to occur in approximately 40 per cent of premature labours. It is important, therefore, to notify your doctor or the hospital immediately so that arrangements can be made for your transfer to hospital, but be certain that the membranes have in fact ruptured and that the watery loss is neither urine nor bath water which has found its way into the vagina and is being expelled either minutes or hours after the bath. After the 36th week of pregnancy rupture of the membranes is of less importance because of the improved chance of fetal survival. However, even at this stage of pregnancy the doctor, midwife or hospital should be notified in order that the necessary arrangements can be made either for your immediate admission or for your delivery.

4 **Mistiness, difficulty and blurring of vision.** In the second half of pregnancy this may be a symptom of pre-eclampsia or of raised blood pressure and if it occurs you should go to bed and notify your doctor at once.

5 **Continuous severe headache** which is not relieved by paracetamol, codeine or other simple headache remedies. Such a headache usually occurs either above and behind the eyes or over the back of the head. A severe headache over the front or the back of the head accompanied by some disturbance of vision may be a symptom of severe pre-eclampsia or raised blood pressure. It is emphasized that this type of headache continues for several hours and does not respond to the usual remedies. The headache which is felt as a pressure on the top of the head is not usually significant.

Symptoms not so urgent as the above five, but which warrant early notification to your doctor, midwife or hospital, are:

1 **Temperature.** A rise in temperature to 101°F (38.5°C). Even if its cause is obvious some form of treatment will usually be necessary.

2 **Frequency and pain on micturition** usually indicate the onset of a urinary tract infection and if they persist for several hours then treatment is indicated as soon as this can conveniently be arranged. Infections in the urine are discussed in Chapter 21 and are particularly common during pregnancy.

3 **Swelling of the hands (including fingers), face and ankles,** known as oedema, may occur at any stage of pregnancy and is frequently associated with pre-eclampsia, a raised blood pressure or excessive weight gain. A certain amount of swelling of the ankles is common in pregnancy, especially during hot weather, but excessive swelling of the ankles such that shoes cannot easily be put on is a warning sign. Swelling of the hands and fingers may cause stiffness of the fingers, especially in the morning and often a sensation of pins and needles in the hand.

4 **Absence of fetal movements.** It cannot be emphasized too strongly that babies frequently stop moving for quite long periods during pregnancy. It is fairly common for a baby to stop moving at about the 22nd or 24th week for several days, and frequently for up to 24 hours during the latter part of pregnancy. However, if your baby does not move for longer than 48 hours tell your doctor as soon as it is convenient to do so.

5 **Excessive vomiting.** A certain amount of sickness or vomiting is very common in the first 14 weeks of pregnancy. If, however, vomiting becomes so severe that no fluid or food can be retained then help should be sought. Sickness usually ceases after the 14th week, although occasional bouts of vomiting may recur. During the last three months of pregnancy most women vomit occasionally, but repeated, recurrent and severe vomiting is unusual and should be reported as soon as possible.

German measles (rubella)

German measles, or rubella, is a mild virus disease which may affect any human but does so only once during life. The rubella virus is one of the few organisms which has the ability to cross the placenta and cause direct infection of the fetus. If the mother is infected with rubella during the first 12 weeks of pregnancy (counting from the first day of the last menstrual period) it may disorganize the growth of the early fetal organs and thus cause congenital abnormalities such as deafness, blindness and congenital heart disease, or other types of abnormality. The actual instance or percentage of abnormality in cases of rubella has varied from country to country and still shows considerable variation. This is because the virus, like any other organism, varies in its virulence or ability to attack tissues, and also any community exposed to a virus for the first time will suffer more severely and will have more severe disease than a community in which the virus has become endemic. (An endemic infection is one in which the virus causes occasional outbreaks of disease within a community.)

The incidence of congenital abnormality varies from about 12 per cent in certain areas of Great Britain to about 30 per cent in certain parts of Australia. This means that even at the most conservative estimate a woman who develops rubella during the first 12 weeks of pregnancy has 5 times as great a chance of congenital abnormality in her child as she would otherwise have. At worst the incidence is about 12 times greater and the majority of countries who have legalized abortion under certain circumstances accept this probability of congenital abnormality in the fetus as one indication for termination.

Rubella in childhood is a mild disease that may pass unnoticed. A woman may be unaware that she has had the disease. Even the mildest attack confers immunity so that she cannot again have the infection and her unborn children are protected. Any pregnant woman who has not had rubella, or who is uncertain, must take purely common-sense precautions.

If you are in the first 12 weeks of pregnancy you should studiously avoid any person who has, or has been in contact with, German measles. You must not feel afraid or embarrassed to refuse an invitation to visit people who have been in contact with rubella. If you explain that you are pregnant they will immediately understand and would not expect you to expose yourself to any possible danger. It is mainly children who develop rubella and the above comments are particularly applicable to children who are at a school in which rubella has occurred.

If you have young children who have not had rubella, they should not visit or entertain their friends if there is any possibility that these have, or have been in contact with, rubella. If rubella is going round their school, keep them at home until you have consulted your doctor.

As a general precaution women should encourage their daughters to have rubella between the ages of 3 and 16. This usually means specifically sending them to play with infected children. Once a girl has had rubella she cannot again be infected. Rubella inoculation of young girls and young married (non-pregnant) women has become established practice. This gives a mild attack of the disease which bestows permanent immunity.

If you have been in contact with someone who has rubella, who has recently had rubella, or who develops rubella within two or three days of seeing you, consult your doctor. A blood test is usually done to ascertain whether you have previously had the disease, when sufficient antibodies will be detected circulating in your blood to protect you from a second attack.

If you actually develop the disease at any stage of pregnancy you should consult your doctor immediately. The very mild rash which is usually the main physical sign disappears after 12 or 24 hours. If you develop the disease after the 12th week of pregnancy it will be less serious from your baby's point of view, but if you do develop the disease before the 12th week of pregnancy it is essential that the diagnosis should be confirmed by your doctor. If you fail to see your doctor when you have the rash it is still possible for the diagnosis to be confirmed by a blood test taken about two weeks later. This will show a high level of antibodies due to recent infection.

If it is confirmed that you have suffered from rubella in early pregnancy then the future of the pregnancy must be decided. Termination can be considered under the Abortion Act of 1967 for the reason that 'there is a substantial risk that if the child were born it would suffer from such physical or mental abnormalities as to be seriously handicapped'. It may be that you do not wish to consider this, but if you do your doctor will discuss it with you. He will base his advice on careful consideration of the many aspects of the problem: the religious grounds, your age, the number of children that you have, how long you have been married, the ease or difficulty which which you establish a pregnancy, your own health and that of your children and husband. Termination of pregnancy is not to be entered upon lightly and obviously a serious discussion will need to take place between yourself, your husband or partner and the doctor. If an antenatal test shows that you have never had rubella, you can be immunized after your baby has been born to avoid any future worry.

When to call the doctor

The main indications for calling your doctor or getting in touch with the hospital are set out on pages 170–71, where there is a list of the ten warning symptoms together with an explanation of their urgency. Of course every symptom must be judged on its merit and it is just as wrong to suggest that you should call your doctor if you have a pain in your little finger as it is to suggest that you should not call him when you start bleeding profusely at the 26th week of your pregnancy. The guidelines have been laid down and the rest is really up to common sense. Make a careful note of your doctor's surgery hours and the fact that during his surgery he usually makes out a list of the patients whom he is going to visit at the end of his morning surgery. Your community midwife probably leaves to go on her morning rounds at about 8.30 a.m. There is always someone on duty at the hospital, but unless it is urgent or you are unduly worried they would obviously prefer to see you during antenatal clinic hours even if you do not have an appointment.

X-rays

Everyone is exposed to what is known as background irradiation which is the amount of irradiation that they receive from the atmosphere. Since the effect of irradiation upon the body is cumulative, this must be added to the irradiation received from man-made sources, of which, in a civilized community, the most important is medical X-rays. It is a basic principle therefore that no one should be subjected to an X-ray unless there is a valid reason for the investigation. X-rays used for ordinary purposes of diagnosis are at such a low dose that they do no harm to ordinary tissues. Any X-rays upon the gonads (sex organs) may, however, cause disturbance of the very sensitive genes (see Chapter 1) within the chromosomes in the reproductive cells of both the testis and the ovary and this may ultimately lead to abnormal formations, known as mutations. Such mutations may give rise to abnormalities in the offspring of later generations, even though the offspring of the present generation are perfectly normal. The developing gonads (testis and ovary) in the fetus are particularly sensitive to the damaging effects of X-rays and this is the main reason why X-rays should, if possible, be avoided during pregnancy.

Some authorities consider that X-rays of the fetus during pregnancy may lead to the development of leukaemia in childhood. This is not certain, but they certainly are of no benefit to the fetus and should be used only if the information obtained outweighs the disadvantages. In very early pregnancy inadvertent high doses of X-rays may lead to abortion. For this reason, women should avoid X-rays after the 10th day of their menstrual cycle.

X-rays of the chest taken during early pregnancy are usually performed with the abdomen protected by a lead screen. In this way the fetus receives no irradiation and cannot be harmed. Similarly there is no danger to the fetus from necessary dental X-rays during pregnancy.

Immunization during pregnancy

There is no objection to the standard immunization and vaccination procedures during pregnancy but for obvious reasons they should be avoided during the first 14 weeks. A smallpox vaccination certificate is valid for 3 years so if you are contemplating pregnancy, make sure it has not expired. If it has, or is due to expire within the next year, then revaccination before starting pregnancy is a wise precaution.

Primary smallpox vaccination, which is vaccination for the first time in a person's life, should not be performed at any stage during pregnancy unless the woman has been in contact with smallpox or there is an epidemic. If you have never been vaccinated against smallpox, you are strongly advised not to go abroad during pregnancy. Get yourself vaccinated after your delivery—and then travel.

Infantile paralysis (poliomyelitis) may be particularly severe if contracted during pregnancy, so make sure you have had your poliomyelitis vaccination when contemplating pregnancy. If you have not been immunized against poliomyelitis, have this done as soon as possible.

Similarly, vaccinations against typhoid, paratyphoid, cholera or yellow fever may be given after the 14th week of pregnancy but are better avoided. There is no increase in the incidence of congenital abnormality or in the rate of abortion when immunization and vaccination have been performed during pregnancy.

Drugs

Drugs in pregnancy are discussed in Chapter 14. Generally, all drugs should be avoided during pregnancy except those that have been specifically permitted by your doctor or midwife. Tablets for nausea or early morning sickness will be prescribed if you are suffering to such an extent that you require treatment. Alkalis may be taken for indigestion; codeine or paracetamol for any headache or other aches and pains.

If you are contemplating pregnancy and are taking any drugs, tranquillizers or sleeping tablets, it is wise to ask your doctor about them before the onset of your pregnancy. If you are already pregnant, you should tell him, or the doctor at the antenatal clinic, as soon as possible. Thereafter you should not take any drugs unless they have been prescribed either by your doctor or by the antenatal clinic.

12 Minor Complaints in Pregnancy

Most pregnant women suffer at times from a number of very minor complaints. The majority of these are not significant but an occasional symptom may be of importance. This chapter sets out a list of these minor complaints or occasional complications, their appropriate treatment and when medical advice should be sought. It may appear unduly long, so that some people will assume there is a vast multitude of minor complications and complaints during pregnancy, but it is as well to state at the beginning that the majority of symptoms and complaints listed here are in fact of no real significance. Complaints such as headache, stuffy nose, constipation, tiredness or backache occur equally in the non-pregnant, but in pregnancy their very presence may cause worry and anxiety. It is hoped that after reading these pages the expectant mother will feel reassured about insignificant symptoms and will also appreciate warning complaints and seek medical advice for the necessary treatment.

Horror stories have no place in modern maternity care. Pregnant women are often assailed by stories, which are frequently grossly exaggerated, from their supposed friends, well-wishers and relations, about some of the complications, symptoms and complaints of pregnancy. Some of these conditions are mentioned in this chapter and it is hoped that by referring to them the pregnant woman will be reassured of their significance or lack of importance.

In this book importance has been given to a long list of minor complaints, whereas very little is said about such things as prolonged labour and difficult deliveries. This is because these latter complications are now comparative rarities and attention has been directed to, and will be increasingly focused upon, those minor complaints or ailments of pregnancy which make the life of the pregnant woman less comfortable and happy than it might otherwise be.

Inevitably there is some overlap between different sections (or even chapters), especially when discussing such common symptoms as headache and nausea. Repetition cannot be avoided if a reasonable explanation is to be given about symptoms that might occur at any stage during pregnancy or after delivery.

Nausea

Nausea in early pregnancy is an almost universal symptom. The degree of nausea varies not only from woman to woman but also from pregnancy to pregnancy in the same woman. It is most common in the morning, but may occur at any time of day and may even last throughout the day. Sickness may ensue if the nausea becomes severe. Pregnant women are seldom worried by either nausea or sickness at night, although if they get out of bed suddenly they may suffer these symptoms.

The exact cause is not known and is probably a combination of several factors:

1 Hormone changes in early pregnancy undoubtedly exert an influence upon the metabolism of the body and probably predispose to both nausea and sickness.
2 The metabolic and chemical changes which take place in early pregnancy probably also predispose to nausea.
3 The hormones which exert their major effect during the early part of pregnancy are formed mainly from the corpus luteum in the ovary and at about the 12th to the 14th week of pregnancy the production of these hormones is taken over by the placenta. There may be a slight difference in the exact nature of the hormones so produced, but this has not yet been detected.
4 During early pregnancy progesterone causes relaxation of involuntary muscle and thus dilatation of the blood vessels resulting in a fall in blood pressure. It is common for a fall in blood pressure to make people feel faint and occasionally nauseated, and this may be an additional factor.

Psychological factors. It has long been considered that psychological factors are a very potent cause of both nausea and vomiting in pregnancy but it is extremely difficult to pinpoint the exact part they play. Some of the most well balanced and stable women complain of extreme nausea and almost continuous vomiting, while in others the psychological element plays a large part. Anxiety, fear, worry, apprehension, all have an important effect, and one only has to consider the plight of the unmarried girl with an unwanted pregnancy, afraid to discuss it with her parents or friends, to appreciate the psychological problems which may exert themselves during the early stages of pregnancy.

Nausea is one of the earliest symptoms of pregnancy. The sensation of nausea or feeling of sickness takes many slightly different forms not only in different women but also in the same woman during different times of the day or different stages of pregnancy. It may be a simple sensation of fullness in the upper abdomen, or so severe as to come in repeated waves, each one associated with the desire to vomit.

Nausea results in several other minor side effects. There is usually a reduction or loss of appetite accompanied by some weight loss during the first three months of pregnancy. The amount lost depends upon the severity of the nausea.

Some types of nausea are associated with the desire to eat whereas others are associated with a marked objection to food. Even when hungry, a woman who is nauseated will usually find that a comparatively small amount of food will satisfy her hunger and she will sit down to quite a large plate of food and find she can only manage to eat a small amount because of the fairly rapid onset of a sensation of fullness. Some women find that eating a small amount of food actually relieves nausea, whereas others are relieved only by self-induced vomiting, such as by tickling their throat.

Nausea is often aggravated by fatty foods or the smell of fat, especially cooking fat, and these should be avoided.

Other factors that specifically create nausea vary from person to person as well as from pregnancy to pregnancy, but smoking and tobacco smoke are classic examples. Strangely enough, coffee is frequently accused and many women will 'go off' all types of alcohol in early pregnancy.

The symptoms, therefore, of 'nausea' vary from a vague sensation of loss of appetite to an almost paralysing feeling of abdominal discomfort and desire to vomit. The more severe the nausea, the more likely is vomiting to occur. There are no hard and fast rules for the onset of nausea or its progress but one simple consolation is the old adage 'the more the nausea, the better the pregnancy' and it is true that the more nausea you have the less likely are you to miscarry. The converse that a person with no nausea is likely to miscarry is certainly not true, but most obstetricians nevertheless like their patients to have some nausea and sickness during the first three months as it does indicate a more stable pregnancy.

Most pregnant women require no specific treatment for nausea other than simple reassurance that it is normal in early pregnancy and will usually disappear at the end of the 14th week. With these assurances they are quite happy to put up with the minor discomforts involved, and find that simple regulation of their diet and daily activities reduces its severity.

The effects of nausea and vomiting upon different women vary. Some accept nausea without complaint, while others complain bitterly. Similarly, vomiting elicits a very different response from different people. Some state that vomiting relieves their symptoms, while others complain bitterly of the discomforts of being sick. There is no simple remedy or cure, but minor changes in routine and diet help different women. Remember:

1 It is a normal phenomenon in early pregnancy.
2 The symptoms will go at about the 14th week.
3 Get up slowly and only after a small amount of tea and dry toast or tea and biscuit has been taken.
4 Take frequent small meals with a small quantity of liquid and drink between meals.

5 Avoid fats and fatty foods.
6 Avoid those things which cause nausea.
7 Avoid wearing very tight clothing.

If the nausea and vomiting persist beyond the 14th week, become excessive or recur later in pregnancy, you must inform your medical adviser.

Drugs of all types are avoided if possible during the first three months of pregnancy, but if nausea becomes severe then it can usually be controlled by an antihistamine drug. Most of these are perfectly safe and Avomine is the one that is most frequently used, but you should not take any of these unless they are specifically prescribed by your doctor. If you are given pills for your nausea, remember that the action of most of them lasts for up to about 12 hours, so that you should take a tablet at bedtime to control morning nausea, and a tablet in the morning to ease nausea in the evening. Some antihistamines make people feel sleepy so you should ask your doctor if you may drive while taking them.

Morning sickness

Morning sickness or vomiting is a classic symptom of early pregnancy and the majority of women probably vomit at least once at some stage during this time. Vomiting does not usually disturb every morning of early pregnancy. The term 'morning sickness' usually refers to the nausea that is common in early morning rather than to actual vomiting. Vomiting is not always confined to the early morning. It may occur at any time of the day or even throughout the day. Some women suffer from vomiting only in the evening.

Vomiting in early morning takes the form of retching because the stomach is empty and only a small quantity of mucus can be produced. Morning sickness may also be brought on by coughing or by the smell of cooking, especially cooking fatty foods, or by eating, especially food containing fat.

The action of vomiting is most uncomfortable and anyone who vomits several times in rapid succession may afterwards suffer from some residual soreness in the abdominal muscles. This will go after a few hours and is of no significance. Vomiting does not harm the baby or the pregnancy, although a person who vomits severely may feel as though she is pressing the whole pregnancy down and out of the pelvis. This never happens; vomiting itself is never a cause of prolapse.

Some women induce vomiting to relieve nausea, especially when it becomes severe.

There are no golden rules for the treatment of morning sickness as each woman is different and her symptoms will vary from day to day and week to week. The intelligent use of the basic principles for the treatment of nausea usually control most, if not all, of the actual sickness.

Occasionally, however, it may be necessary to give drugs, of which the antihistamines are the most useful and most frequently used. Some have been especially developed for use in early pregnancy, whereas others are not advised. Before taking any drugs you should consult your doctor and only take what he prescribes.

One of the secrets in the control of nausea in early pregnancy, and therefore the control of vomiting, is small frequent meals avoiding anything containing fat and any particular foods which cause nausea to the individual concerned. Two or three plain biscuits should be taken to the bedroom at night and placed in a tin beside the bed. These may be eaten at any time on waking during the night and in the morning before any attempt is made to get up, together with a cup of warm sweetened tea. Getting out of bed should be delayed for 15 or 20 minutes after this. About an hour after rising a light breakfast may be eaten consisting of a small quantity of cereal with sugar and a little milk, followed by boiled or poached egg with toast and marmalade, marmite or honey, but no butter. Tea or coffee should not contain much milk. If severe nausea and vomiting persist a light meal or small snack should be taken approximately every two hours throughout the day consisting of unbuttered toast or biscuits, together with whatever fluid is considered least likely to provoke vomiting. Clear soups and Bovril may be drunk as beverages. Butter and fatty foods should be avoided if possible. Milk, while being an extremely good food, is particularly liable to cause nausea and vomiting at this stage of pregnancy and should be avoided if it does. It is important to drink as much fluid as possible without causing vomiting and also to eat a reasonable quantity of sugar, or to add glucose or sugar to the fluids.

Most pregnant women lose weight in the first three months of pregnancy. This weight loss may be as much as 4 kg or even 7 kg. A 4 kg loss in a woman of average weight is of little importance (or 7 kg in a woman who is overweight). Weight loss in excess of this is usually associated with persistent vomiting and medical advice should be sought. The nausea and vomiting should diminish between the 12th and 14th week of pregnancy and disappear after the end of the 14th week, after which weight will be regained rapidly. If the essential fluid intake and glucose or sugar intake are satisfactorily maintained in early pregnancy, the small weight loss is of no importance.

An example of a daily diet for a patient who is suffering from severe nausea, with or without some vomiting, is given below:

Before rising. Two dry biscuits or one slice of unbuttered toast together with a cup of warm tea containing sugar but little milk.

Breakfast (one hour after rising). Breakfast cereal with a small amount of milk and sugar. Unbuttered toast, biscuits or boiled or poached egg. Tea or coffee with sugar and a small amount of milk.

Mid-morning. Milk or Bovril together with toast or biscuits.

Lunch. Soup. Boiled chicken or steamed fish. Purée vegetables. Fresh fruit or stewed fruit with a little sugar. Orange juice, lemon juice or water.

Mid-afternoon. Tea, coffee or orange juice, together with sweet biscuit or sponge cake.

Tea-time. Unbuttered toast, sweet biscuits, sponge cake, tea or coffee with little sugar, or any other form of beverage which does not contain much milk.

Supper. Meat, fish or eggs which have not been fried, together with boiled vegetables or fresh salad. This may be followed by fresh or stewed fruit and the meal may be finished by biscuit and tea or coffee.

Late evening. Biscuit with unbuttered toast together with a glass of fluid, preferably plain water.

It is often found that iced foods and particularly drinks are less nauseating than warm ones.

Many women are fortunate enough not to experience any nausea or vomiting in early pregnancy, while others feel only occasional nausea. It is only the unfortunate few who experience severe nausea or recurrent vomiting. Even those with severe nausea find that the nausea is worse at different times of the day and that some days are particularly worse than others. It is noticeable that any stress, strain or difficulties will tend to make the nausea or vomiting worse, and it is characteristic of some pregnancies that the symptoms become more severe in the evening while rarely present in the morning. The reason for this is unknown and it is untrue to suggest that it is to impress the husband or partner when he returns home from the day's work! There was always stated to be quite a marked psychological factor in the causation of nausea and vomiting. This is probably not true. The most sensible people can suffer from severe nausea and vomiting which will not respond to psychiatric treatment or to psychiatric drugs.

There is very longstanding and extremely good advice that the more a woman has to do in pregnancy the less will she be aware of her nausea and vomiting. It is true that women with the most severe nausea and vomiting are frequently those who have the least to keep them occupied and it is, therefore, most important to keep busy either at work or in the house, encouraged by the knowledge that these symptoms will disappear at the end of the third month of pregnancy.

Do not indulge in self-pity. Do not upset yourself by cooking fatty meals or fried food for the rest of the family, who for a while will have to live on a simple and plain diet and put up with it. A limited amount of exercise, especially outside, is extremely good, but violent exercise usually provokes a further bout of nausea and possibly vomiting.

Excess vomiting (hyperemesis)

Occasionally a woman vomits with extreme severity, and any person who vomits several times a day should notify her doctor. Severe vomiting in early pregnancy may require hospital treatment for a few days because the body cannot obtain enough sugar for its daily needs and it then starts to make special acids known as ketones. Their presence in urine is usually an indication that the vomiting is particularly severe and is sufficient indication for admission to hospital. Immediately on admission to hospital most women are given only fluids by mouth, usually sweetened with sugar or glucose. If they continue to vomit on this strict regime, glucose and other fluids will be fed directly into the circulation via a vein in the arm and they will be given nothing by mouth until all vomiting and nausea cease. With this very strict regime the symptoms will rapidly disappear. The patient who is placed on an intravenous infusion is usually given only sips of water by mouth until such time as she feels hungry. She is then allowed very small quantities (30 to 60 g) of fluid each hour by mouth. If vomiting does not recur the amount of fluid is gradually increased until eventually she can take a light diet. The intravenous infusion is then discontinued.

Only a small and ever decreasing number of pregnant women suffer in this way and are admitted to hospital for treatment. Severe vomiting is not an indication for medical termination of pregnancy except in very rare instances. It used to be a common means whereby a woman with an unwanted pregnancy tried to obtain an abortion, and as soon as she was convinced that the pregnancy would not be medically terminated the sickness would cease quite quickly. With modern drugs and intravenous drip therapy there is no reason to terminate any pregnancy for severe nausea and vomiting in the absence of any other disease.

While there may occasionally be a large psychological factor in the causation of hyperemesis in early pregnancy, the assistance of psychiatrists in the treatment of this condition has not been as helpful as anticipated, and their help is usually sought only for the treatment of previously existing psychiatric disorders. The family doctor is often far better able to understand the stresses and strains which may accentuate ordinary nausea and sickness into excessive vomiting.

You should inform your doctor if vomiting does not cease soon after the 14th week or if it recurs later in pregnancy.

Heartburn

Heartburn is not to be confused with simple indigestion. It is a searing, burning sensation felt in the lower part of the chest just beneath the breast bone, and is frequently associated with bringing up or regurgitating small quantities of very sour acid fluid.

This symptom may occur normally in many women, especially those suffering from gastric or duodenal ulcer, but it is common during pregnancy and does not indicate any ulceration of either the stomach or the duodenum, or anything to do with the heart or the lungs. During pregnancy the effect of progesterone relaxes the valve at the upper end of the stomach which allows regurgitation of the normal acid contents of the stomach into the lower end of the oesophagus or food pipe which leads from the mouth to the stomach. This tube is not normally resistant to acid and constant regurgitations of acid causes severe inflammation in its lower end, and further regurgitation of acid upon this inflamed area results in the sensation of heartburn.

The enlarging uterus also tends to push against the stomach, which tends to cause further regurgitation. In addition, it pushes out the lower ribs, to which the diaphragm is attached, and this has the effect of slightly opening the aperture through which the oesophagus passes into the stomach, enabling regurgitation to occur more easily. In order to try and relieve this burning sensation some people swallow air (aerophagy) and then belch it up again. This only makes the symptoms worse, because the air brings up still more acid with it which further irritates the oesophagus.

In the non-pregnant state the contents of the stomach are not allowed to enter the lower end of the oesophagus, except when there is a defect at the place at which the oesophagus passes through the diaphragm into the stomach. This defect is known as hiatus hernia. During pregnancy any woman who suffers from a hiatus hernia is likely to have an exacerbation of symptoms, particularly heartburn.

Towards the end of pregnancy, if there is excessive pressure applied to the lower ribs, heartburn may become particularly severe. This may be noticeable in women who suffer from hydramnios, which is an excessive quantity of fluid, or have a multiple pregnancy. It is also particularly noticeable in women who have breech presentation and will often be relieved when the presentation is corrected.

If heartburn becomes a constant or serious problem you should notify your doctor. Since most of the causes of heartburn are dependent on the pregnancy itself it is difficult to treat. Part of the cause is the acidity of the stomach contents, so if this can be neutralized by an alkali the pain should be partially or totally relieved, while the other cause is the regurgitation of stomach contents into the oesophagus. Both aspects should be treated.

Swallowing large quantities of strong alkaline mixture to correct the gastric acidity will, however, only relieve the symptoms for a short time and in the end succeeds in making them worse because the stomach reacts to the administration of alkali by producing even more acid. The correct treatment is to take a small quantity of alkali to neutralize the stomach contents and then to suck an alkali tablet so that there is a constant stream of dilute alkali passing down the oesophagus. This will immediately neutralize any regurgitation of gastric contents and thus give the oesophagus time to heal. Once the inflammation has subsided the heartburn will cease. Any of the well-known alkali tablets are satisfactory for this purpose. A quarter of the tablet should be bitten off, chewed and swallowed, and the rest pushed between the cheek and gum where it can dissolve slowly over the next three to four hours.

Milk of Magnesia is also very effective in relieving heartburn. Another very effective method is to give a mixture of aluminium hydroxide gel and magnesium hydroxide (Mucaine). These substances form a film over the lower part of the oesophagus which is impenetrable by the gastric acid, thus allowing time for the inflammation to subside.

Spicy foods should be avoided and small meals should be taken. Large meals just before retiring to bed should be especially avoided. Heartburn is also associated with extra weight gain or an excess intake of carbohydrate and these factors should be checked.

At night when relaxed and lying flat in bed, heartburn may be particularly severe. A simple remedy is to raise the head of the bed, or to sleep with three or four pillows instead of the usual one or two. This prevents slow regurgitation of gastric fluids during the night and will frequently relieve the nocturnal heartburn. Any activity or position that tends to allow regurgitation of stomach contents up into the oesophagus must be avoided, such as lying flat, or especially lying with the head down or bending with the head below the chest (playing with a young child on the floor).

Ptyalism or excess salivation

Ptyalism is a rare complication of pregnancy and is caused by an apparently excessive amount of secretion of the salivary glands into the mouth. It is often accompanied by an offensive taste. This is a most annoying complication of pregnancy and is extremely distressing for those women who suffer from it. The excess salivation floods the mouth and becomes so profuse that the woman is unable to swallow it and is forced to spit out a large quantity, usually into a handkerchief which she carries and which may become absolutely sodden with saliva within twenty to thirty minutes.

The amount of saliva produced during 24 hours by a normal person (and a normal pregnant woman) is about 1.5 litres. Swallowing such a large quantity of saliva is done unconsciously like breathing or blinking. Ptyalism varies in its severity but it is easy to imagine the distress of someone who is constantly dribbling anything up to 1 or even 1.5 litres of saliva in 24 hours.

It is now accepted that this condition is not, in fact, caused by any excess production of saliva but is the result of a hysterical inability to swallow the normal amount of saliva being produced. Ptyalism is very difficult to treat and almost impossible to cure. The only real chance of cure is to discover why the woman has developed this psychosomatic symptom. Attempts to reduce the amount of saliva produced, by the administration of atropine and similar agents, will most certainly fail to relieve the symptom, because even a slight reduction in the amount of saliva produced will not affect the apparent inability to swallow fluid within the mouth. The condition may improve as pregnancy advances, but usually persists until delivery when it is spontaneously relieved. Fortunately ptyalism is becoming less common and is now a rare complication of pregnancy.

Frequency of micturition

Increased frequency of micturition is one of the earlier symptoms of pregnancy and may, in certain circumstances, persist quite normally until delivery. Most pregnant women will become aware of this when they have to get up at night to pass urine and on reflection will also be aware of an increase in urinary frequency during the day. The frequency may be caused by the vascular congestion around the bladder neck which is being compressed by the uterus enlarging in the pelvis. There is no recognizable way of improving or reducing the day frequency. The night frequency may occasionally be helped by reducing the amount of fluid drunk after 8.0 p.m. Most women, however, only get up once during the night and do not consider this one disturbance justifies reducing their fluid intake.

Later in pregnancy a urinary tract infection may cause increased frequency and some urgency to pass urine, or actual pain before, during or after the act of passing water. If frequency of micturition is associated with pain, burning, or the passage of blood then an infection of the bladder or urinary tract is likely and medical advice should be sought. Certain antibiotics may be used safely.

As pregnancy advances beyond the 30th week the baby's head is either becoming engaged in the pelvis or sitting in the pelvic brim. In either of these positions it irritates the bladder and may result in a marked increase in urinary frequency which is not associated with any pain, discomfort, or burning. The frequency may reach disturbing proportions such as once every two hours, or even once every hour, but providing there is no pain it is unlikely that any infection is present. There is no specific treatment for frequency when it is caused by the pressure of the head upon the bladder.

Right at the end of pregnancy, when the fetal head is engaged in the pelvis, frequency of micturition may recur. At this stage there is no room in the pelvis for the bladder as well as the baby's head, and the bladder is pushed up into the abdomen where, as it fills, a swelling is seen in the lower abdomen. Again there is no treatment for frequency at this stage of pregnancy. However, if a urinary tract infection is suspected medical advice should be sought, as its treatment at this stage of pregnancy is of paramount importance.

Urgency of micturition

During the last 6 or 8 weeks of pregnancy the baby's head or feet may bounce against the bladder causing a sensation of the utmost urgency to pass urine. This is only an occasional problem but can be most disturbing and disconcerting.

Stress incontinence

This is the term used for the lack of control, or weakness, of the bladder. Very often during the later weeks of pregnancy the control of the bladder becomes increasingly difficult and occasionally small amounts of urine may escape when they are not intended to do so. This may sometimes happen if the baby gives the bladder a powerful kick, or as a result of the mother coughing, sneezing, straining, lifting or carrying—in other words when anything raises the pressure in the abdomen.

Difficulty in control of micturition

Some difficulty in control of micturition may occasionally be noticed after delivery and especially if the labour has been long or the delivery difficult. Postnatal exercises, especially pelvic floor exercises, will soon overcome this and the bladder will rapidly return to normal.

Constipation

The woman who goes to the lavatory every day does not necessarily empty her bowel completely or satisfactorily. A normal stool is soft and well formed and is passed easily without straining or undue discomfort. A tendency to constipation develops very early during pregnancy because the hormone progesterone causes relaxation of the intestine, therefore reducing its power to propel its contents towards the rectum and the anus. Hence, the intestine tends to dilate and constipation ensues. The onset of constipation is usually the result of habit. Women who for years have failed to obey the call to defecate when the rectum is loaded and ready to be emptied have gradually ceased to appreciate the sensation of the desire to defecate. In due time, therefore, the rectum becomes distended with faeces but the owner receives no signal that the rectum requires emptying. Faeces which are kept in the lower part of the intestinal tract for an indefinite period become hard and inspissated, so that great strain and energy are required to pass them. This vicious cycle must be broken, and it can be broken relatively easily by obeying a few simple rules and regulations.

Firstly, the bowels must be opened every day. Secondly, every call to defecate must be obeyed, no matter how inconvenient it may be. Thirdly, an adequate fluid intake is essential. At least 2 litres of fluid should be drunk each day. The majority of pregnant women fail to drink a sufficient quantity of fluid. Fourthly, a reasonable amount of roughage, fresh vegetables and raw, fresh fruit, should be eaten each day. If these simple rules are obeyed, most pregnant women will be relieved of their constipation.

If aperients are required they should be prescribed by the doctor. The correct amount of any aperient is that amount which will enable the bowels to be opened normally each day. Never take too large a dose which will result in attacks of diarrhoea, inevitably followed by two or three days of constipation whilst the intestine refills, and this is again inevitably followed by the administration of a violent purgative and a further bout of diarrhoea. Strong purgation also predisposes to abortion.

Some iron tablets may cause constipation and if this happens it should be discussed with your doctor with a view to changing to another variety which does not disturb the bowel.

Flatulence

Flatulence is a common complaint especially in early pregnancy and is usually caused by the swallowing of air (aerophagy) to relieve the nausea so common in the first three months of pregnancy. Flatulence and gas distension of the intestine may result in a feeling of distension and also a frequent desire to pass flatus. It is also possible that the constipation so often present during pregnancy is a further factor in producing flatulence. A very mild purgative, such as Milk of Magnesia, which encourages intestinal movement may help, not only in the dispersal of the wind but also in discouraging its further formation within the intestine. Women who suffer from flatulence should avoid gas-producing foods such as onions, beans, peas, carbohydrate and heavily fried foods. By learning not to swallow air the gaseous distension of the abdomen will frequently be alleviated.

In later pregnancy flatulence may be associated with heartburn, where aerophagy is a common reaction to the pain.

Vaginal discharge

Vaginal discharge may occur throughout pregnancy as a result of increased blood supply to the vagina and cervix. The term discharge is intended to mean the passage from the vagina of a simple clear mucoid or white discharge without any soreness, pain or irritation. This occurs normally during pregnancy and may also occur at puberty, at the time of ovulation, for a few days before or immediately after a period, as a result of sexual excitement, and in some women while taking contraceptive pills. Apart from these circumstances it should always be examined, in particular during pregnancy, especially if it becomes offensive, causes irritation or soreness. At some stage of pregnancy more than 50 per cent of women develop a so-called 'erosion' or ulcer on the cervix. This is a result of the rapid rise in hormone levels during the early stages of pregnancy and such an erosion increases the amount of vaginal discharge that may already be present, but it should be clear and mucoid causing no other symptoms.

Occasionally the discharge becomes yellowish and smelly and this is nearly always because the cervical erosion has become infected, although it may mean the vagina is infected while the cervix is quite healthy. The discharge will almost certainly then become more profuse and cause soreness in the vulva. If this happens you should report it when you next visit the clinic so that it can be treated.

A cervical erosion usually heals spontaneously within a few weeks of delivery; if it does not, the discharge will continue and special treatment will be required to cure it.

Vaginal irritation

Vaginal irritation is nearly always associated with irritation of the vulva. A very mild discomfort may occur in the early stages of pregnancy as a result of pelvic congestion, but this is barely noticeable and always transient. It is otherwise caused by a vaginal infection or an infection of a cervical erosion. Such infections are caused by ordinary bacteria that may similarly infect the skin or throat. They are not dangerous and will not cause any damage to your baby or harm to yourself. They are just very annoying. The irritation is caused by inflammation set up by the infection; the discharge will be yellow and offensive.

An offensive and infected discharge should be reported when you next visit the clinic. The exact diagnosis may be doubtful and a small amount of the discharge will then be taken for culture in the laboratory. Inserting antibiotic pessaries or chemical cream into the vagina at night will cure the infection and relieve the symptoms.

Thrush infection (monilia)

Pregnant women are very susceptible to this particular type of infection which frequently produces a distressing amount of irritation and soreness. It is easily and simply treated by using a fungicidal cream or pessaries. If you have had a thrush infection during pregnancy, keep a reserve of fungicidal cream or pessaries since the infection has a habit of recurring later in the pregnancy for no apparent reason

Trichomonas vaginitis

Trichomonas vaginalis infection may also produce very severe irritation and soreness, but can be cured quite easily with appropriate treatment.

Tiredness in pregnancy

Tiredness, weakness and lassitude are normal symptoms in early pregnancy and are nature's way of slowing down the pregnant woman to help preserve the pregnancy. From a purely biological point of view it seems obvious that the more a pregnant woman can rest in early pregnancy the better chance does the pregnancy have of surviving, and a sensation of tiredness or lassitude can be accepted as a natural phenomenon. It is quite wrong to fight against it. You do much better to give in gracefully and to take more rest. It will nearly always be found that one or two hours' rest in the afternoon and an extra hour or two's rest at night will suffice.

Women who are having their third child frequently complain of feeling more tired and lethargic than they did with their first one or two. This is not surprising since they now have one or two children to look after, whereas with their first pregnancy they did not have this demanding task to face as well as a pregnancy itself.

It really is most important that your husband or partner and other members of the family should realize that tiredness, weakness and lassitude are a normal part of pregnancy. They are usually more severe in the first three months and your husband or partner must understand that this, together with a certain amount of nausea, may stop you from being the energetic individual that he is accustomed to. He may have to cancel appointments or social engagements, but this is immaterial. Rest is essential. If you do not rest then you will become depressed and bad tempered, and quite honestly it just is not worth it.

Extra rest does not necessarily mean sleep. If you are working and are unable to rest in the afternoon, you should try to get at least 10 hours in bed at night, even though this does not mean 10 hours' sleep.

Most of the tiredness and lassitude will go at the end of the 14th week and, with the return of some of your former energy, you will feel much happier. Tiredness may again return towards the end of pregnancy, when it is only natural.

Shortness of breath

Many pregnant women complain of intermittent shortness of breath at all stages of pregnancy, but it is more common towards the end when the enlarging uterus pushes the abdominal contents upwards underneath the ribs. The diaphragm is thus forced up into the chest. This incursion upon what is really the thoracic cage means that the diaphragm cannot descend as far as usual and, therefore, the respiratory movement of the chest becomes less efficient. This causes inefficient breathing and shortness of breath on the slightest exertion may easily occur. It should not be sufficient to incapacitate a person during normal day-to-day living and if it becomes noticeable while walking gently on the flat or after climbing one flight of stairs, you should tell the physician or midwife when you next visit the antenatal clinic.

Shortness of breath may occur at night while lying fairly flat in bed and can usually be relieved by propping the head and shoulders up on two or three pillows which reduces the pressure of the enlarging uterus on the diaphragm.

Women having their first baby usually notice 'lightening' at, or about, the 36th week and this is the result of the baby's head descending into the bony pelvis, causing the upper part, or fundus, of the uterus to descend anything up to 5 or even 7.5 cm. The consequent reduction of pressure on the diaphragm allows it to descend further and thus increase its efficiency. Shortness of breath which is present before the head engages may easily be relieved when this happens.

If shortness of breath is sudden, or associated with any upper respiratory tract infection, cold, fever or bronchitis (or even with a severe cough) you should notify your doctor as soon as possible.

Fainting

Most women feel faint on some occasion during early pregnancy and a few may actually faint. The feeling of faintness results from the lowering of the blood pressure which is due to two main factors. Firstly, the effect of progesterone which dilates the smooth muscle of the blood vessels and therefore predisposes to pooling of blood in the lower parts of the body, and, secondly, the sudden and rapid demands of the uterus for an increased blood supply. If the blood pressure falls below a certain level the blood supply to the brain is reduced, causing faintness. When people faint they fall to the ground, so that their brain is once more on a level with their heart instead of being several inches above it and the blood supply is automatically restored.

Faintness or fainting is particularly noticeable during the first three months of pregnancy when the blood pressure is lowered beneath its normal level and is likely to fall even further if blood is allowed to 'pool' in the legs during prolonged standing such as in bus or shopping queues. It can be prevented by not standing still for any length of time or, if it is necessary, by moving and exercising the feet and legs to ensure the return of blood from the legs to the heart.

Fainting is especially likely to occur when suddenly standing from a sitting position because the automatic reflexes of the body which adjust the blood pressure to the sudden changes of posture are rather slow to react, and the brain has a temporary lack of blood.

The actual feeling of faintness is not harmful and recovery is rapid, nor does fainting itself harm either the baby or the mother, although she may injure herself when she falls to the ground. Injuries, however, are rarely serious, unless a woman falls on some sharp or hard object. A pregnant woman should practise her immediate reaction to a sensation of faintness. Immediately she begins to feel light-headed she should sit down if she has been standing, or lie down if she has been sitting. She should immediately take several deep breaths as rapidly as possible. This movement of the chest will help the return of blood to the heart and the blood pressure will rapidly return to normal. The old-fashioned precaution that a pregnant woman should carry a bottle of smelling salts in her handbag is extremely good, but taking several deep breaths has the same effect as inhaling smelling salts.

Most pregnant women rapidly appreciate the conditions which make them feel faint and avoid such situations. The classical example is a young woman, eight weeks pregnant, who, not having eaten any breakfast, leaves home to stand for five minutes in a bus queue.

Backache

Backache is a very common symptom throughout pregnancy. It is explained very easily on theoretical grounds. The placenta produces the hormone progesterone which causes softening and eventual stretching of the tendons and ligaments in the body. This is most important in the pelvic joints, but the hormone also acts upon the spine, causing relaxation of the ligaments supporting the spinal column. The characteristic posture adopted by most women in pregnancy places a considerable strain on the lower joints of the spine, especially the one between the spine and the pelvis. The relaxation of the ligaments results in excessive mobility of this joint and strain upon the surrounding structures with the resulting aching discomfort. This is made worse by bad posture or by excessive exercise, either of which alone may cause backache. Backache may also be increased by an excessive gain in weight, repeated changing from high to low heels, or previous injury or damage to the back.

The most important aspect of the treatment for backache is preventive.

Correct posture is essential; this may be attained by pressing the whole length of the spine against a flat wall and trying to maintain that posture. Adequate rest, especially during the last three months of pregnancy, is of immense importance. Some people prescribe supporting corsets for the back, but unless there is any underlying disease of the spine it is unlikely that they are of anything but temporary value. Massage and application of heat in the form of an electric pad, or radiant heat may also give some relief. The application of liniments is no more beneficial than the massage used to rub them in.

Very occasionally backache is associated with damage to an intervertebral disc. Prolapse of an intervertebral disc is an organic disease of the back and can cause backache, sciatica or lumbago in the non-pregnant state. When this occurs in pregnancy the symptoms may become very severe. Any woman who has a predisposition to lumbago or has had a slipped intervertebral disc must be extremely careful during her pregnancy to avoid excessive weight gain or back strain. In the event of true lumbago she should go to bed and rest there until medical advice has been sought. Occasionally the pain involves the sciatic nerve and travels through the centre of the buttock, down the back of the leg behind the knee and even as far as the ankle. This sort of irritation of the sciatic nerve nearly always indicates some pressure is present and that the nerve is being distorted or inflamed and medical advice should be sought. The usual treatment of this is complete bed rest, lying flat upon a hard, rigid bed or on an ordinary mattress with fracture boards underneath. If boards are not available the top mattress can be placed on the floor.

Sacro-iliac pain

Sacro-iliac pain is a classical low backache of pregnancy. The pain occurs in the sacro-iliac joint which is at the top of the buttocks about 3 in from the mid-line and extends downwards into the buttock itself. The pain of sacro-iliac strain is usually located exactly over the joint and is quite distinctive, whereas that of low backache or a slipped intervertebral disc is generally in the mid-line. In sacro-iliac strain there is usually a single area of maximum pain and pressure upon this area can be extremely painful whereas sciatic pain is usually along the distribution of the sciatic nerve. Generally, sacro-iliac strain produces an intense local pain which may become worse on rotary movements of the spine upon the pelvis, as turning over sideways in bed, which tend to open and close the joint. This condition can be quite crippling and may easily prevent satisfactory walking. It may cause a very pronounced limp and may be so severe as to make life absolutely miserable.

The usual treatment is manipulation. It is usually accompanied by many creaks and cracks which are caused by the breaking down of tiny adhesions within the joint, thus resulting in a much more mobile joint which by

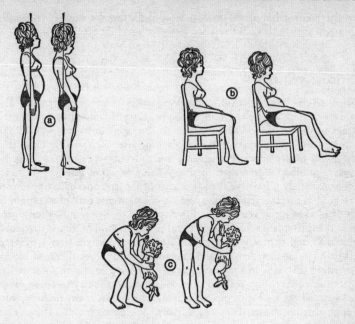

Fig 20   Posture during pregnancy

virtue of its mobility is no longer painful, although complete relief may not be felt for two or three days. The results can be quite dramatic, and the gratitude of someone who has been relieved of severe sacro-iliac pain has to be seen to be believed.

Everyone agrees that bad posture causes backache, but good posture is very difficult to achieve and almost impossible to maintain all the time. The main problem of posture in pregnancy is the obvious effort in maintaining a good upright posture in early pregnancy if you are feeling nauseated, tired and somewhat miserable, and in late pregnancy when you have a large abdomen sticking out in front. It is so much easier just to relax and let it stick out. However, good posture must be maintained both in early and in late pregnancy. The great secret is to stand as upright as possible holding the abdomen and buttocks in and pushing the chest out as shown in fig. 20. Lounging or slouching in chairs is just as bad for your back as standing badly

Excess weight gain

Excess weight gain obviously places undue strain on the back and will eventually result not only in bad posture but also in backache. The importance of control of weight gain in pregnancy cannot be too forcefully repeated.

Varicose veins

Varicose veins may develop in the legs at any stage of pregnancy. The veins in the leg, as elsewhere in the body, carry the blood back from the tissues to the heart, whence it is sent to the lungs to be oxygenated and then sent once again to the body through the arteries. Veins are fairly thin tubes with muscular walls which are normally capable of controlling the pressure of blood within their lumen. When a person is standing the heart is approximately 4 ft above the lower part of the leg and a head of pressure may build up in the veins of the legs. A constant pressure of a column of 4 ft of blood on the veins in the lower part of the leg would after a time cause them to dilate, distend and become distorted. The veins, therefore, contain a number of valves which are situated at approximately 6 in intervals throughout their length, and effectively divide the column of blood, preventing the veins in the lower part of the leg from being subjected to a pressure equal to the column of blood rising to the heart. These valves are small, elliptical-shaped pieces of tissue which close if any back pressure is applied from above. They are in pairs, one on each side of the vessel and they meet in the middle. If the veins dilate at the site of the valve, the valve cusps will fail to meet and blood will be allowed to pass back. When this happens the valve is said to be incompetent and pressure from above will be transmitted through the valve to the area of vein beneath. This will increase the pressure in this particular area and will place an undue strain upon its muscular wall. If this strain becomes too great the muscle in the wall of the vein becomes tired and allows the vein wall to dilate and stretch. The vessel will, therefore, become not only wider but also longer than normal and this distended tortuous vein is known as a varicose vein.

So long, therefore, as the valves in the vein remain satisfactory and competent it is unlikely that a vein will become varicose. The hormone progesterone causes smooth muscle to relax and this includes the muscle of the vein walls which will then dilate. If this occurs at the site of a valve it will become incompetent and lead to varicosity. Standing for long periods also predisposes to varicose veins in the legs.

As pregnancy advances and the uterus increases in size it presses on the veins in the pelvis, tending to create an obstruction to the flow of blood from the legs to the heart and thus increasing the pressure within the veins of the legs. The last factor frequently causes eventual breakdown of the valvular system in the superficial veins of the legs and the formation of varicosities.

Excess weight gain is an important factor in causing veins to dilate

There is also a hereditary factor in the formation of varicose veins which may be transmitted by either the mother or the father. Any woman with a predisposition to varicose veins is more likely to suffer from them during pregnancy. Once varicosity has commenced in the veins of the lower limbs it becomes a progressive condition which deteriorates gradually during pregnancy.

Varicose veins are unlikely to form during the first pregnancy, or if they do they only appear in the pregnancy to a mild extent. They improve after delivery since the obstruction due to the enlarged uterus is removed, the progesterone level is no longer high and the weight is reduced; the improvement will usually continue for up to six months. They become gradually more severe with each successive pregnancy and, as their severity increases, so does their perseverance between pregnancies. While mild varicose veins may regress completely after the end of pregnancy, severe varicose veins will only partially regress so that their treatment by either injection or surgery becomes necessary. The first veins to be involved are usually those on the inside and back of the calf, and frequently the right leg is affected earlier and more extensively than the left. They may also start above the knee on the inside of the thigh. Severe varicose veins in the legs are unusual before the end of a third pregnancy and many women manage to get through four or even six pregnancies without any varicose veins appearing.

Occasionally varicose veins first appear as very small spidery networks in the skin itself. These are the superficial skin blood vessels known as capillaries. The affected veins themselves are distended, soft, turgid cords lying just beneath the skin. The bluish discoloration may show through the skin, but later this may be superseded by brown staining of the skin over the veins.

Varicose veins may be prevented or their development kept to a minimum by (1) avoiding excessive weight gain, (2) avoiding standing still, (3) avoiding crossing the legs, and (4) gentle exercise. Even when standing still the muscles of the legs should be gently contracted intermittently by rocking backwards and forwards on the feet, consciously pressing the knees backwards to extend the legs fully, flexing and contracting the toes, or by gentle movements of the feet. Any movement of the feet or toes which will contract the muscles both in front and behind the leg below the knee will assist the circulation of blood through the lower limbs.

It is essential to avoid wearing underwear with any form of elastic round the upper part of the legs, since this constricts the legs and slows down the venous return from the leg. Similarly tight abdominal underwear will restrict the blood flow from the lower limbs.

When sitting down it is always advisable to raise the feet on a stool, since this will assist the return of blood. The legs should not be crossed because this obstructs the main flow of blood behind the knee.

The symptoms of varicose veins are variable. A mild irritation of the skin overlying the varicosity may be the first indication that a vein is dilating. Many women complain about the unsightly blue or brown colour of the veins. In very severe instances the skin over the lower and inner part of the shin becomes thin and shiny and tends to lose its vitality. It subsequently becomes smooth and red and may eventually ulcerate to form a varicose ulcer. Such ulcers are rare and are usually a manifestation of very severe varicose veins which should have received treatment many years previously.

Dilated veins may cause swelling of the ankles and feet during pregnancy, even in the absence of any other factor. This is not usually severe but may cause some discomfort, especially towards the end of the day, and may also cause shoes to become tight after standing for any length of time.

A dull aching pain in the calf or shin may be caused by varicose veins. This pain is not usually severe but its very persistence may cause considerable annoyance. The discomfort is worse at the end of the day, although it may occur at any time, especially after prolonged standing or exercise.

Severe cramp in the calf of the leg may happen at night. This is thought to be due to calcium deficiency but it has not been proved. Day cramps may be associated with varicose veins.

Varicose veins cannot be cured nor can they be prevented completely during pregnancy. The advice given above will reduce their severity.

If varicose veins have already developed then extra care should be taken to ensure that they do not progress further. Elastic nylon stockings or tights provide support for the outer side of the superficial veins. They assist the venous return from the leg and go a long way towards preventing the veins becoming worse. Such elastic support must be worn all day and should preferably be put on before getting up in the morning or immediately after bathing. It is useless to wear them for just a few hours each day, or to wear them for all but one hour during the day, because during that hour the pressure upon the veins can cause further damage. Elastic support cannot cure varicose veins—all it may do is prevent their further deterioration.

Stockings or tights may be bought in various sizes and only the correct size should be worn. Elastic bandages may also be used to support the legs. These may be 7 or 10 cm wide and when applied should be wrapped once or twice round the foot in order to anchor the bandage before it is wrapped in a spiral fashion up the leg extending to at least 10 or 15 cm above the knee. The difficulty with applying elastic bandages is obtaining an even application so that the edges do not bite into the skin to form localized constrictions. These tight rings cause even worse varicosities below them instead of helping to prevent further dilatation. Special supporting elastic nylon stockings or tights are socially as well as medically acceptable. They should be washed each night. All they require is simple rinsing in a hand basin and they will hang dry overnight.

Varicose veins that persist after pregnancy can be completely removed by surgical operation.

Vulval varicose veins

Varicose veins occasionally form in the vulva during pregnancy, where they are usually to be found in the labia majora. They may cause quite severe aching and irritation during the later stages of pregnancy. Support for veins in the vulva is difficult and probably the easiest method is to wear tights or a pair of tight elastic pants (not constricting the top of the legs, however). The wearing of sanitary pads may also provide support, but is not recommended. Women with varicose veins of the vulva are often very afraid that these may burst and cause profuse haemorrhage, but this is almost impossible except occasionally during delivery. If one does happen to rupture, however, the bleeding can be easily controlled by pressing with the finger on the area of the rupture until medical aid is obtained. Vulval varicose veins usually disappear spontaneously after delivery but if they persist the treatment is by a simple surgical operation.

Piles

Piles, or haemorrhoids, are varicose veins in and around the rectum and anal canal. They are formed in much the same way as varicose veins in the legs, except that whereas in the legs there is pressure by virtue of the distance from the legs to the heart, in the rectum and anal canal pressure may be caused by constipation and straining. They frequently cause bleeding, especially when the bowels are opened.

Piles are caused by:

1 straining to empty the bowel, which may be the result of either constipation or uncontrolled diarrhoea;
2 progesterone, the hormone which relaxes the smooth muscle of all the blood vessels and to which the veins of the anal canal are no exception;
3 a previous history of constipation and straining which may have caused some varicose deformation of the veins prior to the onset of pregnancy and which during pregnancy will become much more marked and obvious;
4 the pressure of the baby's head in the pelvis during late pregnancy which may obstruct the veins and impair the return of blood from the pelvic organs;
5 a hereditary predisposition to the formation of haemorrhoids, although this might basically be a predisposition to constipation.

Pregnancy causes increased pressure within all the veins below the umbilicus and as the uterus enlarges this pressure on the large vein in the back of the abdomen which carries the blood back towards the heart is increased. The lining of the anal canal contains many veins which can enlarge and become varicose in the same way as the veins in the leg. The presence of hard and often bulky faeces, together with straining to pass them, helps to cause enlargement of the varicose veins in the anal canal.

If haemorrhoids become sufficiently large they will spread to include those veins at the margin of the entrance of the anus and if they become larger still they will actually protrude outside the anus. Protrusion occurs at first only momentarily with the passage of a motion, but later they may remain prolapsed after the bowels have been opened.

Bleeding from haemorrhoids may occur at any time during their formation but is more likely the larger they become. It may be slight and only noticeable immediately after the passage of a motion or occasionally become more severe and continue for several minutes. Rarely does bleeding continue for any length of time.

Local irritation around the anus is one of the commonest symptoms of early haemorrhoids. This becomes worse in the presence of constipation. Local soreness and even pain may be present especially when the bowels are open, but frequently occur during constipation as the result of pressure from a large mass of faeces upon the anal canal. When haemorrhoids protrude through the anus and become prolapsed they become intensely sore and very painful.

Occasionally a small thrombosis may occur in one of the piles protruding through the anal margin and this is known as a thrombosed prolapsed pile. The pile becomes swollen and extremely tender. It can be felt as a comparatively small, hard, rounded area just at the margin of the anus and is one of the most painful conditions that can happen during pregnancy. It is a self-limiting condition taking three days for the pain and tenderness to increase, followed by three days in which the symptoms remain fairly constant and then three days during which they disappear. A thrombosed prolapsed haemorrhoid can be sufficiently painful to prevent a person walking and is certainly very painful on sitting down.

Chronic constipation is the biggest factor in the formation of this uncomfortable, and sometimes painful, complication, and it is probably the constipation rather than any inherent hereditary factor which causes the formation of the piles. Constipation is dealt with on pages 186–7. The best treatment of piles is the routine prevention of constipation, before, during and after pregnancy. Slight rectal bleeding should be treated by diligent care of the bowels and avoidance of constipation. If rectal bleeding becomes more severe your doctor should be notified, for although it is difficult to treat piles satisfactorily during pregnancy, he should be aware of the condition and may prescribe some suppositories. Irritation and soreness, which are usually more noticeable at night, are best treated by the application of an ointment to the anal area after defecation and before going to bed.

If the piles actually prolapse and remain prolapsed after defecation they should be replaced as soon as possible. The haemorrhoids can be gently pushed back with the finger, although care must be taken that they are not damaged by the finger nail, and once they have been found to prolapse even more vigorous measures must be taken to ensure that constipation does not recur. If the piles cannot be replaced immediately they may be replaced after lying for a few minutes in a warm bath. If they prolapse again as soon as they have been replaced then the woman should go to bed and rest with the feet up for 30 to 60 minutes after the piles have been replaced. If piles need to be replaced after defecation your doctor should be notified.

The treatment of thrombosed prolapsed piles varies greatly. This intensely painful condition usually occurs during the last 6 or 8 weeks of pregnancy. The local application of Anusol or Proctosedyl ointment will help to alleviate the symptoms. It is often suggested that the local application of cold lead lotion or witch hazel, or some other compress, will help. They do certainly soothe the pain though they do not really help the natural history of the condition. Any further straining and constipation must be rigorously avoided. Your doctor may consider that it is necessary to remove the clot from the pile and this is done quite easily and painlessly after injecting a small amount of local anaesthetic. This results in a dramatic relief of symptoms, but is usually considered only worth performing if it can be done during the first two days that the pile has become thrombosed. The use of an anaesthetic ointment applied three or four times a day will often relieve some of the pain.

It is not usually considered wise to inject haemorrhoids during pregnancy, although some doctors do treat the more severely affected without any ill effect. Operative treatment is usually reserved for persistently prolapsed piles. Most doctors prefer to reserve both injection and operation until some time after the end of pregnancy and will usually persevere with conservative treatment if possible.

Minor degrees of haemorrhoids usually regress spontaneously after the end of pregnancy and require no treatment. It is wise, however, for any patient who has suffered from haemorrhoids in pregnancy to discuss this with her doctor afterwards because any residual haemorrhoids will become rapidly worse during a subsequent pregnancy and it is to her advantage to have them treated before her next pregnancy.

Intertrigo

Intertrigo is a red irritating skin rash where folds of skin are in close contact. It is seen most frequently underneath heavy and pendulous breasts and also in the groins. Intertrigo is more common in women who are overweight and especially in those who either do not wash sufficiently frequently or perspire excessively. It is caused by an excessive quantity of sweat which cannot evaporate because of the close contact of the skin surfaces. The skin first becomes soggy, then sore and inflamed, giving rise to a reddened, scaly irritating rash.

The easiest way to prevent this condition is to avoid putting on an excess amount of weight and to prevent the skin becoming wet and continuously soggy by excessive perspiration. If intertrigo develops it is treated by frequent bathing and washing of the affected areas and gently powdering with ordinary talcum powder. Care must be taken not to apply so much talcum powder that it becomes caked. If the irritation is annoying either calamine lotion or hydrocortisone ointment (on a doctor's prescription) can be applied twice daily.

Pigmentation

Breasts

Pigmentation of the nipples and the areola commences at about the 14th week of pregnancy. The amount and area of pigmentation vary from person to person, but is generally more obvious in women who have dark hair and less marked in women who have fair hair and skin. Women with red hair, who so frequently have very delicate skin, usually have very little pigmentation of both the nipple and the areola. In very dark people this pigmentation may spread beyond the areola on to the breast itself. This secondary areola usually appears about the 18th or 20th week of pregnancy. It may occasionally involve most of the skin over the breast. Pigmentation of the secondary areola will disappear very rapidly after delivery except in those women who have very dark colouring when it may remain for several weeks or even months.

Pigmentation on the primary areola tends to be of a more permanent nature. The nipple and the areola may become lighter very shortly after delivery but some brown pigmentation may become permanent in women who have had more than one child. Breast-feeding does not affect the permanence of this nipple and areola coloration.

The linea nigra

The linea nigra is the dark line which develops down the centre of the abdomen commencing at the 14th week of pregnancy. Similar to other areas of pigmentation in pregnancy, it is most noticeable in brunettes, less noticeable in fair-haired women and frequently absent in red-headed women. Except in those of the very fairest complexion, the linea nigra always accompanies pregnancy, and extends as a pigmented dark line of varying width up to 1 cm from the pubic hair to the umbilicus. The umbilicus itself flattens and pigments as pregnancy advances The linea nigra may extend above the umbilicus to the lower part of the rib cage.

The linea nigra has no special significance to either the mother or the unborn child. It cannot be washed or scrubbed away because it is caused by dark, or pigmented, cells within the substance of the skin itself. It begins to fade soon after delivery but may take several months to disappear completely. Occasionally the pigmentation in and around the umbilicus remains for several years.

Other areas of pigmentation

Any pigmented birthmark, mole or scar is likely to become darker during pregnancy. This applies particularly to freckles, which may also enlarge. This effect becomes even more obvious if they are exposed to the tanning effect of the sun. Any scar, particularly on the abdomen, which has been present for less than one year at the onset of pregnancy may undergo quite severe pigmentation.

The increase in the pigmentation and the number of freckles both on the face and the body will begin to disappear shortly after delivery, and the condition of the skin will return to normal within a few weeks. Occasionally larger moles or darker areas of pigmentation may persist for longer.

The butterfly mask of pregnancy

There is a characteristic area of pigmentation that occurs on the face in late pregnancy, especially if it has been exposed to the sun. It has a butterfly-shaped distribution where the pigmentation spreads from the nose over the cheeks like the wings of a butterfly. An area of pigmentation may also occur on the forehead. While the mask of pregnancy may sometimes be attractive, its characteristic blotchy and irregular colouring is more likely to annoy its owner.

It has no special significance. There are many old-fashioned stories concerning either its value or its disadvantage to its owner, but none of these have any medical or scientific basis.

Women should not bleach the mask of pregnancy. Such attempts usually result in more blotchiness, and as the surrounding skin is also bleached so the mask itself becomes even more obvious. The mask will begin to fade a few days after delivery and may disappear completely in three or four weeks. Occasionally, however, it persists for several months.

Stretch marks

Why do stretch marks occur? There are many erroneous theories about their origin but there are only two main reasons. The first is the amount of progesterone produced by the pregnant woman and the second, the amount of weight gain.

A large number of old-fashioned remedies are advised to prevent stretch marks, none of which are guaranteed to work. They range from eating certain special vegetables and herbs to massaging the abdomen with liniments and oils.

It is commonly thought that some women have a particular type of skin which possesses great elasticity and will therefore not form stretch marks, whilst others have skin which contains little or no elasticity and will develop stretch marks regardless of what they do to avoid them. This is erroneous.

Many girls at the time of puberty develop stretch marks on the breasts, buttocks and thighs, and occasionally on the upper arms. These are associated with the rapid production of hormones and a rapid weight gain at that time. The production of oestrogen and progesterone at puberty is usually associated with an increase of appetite, but they also cause better utilization of the food, so that it is more readily deposited as fat in the breasts and in the subcutaneous tissues of the buttocks and thighs. Stretch marks form if the skin is stretched beyond its normal elasticity. They are originally brightish red or livid and while they may lose their colour over several years, the scars never completely disappear. A similar process works during pregnancy when stretch marks occur on the breasts, especially in women who normally have small breasts that enlarge rapidly and dramatically with the onset of pregnancy. Nothing can be done to prevent these. They also appear later on the anterior abdominal wall. Stretch marks over the buttocks, legs and upper arms during pregnancy are always associated with gross increase in weight.

During what doctors might call a 'good pregnancy' a great deal of hormone may be produced which predisposes to fluid retention and a very rapid increase in weight. A woman does not know if she has a large amount of circulating hormone, but she does know that anything she eats 'turns to fat' and she must be particularly careful with her diet if she is to avoid excessive weight gain. A woman who gains only 9 kg throughout a pregnancy will almost certainly not develop stretch marks whereas a woman who gains 18 kg almost certainly will.

Oiling the skin of the abdomen will not prevent stretch marks although many people swear that it will. The woman who religiously oils her abdomen to prevent stretch marks is usually one who is most careful with her diet and her weight and, though she may attribute her lack of marks to oiling her skin, it is in fact due to her lack of obesity. However, the skin does tend to become dry and scaly during pregnancy and the daily application of oil over the whole body will do a great deal to preserve its normal texture

If over-distension of the abdomen occurs as the result of a twin pregnancy or polyhydramnios then stretch marks are extremely difficult to avoid. Some women do avoid them by rigid control of their weight gain, which during twin pregnancy should be restricted to 13 kg.

The first stretch marks appear literally overnight and are rapidly followed by others if weight gain is not carefully controlled. Once stretch marks have appeared they will remain for ever. It takes several months following delivery for the marks to lose their livid coloration and eventually they have a light silvery colour, but, probably even more important, the skin that has been stretched will never properly return to its former elasticity and texture.

Taste

A change or alteration in taste is not really a minor ailment of pregnancy but, like so many things that happen in pregnancy, it is difficult to know under what particular heading this should be described.

Even before the suppression of the first period some women can diagnose their pregnancy because they notice a strange taste in their mouth, or a different taste appreciation for certain foods. The classic taste is metallic, persistent, quite definite and unfortunately usually lasts throughout pregnancy.

Other women notice that their tastes change and that, whereas they had previously liked coffee, it now tastes horrible; similarly, some women may show dislike of spicy foods and alcohol. Unfortunately, most of the changes result in a liking for sugar and sweet things, which makes dieting even more difficult.

Changes of taste are not the same as cravings or 'pica', although some alterations of taste are quite out of character and occasionally quite bizarre. Gingivitis or other infections in the mouth will not only alter taste but may also create an unpleasant taste in the mouth and cause the breath to become offensive. When they are treated the symptoms will go.

Bleeding from the gums (gingivitis)

The gums respond to hormones in pregnancy as do most of the other organs in the body. A certain amount of congestion is the result of an increased blood supply. This causes thickening of the gums, especially where they lie immediately against the teeth, so that tiny little depressions are formed between the gum and the tooth. Food particles, other debris and stale saliva will collect in these hollows as well as in the spaces between the teeth. Bacteria inevitably grow and multiply in these conditions and very shortly begin to cause infection. Infection of the gum immediately adjacent to the tooth is known as gingivitis. It further increases the blood supply to the mouth, makes the gum sore, tender and liable to bleed very easily. Infection between the gum and the tooth is the whole basis for dental caries in pregnancy as discussed on pages 160–1. It is true that the baby may take calcium from the mother's bones but he cannot remove any calcium from the teeth and thereby predispose them to dental caries. The dental caries result from gingivitis due to poor mouth hygiene.

Treatment of bleeding from the gums should ideally be preventive by regularly consulting your dentist and being most meticulous about oral hygiene. Proper brushing of the teeth with a not too hard brush in an upwards movement from the gums to the crown, and not vigorous sideways abrasion, is essential. If bleeding does occur, you should see your dentist as soon as possible so that treatment can be started before any permanent damage has been done.

Nasal congestion

Nasal congestion or stuffiness in the nose is a common complaint during pregnancy. Congestion is due to the increased blood supply to the mucous membrane and an increase in the secretions of the nasal passages, and does not require any specific treament unless it becomes intolerable to the patient. She should then consult her doctor who may advise her to insert drops or to use a nasal spray for a short time. These should not be used without first consulting a doctor, because these drops or sprays contain decongestants which cause a constriction of the vessels in the nose and which, although very good for the nose, may adversely affect other parts of the body if they are absorbed into the blood stream. Their excessive use may make the whole condition much worse.

Nasal congestion is a direct result of pregnancy and will, therefore, be relieved when the pregnancy ends. If it persists you should seek expert advice.

Nose bleeds in pregnancy

Bleeding from the nose is more common in pregnancy and is particularly noticeable during autumn and winter. Nose bleeds are usually transient with the loss of only a small amount of blood and they cease spontaneously after a few minutes.

In pregnancy they are not an indication of a rise of blood pressure and all the old wives' tales associated with recurrent nose bleeds and injury to the fetus *in utero* are absolutely groundless.

The mucous membrane lining the nasal passages has a greatly increased blood supply during pregnancy which makes it become thicker, congested and more easily damaged. It may be injured by trauma, of which the classical example is picking the nose with the finger, or result indirectly from living in a dry centrally heated atmosphere when the secretions in the nasal passages become hard and encrusted on them, and their removal may damage the mucous membrane.

Nose bleeds should be treated by applying pressure with a handkerchief to the affected nostril or by gently pinching the nose. If the nasal passages are dry and cracked, a small amount of white vaseline or lanolin should be inserted into each nostril on a fingertip and gradually massaged into the nose by gently rubbing the nostril. This should be repeated each night. If this does not stop the bleeding, or if the bleeding recurs, you should consult your doctor.

Headache

Headaches may occur at any time during pregnancy, just as they occur in the non-pregnant woman. They are not more likely to occur than at any other time, although occasionally the worry and concern that a woman may have during pregnancy make them more frequent. Some women complain of quite severe headache with the nausea of early pregnancy. Headaches may be treated by simple remedies such as rest or taking aspirin or paracetamol. Codeine is not usually recommended because it tends to increase constipation.

Migraine sufferers are usually slightly better when they are pregnant, but there is no hard and fast rule.

Headaches associated with common causes, such as flu or too much alcohol, are the same as in the non-pregnant and the normal remedy of aspirin with a pint of water is all the treatment usually required.

Headaches which occur in the front of the head, usually situated above the eyes, must always be treated carefully, partly because they may be associated with migraine or eyestrain, but also because they may be particularly difficult to relieve by simple aspirin treatment. If the pain is not relieved after about an hour then you should rest in bed.

The serious, but extremely rare, condition of eclampsia (Chapter 18) is also associated with a very severe frontal type of headache, which is not relieved by paracetamol or any other type of drug. It is a very severe pain and is associated with flashes of light, changes of vision, irritability and vomiting.

Pressure headaches, where there is a sensation of a heavy weight pressing on the top of the head, are usually caused by nervousness or emotional problems and nearly always respond to tranquillizers or similar treatment. These should only be taken on advice of a doctor.

Muscle cramps

Cramp in the muscles of the thigh, calf and foot, more especially in the calf, become fairly frequent during the last quarter of pregnancy and usually occur at night. They can be intensely painful and suddenly wake a woman from sleep with a sensation of severe cramping pain in the calf extending down to the foot. The muscles of the calf are felt tightened into a hard knot and the pain may be sufficient to make the woman cry out immediately she wakes. The treatment is rapid, firm and almost violent massage of the affected muscles as well as movement of the foot both upwards and downwards helping it with one hand. During a cramp the foot is nearly always extended and pressed downwards, and one of the secrets of relieving the pain is to bend the foot and toes upwards. The combination of movement of the foot and massage of the calf usually relieves the pain although it may take a few minutes. After the acute pain has ceased a fairly severe ache remains. Tenderness persists in the calf for several hours and frequently lasts for two or three days, making walking difficult. Such muscle cramps do not damage the leg or its muscles, but they can be extremely painful and their demoralizing effect quite considerable.

It was generally thought that cramps were due to a low level of usable calcium in the blood. The standard treatment for frequent cramps was to take calcium tablets two or three times a day. However there is no definite evidence that such treatment is useful. On rare occasions muscle cramps are the result of a persistent low salt diet. If a woman has been on such a diet and her cramps are not relieved by taking calcium, she may be given more ordinary salt to eat. Generally speaking, the intake of salt during pregnancy should be diminished or reduced and pregnant women are warned against taking large quantities of salt. Taking extra salt for the treatment of cramps must, therefore, only be under the direction of a physician.

Pelvic discomfort

Pelvic discomfort is nearly always present towards the end of pregnancy and may take one of a variety of forms. In a woman having her first baby it usually begins at about the 30th or 32nd week with the softening of the ligaments which hold together the bones of the pelvic girdle. This results in some relaxation of the joints and the resulting extra unaccustomed movements may cause severe aching which is most noticeable after exercise or at the end of the day. It is best treated by rest; lying down for half an hour or so usually relieves the discomfort. At the 36th week of pregnancy in a woman having her first baby the baby's head usually engages in the pelvis causing aching or generalized heaviness in the pelvis. The head may press upon nerves, causing pains in the groins that sometimes radiate down the front or inner side of the thigh as far as the knee and which are most noticeable when walking or after exercise. Occasionally pain may occur in the back of the pelvis and radiate down the back of the leg. These pains, being due to pressure on nerves, are intermittent and there is no need to be concerned, but if they become severe or continuous you should report them to the antenatal clinic when you next attend.

The bones in the front of the pelvis are joined together at the symphysis pubis and this joint, like the others in the pelvis, is softened and tends to separate towards the end of pregnancy. Pressure upon it may cause some tenderness and on rare occasions it becomes painful. This will be noticed particularly after exercise or when moving the weight from one leg to the other. Although occasionally pain in the symphysis pubis may be quite severe, it causes no harm. It used to be treated by very tight binding of the pelvis to try and prevent movement in the joint; it is now accepted that this does not relieve the pain and that there is no specific treatment for its relief other than rest, avoiding exercise, reassurance and the administration of aspirin or paracetamol. These should not be taken excessively in late pregnancy.

Abdominal pain

Abdominal pain may occur during pregnancy from any condition which might cause abdominal pain in the non-pregnant state. It is impossible to consider all the causes of abdominal pain that might occur throughout pregnancy. Generally speaking, however, pain is a frightening symptom. It can be considered under three different headings:

Well-known pain. This type of pain or discomfort has been noticed before the onset of pregnancy. It may be, for instance, associated with constipation. Such a pain need not worry you but should be mentioned to your doctor or at the clinic at your next appointment.

Pain of gradual onset. There are several specific discomforts or pains which occur during pregnancy commencing very gradually, so that it is several days or weeks before a pain of noticeable severity has developed. This type of pain does not indicate any serious condition and should be discussed at your next visit to the clinic.

Pain of sudden onset. This type of pain has never occurred previously and is, therefore, likely to be associated with the pregnancy. Such severe pains are associated with miscarriage, ectopic pregnancy, fibroids and ovarian cysts, although it is surprising how much pain constipation or fetal movements can sometimes cause. Severe pains of sudden onset should be reported as soon as possible.

Round ligament pain

This is a specific pain or discomfort that occurs during pregnancy caused by the stretching of the round ligaments supporting the uterus. These ligaments pass from the upper and outer part of the uterus down the lower side of the abdomen into the groin. Round ligament pain usually begins about the 16th or 20th week of pregnancy, although it may not begin until the 28th week, and usually continues until about the 32nd week when it disappears spontaneously. It is recognized as being an aching, dragging, nagging pain, usually more severe on the right side than the left, just to one side of the uterus. Occasionally sharp stabs of pain may be felt and the pain may be particularly annoying when a woman stands up after sitting for any length of time. It can be confused with an acute or chronic appendicitis and should be mentioned when you next visit the clinic.

There is no specific treatment for round ligament pain. Reassurance is all that can be given. The pain will not do the patient or her baby any harm. It does not usually become sufficiently severe for pain-killing drugs to be given.

Costal margin pain

The costal margin is the lower border of the chest wall. Towards the end of pregnancy pain may be felt here, at the junction of the lower edge of the ribs and the abdominal wall, just below the breasts or occasionally to the side. This is caused by compression of the lower ribs by the enlarging uterus and usually begins at the 30th, 32nd or even 34th week of pregnancy. It is more common on the right than the left side because the uterus usually enlarges more to the right and presses more on the right ribs. It can, however, occur on the left or may sometimes be present on both sides and can be sufficiently severe to cause a great deal of discomfort. The pain tends to be more severe when sitting than when standing or lying flat, because in the sitting position the ribs are compressed even more by the enlarging uterus. There is little that can be done to relieve it other than to avoid sitting in a slumped or slouched position.

Occasionally the ribs become very sore and the pain becomes quite severe. There is no definite cure other than delivery. The pain disappears spontaneously as soon as the uterine fundus stops pressing on the lower ribs. If it is the first baby, this happens when the head engages in the pelvis and lightening occurs at about the 36th week—otherwise the discomfort may continue until labour begins.

Reassurance and a promise that the pain will go at delivery do not seem to offer very much in the way of treatment, but most women learn to live with it after they realize that it will not harm either them or their baby.

Oedema (swelling of the ankles and feet)

Part of the natural weight gain of pregnancy is due to the retention of water within the body. The amount of water retained varies from woman to woman and also between different pregnancies in any one person. It is impossible to give any reliable figure for the exact amount of water retained at any stage during pregnancy. Salt is one of the main factors which allow the body to hold extra fluid within the tissues and the majority of obstetricians therefore limit the amount of salt taken by their patients. An excessive amount of fluid retained in the body tends to gravitate into the feet and ankles during the day, or on to the skin overlying the lower part of the back when a person is lying in bed.

A minute amount of swelling of the ankles is common in most people, pregnant and non-pregnant, towards the end of the day but hardly noticeable. Obvious, unnatural swelling of the ankles, generally known as oedema, can be easily recognized because of its 'pitting' nature. If pressure is applied to an area of oedema with a finger or thumb for 20 or 30 seconds, the fluid in the tissues being compressed will spread into the surrounding area, and when the pressure is removed a depression will remain which can be both seen and felt easily. It is one of the classical signs of pre-eclampsia. In fact, the majority of women develop pitting oedema at some stage during their pregnancy.

Oedema of the ankles results not only from the retention of large amounts of fluid in the body but also during hot weather and by prolonged standing which allows pooling of fluid in the lower parts of the legs. The oedema or swelling usually disappears during the night, when the feet are raised, but reappears during the following day. It is a gravitational problem and rest during the day with the feet raised will tend to reduce swelling.

Severe oedema or swelling may be associated with considerable discomfort in the lower leg and ankle. It also causes pain and discomfort when wearing shoes, because they constrict the feet which not only become hot and swollen but also tend to swell to a greater extent at the edge of the shoe, or in the region of the straps, thus causing them to cut into the skin.

Any pregnant woman who develops recognizable oedema of the ankles or feet should consult her medical adviser or midwife when she next visits the antenatal clinic. Oedema is not dangerous but it constitutes an abnormality of pregnancy and merits serious consideration by those looking after her. Also their advice upon diet or any other factors related in the management of the pregnancy may be necessary.

The management of oedema of the ankles varies according to its severity. A very mild amount occurring only at the end of the day, especially in warm weather, requires no treatment. Slightly more oedema occurring at the end of the day in cold weather may require only extra rest during the afternoon. As the amount of oedema increases it can be controlled by a more rigid diet and careful supervision of the woman's weight gain, and sometimes by eliminating spices and pickles from the diet. Even more severe oedema demands strict rest at home and the doctor may prescribe diuretic drugs which squeeze extra water out of the body. The prolonged use of diuretics or salt intake restriction is an inappropriate form of treatment.

If oedema of the feet remains severe or there is an accompanying rise in blood pressure, the woman will be admitted to hospital for further observation and treatment.

Swelling of the face

A certain amount of swelling of the face is natural during pregnancy. One of the earliest methods of diagnosing pregnancy in social circles is to notice a fullness of the face especially in the region of the cheek bones and around and beneath the jaw bones. A certain amount of generalized enlargement of the face results from the deposition of subcutaneous fat and fluid that occurs as pregnancy advances. This is normal and may sometimes be very pronounced. Occasionally, however, there is true oedema of the face when the wrinkles of the forehead are eliminated, the eyelids become heavy and rather baggy, the skin on the cheeks becomes distended and shiny, and jowl forms in the skin under the jaw bone. Such marked facial alterations usually accompany excessive weight gain or fluid retention. While not being one of the diagnostic signs of pre-eclampsia, they are usually associated with it.

The treatment of this condition is by strict and rigid dietary control, or the administration of diuretics, to remove the extra fluid. The increases or alterations of the facial contour will always return to normal after delivery, providing of course that the woman's weight returns to normal. Any permanent increase in her weight will also result in permanent alteration in her facial contour.

Swelling of the fingers

A certain amount of swelling of the fingers seems to occur during most pregnancies, for which the reason is unknown. The knuckle joints of the fingers tend to become much larger so that rings which could easily be removed can only be removed with difficulty towards the end of pregnancy or after delivery. There is rarely any pain or discomfort with such swelling. Oedema of the fingers, however, may also occur during the latter stages of pregnancy causing rings to become excessively tight, and is usually associated with fluid retention. This type of oedema is not due to gravity because the hands are not always hanging down. Oedema of the hands becomes more marked during the night and is therefore most noticeable early in the morning, when the fingers are stiff and may have a tingling sensation. It may be necessary to work the fingers before they are sufficiently supple to handle ordinary kitchen utensils. Stiffness or swelling of the fingers should be reported to the doctor or midwife at the next visit to the antenatal clinic. Rings which have become uncomfortably tight may be removed after soaking the hands in cold water and wiping the ring and its finger with soap. There is also a very ancient but effective method of doing this by winding a piece of string gently round the finger starting at the tip and gradually working the way up towards the ring. This squeezes the fluid out of the finger and towards the hand, and when the string is removed the ring can be slipped over the now normal finger.

Severe swelling of the fingers may occur as a symptom of pre-eclampsia, but should generally be regarded by pregnant women as a warning and not as a symptom of serious disease. Oedema of the fingers may be treated in the same way as oedema of the ankles, mainly by diet, but sometimes by diuretics.

Carpal tunnel syndrome

Pain in the wrist and pins and needles extending from the wrist down into the hand is a condition known as carpal tunnel syndrome. The carpal tunnel is in the front of the wrist and carries the tendons and nerves to the palm of the hand and fingers. When the hand and fingers swell the area of the carpal tunnel also swells but, as it is bounded by bone on one side and a fibrous ligament on the other, any swelling results in pressure on the tendons and nerves within the tunnel. The pressure causes irritation of the median nerve as it traverses the tunnel, resulting in the sensation of pins and needles extending downwards into the thumb and fingers, but never affects the little finger. This is most frequently noticed in the early morning before movement of the wrist has dispersed any fluid, and is usually accompanied by stiffness of the fingers and joints of the hand. As the hands are moved, the joints become more supple and the numbness and tingling pass. If it continues throughout the day it should be reported to the doctor.

Carpal tunnel syndrome is the classic reason why a pregnant woman drops things in the early morning.

It is a warning rather than a dangerous symptom, although the discomfort may make the woman seek medical advice. The management is exactly the same as that for oedema of the ankles and fingers, namely dietary control and sometimes diuretic treatment. It always disappears a few days after delivery.

Occasionally, if there is no swelling of the fingers or of the ankles, the symptoms may be due to a deficiency of vitamin B and not pressure on the nerve. The symptoms may respond to the administration of vitamin B, so all vitamin pills given by the doctor or clinic should be taken regularly.

Discomfort in bed

Towards the end of pregnancy it may be extremely difficult to find a comfortable position in bed, especially if you normally sleep on your back or abdomen. The growing uterus will obviously prevent you from sleeping on your abdomen and will also make sleeping on your back rather uncomfortable. If you turn on one side then your enlarged uterus will tend to drag you over into an uncomfortable position. You may find that sitting up with two or three extra pillows is the most comfortable position and the one in which you will sleep longest, or lying on your side with a pillow under the abdomen may be sufficiently comfortable for a good night's sleep.

One of the main prescriptions for a good sleep is a firm bed. There is nothing worse than a mattress that sags into a hollow in the middle and, if it is not practical to buy a new mattress or bed, the hollow can be counteracted by putting some 15 cm wide wooden boards across the bed under the mattress.

Heartburn is often worse at night and discomfort can be eased, or even cured, by raising your head on two or three extra pillows or by lifting the head of the bed about 15 cm with bricks or similar objects under the legs at the head end. Make sure it is secure!

Insomnia

Insomnia is the inability to sleep. Many pregnant women find that mild insomnia may affect them in different ways, mostly during the last third of their pregnancy. Firstly, they have difficulty in getting to sleep. Secondly, they wake after two or three hours of sleep and find that they cannot sleep again. Thirdly, they have problems with their temperature control. Fourthly, they may suffer from frequency of micturition.

The movements of the baby sometimes become more vigorous at night than during the day. This may be actual fact or simple imagination, but in either event they become more noticeable and may be sufficiently violent to wake the mother from comparatively deep sleep. Once she has been awakened her baby is often sufficiently active to prevent her getting to sleep again. The movements of the baby vary as pregnancy progresses and are often most violent at about the 32nd week when the baby is sufficiently strong and still has sufficient room actually to punch and kick. As pregnancy advances beyond the 32nd week the amount of water surrounding the baby gradually diminishes in relation to the size of the baby so that its movements have more of a squirming nature. One type of movement is not more likely to wake, or keep awake, a woman than another, but if the kicks of the 32nd week cause wakening then the squirming movements later on may not do so.

The variation in the metabolic rate of the pregnant woman often causes confusion in her temperature regulation. The body temperature is accurately controlled by a delicate temperature regulation centre in the lower part of the brain which may occasionally fail to function satisfactorily during pregnancy, making a woman feel alternately hot and sweaty, then cold and clammy. This is most commonly experienced during the height of summer or the depths of winter, particularly at night, and more especially in the last 10 weeks of pregnancy.

The treatment of insomnia is basically comfort and peace of mind. Someone who is either uncomfortable or worried will obviously have difficulty in sleeping. If discomfort is due to any actual aches and pains you should mention these when you next visit the antenatal clinic. If there are any worries concerning the pregnancy or its outcome these should also be discussed, and it will usually be found that these fears are groundless. Comfort together with a warm drink when going to bed are the usual household recipes for sound sleep and are just as applicable in pregnancy.

Increased frequency of micturition occasionally results in an inability to sleep through the night. A woman may be wakened by the desire to empty her bladder after which it is difficult for her to return to sleep. In these circumstances she should not drink for one or two hours before going to sleep.

It is difficult to advise any realistic method of enabling a return to sleep having once woken during the night. When people do wake at this time they usually become very 'wide awake'. Their mind becomes active and the harder they try to return to sleep the more difficult it becomes. Perhaps getting up, walking around, making a warm drink or reading a book is the ideal method of trying to reduce the mental activity. When apparent temperature changes such as heat and sweating cause wakefulness it is no use throwing off some of the bed clothes, because in a short while you will feel cold. If the feeling of warmth causes persistent waking or insomnia then the number of blankets ought to be gradually reduced. The amount of bed clothing used by most married couples is a habit arrived at by mutual agreement. If a pregnant wife wakes in the night feeling hot and sweaty and wishes to reduce the number of bedclothes, her husband, who does not feel any of the other inconveniences of pregnancy, should graciously give way even at the expense of feeling cold in the middle of the night. He can always wear a vest! If this is his only discomfort in pregnancy he can hardly grumble.

There is a whole range of sleep inducing tablets available. Some are mild and some are extremely powerful. There is also a large range of tranquillizers. None of these should be taken without the permission of your doctor, and the stated dose should never be exceeded. While some drugs may be harmful to the pregnant patient, there is a large range of tranquillizers and hypnotic drugs which are safe to take during pregnancy so long as they are taken in the recommended dose.

It is most important that you should get a good night's sleep, otherwise you will become tired and irritable during the day and your pregnancy will become rather a bore. Simple sleeping tablets are perfectly safe for you to take during the later weeks of your pregnancy. You need not be afraid you will become addicted to them since your normal sleeping pattern will return after delivery.

Cystitis

Cystitis, or urinary tract infection is one of the most common infections during pregnancy and probably affects about 20 per cent of all women at some stage (see Chapter 21).

The classical symptoms are an increase in the frequency of micturition with discomfort or pain before, during or after passing urine. There may also be a sense of urgency to pass urine which may occasionally contain blood. The infection is usually longstanding or recurrent, and the symptoms may appear gradually over several weeks or even months. However, cystitis may occasionally be sudden in onset when the symptoms of pain and frequency of micturition will appear in just a few hours. An acute cystitis is nearly always associated with a rise of temperature and perhaps also an attack of shivering. There may be pain in one of the loins in the region of the kidney. If an acute cystitis is suspected you should go to bed, send for the doctor and drink as much water as possible while awaiting his arrival.

A special specimen of urine is usually taken for investigation and culture of the organism. Most of these infections are treated by a course of antibiotics and the majority are quickly cured. A urinary tract infection even of the most severe nature will not affect the baby and will not have any permanent effect on the mother provided it is treated properly and cured fairly quickly.

Overstretching of the abdominal muscles

During a normal pregnancy the abdominal muscles become distended and stretched but are always able to return to their former condition after the conclusion of the pregnancy, especially with the help of gentle exercises. Abdominal distension does not start until about the 20th week of the first pregnancy or about the 16th week of a subsequent pregnancy. The abdominal girth should increase to a maximum of approximately 100 cm at term in a normal pregnancy and the muscles are perfectly capable of returning to their normal tone providing this girth is not exceeded.

There are three main factors which contribute towards over-distension of the uterus or abdomen during pregnancy and, therefore, to overstretching of the abdominal muscles. They are obesity, multiple pregnancy and polyhydramnios—an excessive amount of water around the baby. During normal pregnancy the muscles may begin to ache, especially just above the pubic bone, at about the 20th week. This is due to normal stretching and usually lasts for three or four weeks. It is especially noticeable after exercise or towards the end of the day and indicates that the muscles are being placed under a certain amount of stress and that more rest should be taken.

Some people believe that support of the abdomen and abdominal muscles is beneficial at this stage. This is doubtful since the muscles themselves are perfectly capable of maintaining their tone and will not become overstretched during a normal pregnancy. An abdominal support allows the muscles to become slack so that they are in fact more likely to lose their tone later in pregnancy or after delivery. Bad posture undoubtedly causes some overstretching of the abdominal muscles. During pregnancy the weight of the body is thrown forward by the pregnant abdomen which leads to an arching of the back and a prominence of the buttocks and a compensatory leaning back of the upper part of the chest. Later in pregnancy this characteristic posture becomes more marked and the tilting forward of the pelvis leads to the classical pregnant walk or wobble. High-heeled shoes cause the pelvis to tilt further forwards and the back to arch even more. This places an increased strain on the muscles of the abdomen and leads to their overstretching. The correct posture is to keep the bottom tucked in as much as possible, which in turn will flatten out the curve in the small of the back and level the pelvis. This means a woman is standing much straighter and more erect and there is less protuberance of the abdomen.

There is no reason to suppose that wearing a maternity girdle or maternity corset will in any way assist posture during pregnancy. If one is worn it should only support the lower part of the abdomen so as to relieve the sense of weight or heaviness and should not constrict the abdomen above the umbilicus.

Injuries during pregnancy

Most pregnant women fall down at some stage during their pregnancy especially during the last month when their balance is upset by the protuberant abdomen and by the awkward clumsiness generally accompanying the end of pregnancy. Simple falls or accidents usually result in a few bruises, but frequently the falls are in a forward direction, resulting in the abdomen (and uterus) receiving most of the force of the fall. Such a fall may cause great anxiety to a woman in late pregnancy, because of the possibility of injury to her baby and because of the possibility of injury to herself or the onset of premature labour. It is almost impossible to cause physical injury to a baby when it is inside the uterus. This applies at any stage of pregnancy. The only way in which a fetus can be injured by direct violence is by striking the uterus very hard with an extremely sharp object. Ordinary falls, no matter how severe, almost never cause damage or injury to the baby. Occasionally, women in late pregnancy fall downstairs and this may result in multiple injuries both to the back and the abdomen. Even so, it is extremely difficult to damage the contents of the uterus even if the anterior abdominal wall strikes the leading edge of the stairs while falling. In such an accident the first reaction is to see if any bones have been broken and if all limbs and joints move freely it is unlikely that severe damage has been done. Bruising is bound to occur but is not harmful. The pregnant woman should rest quietly for a few minutes in a comfortable chair or in bed. The only indication in early pregnancy that the uterus has been damaged is bleeding from the vagina and if this occurs she should go to bed and tell the doctor immediately. Bleeding resulting from ordinary injuries is rare.

Later in pregnancy a pregnant woman can feel if fetal movements are continuing after an accident. Sometimes after a violent fall fetal movements cease for one or even two hours and then recommence again with their former vigour. If they cease for more than three or four hours the doctor should be notified. The doctor or the hospital should be notified immediately if there is any loss of blood or water from the vagina. If her head has been struck during the fall and the woman knows that she lost consciousness, even for the shortest time, she should notify her doctor as soon as possible.

Virus disease

Obviously all infections should be avoided if possible during pregnancy. The majority of contagious diseases are caused by viruses, most of which can cross the placenta and enter the fetal circulation, so that in early pregnancy (before the 12th week) there is a possibility that they may affect the development of the baby. After the 12th week they rarely harm the fetus but are better avoided even in late pregnancy because they produce unpleasant symptoms.

Visual disturbances

Some women complain that their eyesight changes during pregnancy. There is nothing in pregnancy itself that causes or results in any damage to the eyes.

During pregnancy, however, extra fluid is retained within the body and if this becomes excessive, as in pre-eclampsia, or there is a large gain in weight, some very minor changes may occur in the eyes. A woman with particularly good eyesight will not notice these changes, but if a woman's eyesight is not very good at the onset of pregnancy, then the small changes may be noticeable. Her vision will return to normal after the end of pregnancy.

Contact lenses

If an abnormal amount of fluid is retained in the body during pregnancy some inevitably finds its way into the eyes and produces a very slight change in the shape of the eyeball itself. This may be quite critical to those women who wear contact lenses which may become uncomfortable. The eyes will return to their previous contour after the end of the pregnancy and the lenses will again be comfortable. It is especially important for those women who wear contact lenses not to gain too much weight.

Warning to those who wear contact lenses. Those of you who wear contact lenses must always tell your doctor, your midwife and the staff at the booking clinic in the hospital when you first see them. Doctors have a habit of gently pulling down the lower eyelid to see the colour of the mucous membrane on its inner side which gives them a good indication of the condition of your blood. Unless the doctor realizes that you are wearing contact lenses, he may inadvertently press on the upper eyelid and, although he is unlikely to dislodge the lens, it may cause discomfort.

It is particularly important to remove contact lenses when labour begins, preferably before you go to hospital—but do not forget to take them with you.

Spots before the eyes

Most people occasionally notice a few spots before the eyes which disappear quite rapidly when they blink or move their head. In pregnancy fairly large spots occasionally appear in the field of vision. These may disappear quickly, or may persist and be associated with a severe frontal headache when they are usually caused by a sudden rise in blood pressure. If spots before the eyes persist with a frontal headache it should be reported immediately.

Flashes of light

Women who develop severe pre-eclampsia with a very high blood pressure may notice bright flashes of light before their eyes. Such a symptom usually heralds the onset of eclampsia and is now extremely rare in Great Britain.

Personality changes

There are many different changes that may occur in a woman's personality during her pregnancy (see Chapter 1). Some personality changes together with her variations in emotional response are to be expected and anyone who is interested in pregnancy should make some attempt to understand what these involve and try to appreciate their extent and influence on a pregnant woman.

13 Weight Gain in Pregnancy

The importance of the amount of weight gained during pregnancy cannot be over-emphasized as the welfare of both the mother and her child can be directly related to it.

Most women gain weight during pregnancy but the amount varies not only from woman to woman but also from pregnancy to pregnancy. It is impossible to set down a rigid rule which states exactly how much weight a given person should or should not gain during pregnancy especially since the weight at the onset of pregnancy exerts a big influence on this. A woman of average build and height on unrestricted diet will gain in the region of 12.6 kg throughout pregnancy.

The weight will usually fall in the first three months due to nausea, vomiting and loss of appetite. This actual weight loss may vary from just 5 or 1 kg to as much as 9 or even 14 kg, especially if there is severe vomiting. The gain in weight usually starts about the 12th to the 14th week of pregnancy when the nausea and sickness are naturally relieved and a sense of well-being encourages the woman to eat and drink more than she might do otherwise. Weight gain up to the 20th week, however, is not usually very great. The greatest increase occurs between the 20th and 30th week of pregnancy, and many obstetricians take exception to excessive weight gain in this particular phase because weight gain during this time is associated with a much higher incidence of pre-eclampsia. The speed of weight gain slows after the 30th week and gradually diminishes until about the 38th or the 39th week of pregnancy after which there is very often a fall in weight.

Ideal weight gain

The gain in weight during pregnancy is the result of many factors. There is an increase in the size of the various organs, notably the breasts and the uterus; there is the weight of the fetus itself together with the placenta and the amniotic fluid; there is a natural increase in the mother's circulating blood volume by as much as 30 per cent to supply the demands of the uterus and the breasts as well as the rest of the body. These factors together account for approximately 8 kg and a total gain of 8 to 9 kg is all that should be allowed throughout pregnancy.

The final weight gain associated purely with the pregnancy itself is:

The weight of the baby	3.2 kg
The weight of the placenta	.67
The weight of the amniotic fluid	.91
The weight of the uterus (normally 85 g.)	.91
Increase in weight of the breasts	.67
Increase in circulating volume of blood	1.81
Total:	8.2 kg

Any extra weight is due either to fat or to fluid retention. The scheme to be aimed at is:

0–14 weeks: No weight gain.
14–20 weeks: Total of 2.3 kg.
20–30 weeks: Total of 4.5 kg. This is the most difficult period of pregnancy with regard to restricting weight gain but it is also the most important.
30–36 weeks: Total of 2.3 kg.
36–40 weeks: No weight should be gained, and indeed from the 38th week onwards a pregnant woman will very frequently lose weight.

Excessive fluid retention, and consequent increase in weight, may occur at any stage during pregnancy and results from the presence of a high level of hormones (which may play a part in the cause of pre-eclampsia) or an excessive intake of salt or spicy food, or both factors together.

Early in pregnancy none of these factors are operative and weight remains constant or actually falls. At about the 10th week when the circulating blood volume starts to increase there may be some weight gain. At this stage or shortly afterwards food intake may be increased when nausea and vomiting cease. Towards the 14th week the appetite returns, and women may eat too much of the wrong type of food. There is no truth in the saying that a pregnant woman should 'eat enough for two'. She should, however, have a good adequate diet and supplements such as vitamins, iron and calcium are essential. A weight gain between the 20th and 30th week of more than 4.5 kg predisposes to pre-eclampsia with the resulting harm to both the mother and her baby. The pattern of weight gain changes once more after the 30th week of pregnancy. Sudden and dramatic increases may occur, usually as a result of fluid retention which may be a sign of the onset of pre-eclampsia. The amount of weight gained usually diminishes from about the 35th week of pregnancy and may cease altogether at about the 38th week of pregnancy or as the expected date of delivery is approached. One of the most reliable signs of full maturity is actual loss in weight even though this may amount to only .5 or 1 kg; it may occur at any time after the 38th week and labour usually follows within 7 to 10 days of such a fall. However, if it does not begin there is no need for concern. Weight loss towards the end of pregnancy is due to a reduction of hormones which is considered, by many people, to be one of the causes of the onset of labour.

Fierce arguments rage upon the amount of weight which a person may be permitted to gain in a normal pregnancy. Many consider that it should be between 9 and 13 kg for the average woman of average build. Some women, however, who diet to reduce their weight artificially prior to the onset of pregnancy often discover that the weight previously lost is replaced with alarming ease at the beginning of their pregnancy. Such women may find it very difficult not to gain more than 13 kg. Conversely, some women whose pregnancy commences when they are grossly overweight need gain no weight at all throughout their pregnancy providing they diet carefully for the whole duration. This was well illustrated by a woman who weighed 150 kg before the onset of pregnancy and, suffering from severe nausea and vomiting throughout most of it, weighed 115 kg at delivery. Her baby was absolutely normal and four weeks after delivery she weighed 108 kg. Still perhaps a little overweight!

All weight gained in excess of 8 or 9 kg will remain after delivery and will be distributed over the shoulders, upper arms, chest, abdominal wall and thighs.

Excess weight gain

Every pregnant woman ought to have access to a weighing machine, either at home or in the clinic, where she can check her weight. If she is gaining too much weight it means that she is not adhering to the diet prescribed below. The first thing for her to do is to read through her diet and see what she is eating incorrectly. This is nearly always found to be carbohydrate, in the form of sugar or flour, and their intake must be very carefully checked and reduced accordingly. Most people on a diet tend to nibble between meals, especially cheese, and this is to be discouraged unless such nibblings consist of fruit alone. It is not generally realized that cheese has an extremely high calorie content and will cause an increase in weight more rapidly than most other foods. Its intake should be strictly limited.

Milk is invariably prescribed for most pregnant women and is of inestimable value for those people who are undernourished or whose diet is inadequate. It is true that milk contains a certain amount of vitamins and also calcium, but it also has a fairly high calorie content. A person who is eating a well-balanced and normal diet does not require to drink half a litre a day. Many women adhere rigidly to a basic diet but by eating large amounts of cheese and drinking half a litre or more of milk a day proceed to put on an undue amount of weight.

An unlimited amount of fluid may be drunk throughout the whole of pregnancy, but the calories in the drink must be carefully estimated —always remembering that milky drinks and processed fruit juices have a relatively high calorie content. Tea and coffee may be drunk freely, providing only a small quantity of sugar is added. Alcohol also has a high calorie value and pregnant women should be reasonable in their alcohol intake anyway.

Remember, 9 kg is the limit.

Rich and indigestible foods should be avoided, for example curry, cream, fried food and strong tea, especially as some women are more prone to indigestion during pregnancy.

During pregnancy a woman needs to ensure that she is taking a well-balanced and adequate diet. The list given below shows the foods which are richest in the various nutrients essential during pregnancy, but any normal well-balanced diet contains an ample and sufficient amount of almost all these items.

Diet during pregnancy

Eating the right foods during pregnancy helps to ensure a healthy baby. Don't eat more than usual—the old idea of 'eating for two' is mistaken and pregnancy is far more enjoyable if you avoid putting on too much weight; the aim should be to put on no more than 9 kg during the whole pregnancy.

The baby is a parasite. He will take what he requires from his mother even to the detriment of her general health. For ease of growth and development it is necessary to provide the growing baby with an ample amount of those foods that he requires, and it is essential to supply the mother with sufficient to meet the demands of her baby. A pregnant woman can remain perfectly fit and healthy without gaining an excessive amount of weight.

The human body (and especially the baby) requires a great variety of foods, including minerals, for growth and development, the vast majority of which can be found in a normal balanced diet. The diet should contain (1) an adequate quantity of protein, (2) a reasonable amount of fresh fruit and vegetables, (3) a moderate amount of carbohydrate, (4) a moderate amount of fat and (5) adequate fluid. Under normal circumstances the average person eats a reasonably well-balanced diet.

Protein. The foods which contain protein are all types of meat such as beef, pork, poultry, lamb, veal, kidneys, liver, tripe, heart, sweetbreads. All kinds of fish such as sardines, haddock, kippers, herrings, sole, salmon, shrimps, lobsters, pilchards, oysters, prawns; also eggs, cheese and milk. Some vegetables such as peas, beans, nuts and lentils contain protein.

Carbohydrate is found in large amounts in anything which contains flour or sugar. The main carbohydrate foods are sugar, all bread, cereals, rice, potatoes, spaghetti, macaroni, cakes, pastries, sweets, jams, honey, chocolates, syrup.

Fats. Most of the foods which contain fat are obvious. They include fatty meat, especially bacon, margarine, butter, milk, cream, cheese, mayonnaise, lard, salad dressing, cooking oil, cooking fat, nut and fish oils.

Vitamins. A plentiful supply of vitamins is essential for the baby's growth as well as for the mother's health.

Vitamin A is present in all fish oils, especially cod liver oil, also in egg yolk, offal (such as liver, heart, kidneys), milk, cheese, butter, margarine, most fruits such as bananas, peaches, apricots—especially when fresh (there is not much vitamin A in these fruits when they have been dried or cooked)—vegetables, especially spinach and tomatoes, also turnips, beetroot, carrots, brussels sprouts.

Vitamin B_1 is found mostly in the seeds of plants like beans, peas, nuts and wheat (from which wheat germ oil is made) as well as crude rice and soya bean. It is also found in yeast and uncooked yeast, in eggs, liver, brain, heart, seafoods (especially fish oils) and in proprietary preparations such as Bemax and Marmite.

Vitamin B_2 is present in meat, liver, kidneys, heart and brains and all fish and shell fish and also in nuts, milk, cheese, cream, yeast, whole wheat, peas and beans.

Vitamin C is present in most fresh fruits, especially oranges, lemons, tangerines, grapefruit, tomatoes, blackcurrants, melons, strawberries and also in vegetables such as cabbage, lettuce, carrots, radishes, brussels sprouts, watercress and broccoli, and in milk. Vitamin C is destroyed by cooking or heating.

Vitamin D is present in nearly all fish oils and fish extracts, as well as in most animal fats, eggs, cheese, butter and milk. Vitamin D is essential for the satisfactory metabolism and absorption of both calcium and phosphorus used in bone building. So that the fetus has an adequate calcium supply the pregnant woman must have an adequate level of vitamin D. It should be noted, however, that the amount of vitamin D given to the pregnant woman must be carefully controlled since it is possible to take too much of this particular vitamin. One of the advantages of sunbathing is that vitamin D is formed in the skin by the action of ultra-violet light on it. This does not, however, mean that sunbathing is essential or even a good thing during pregnancy, but there is certainly no harm in it. You should not use an ultra-violet sun-ray lamp during pregnancy, but you may use modern ultra-violet sun beds or other equipment if your doctor agrees. Naturally you must adhere to the manufacturer's instructions.

Vitamin E is thought to be necessary to establish pregnancy, but its value during pregnancy is doubtful. It is found in most germinating seeds and eaten in the form of wheat germ oil and cotton seed oil. Small quantities are also present in eggs, milk, butter, cheese, unpolished rice, wholemeal bread and wheat.

Milk

Contrary to popular belief, milk is not essential for the pregnant woman. It is a very good, and indeed a perfect, food rich in calcium and vitamin C, but if you are taking an adequate well-balanced diet you need not drink it as it only increases calorie intake and, therefore, weight gain. You can get the calcium requirement from other foods or even from tablets. However, for the really undernourished or underprivileged, and those who cannot obtain an adequate diet, milk forms an ideal food.

Sugar and sugar substitutes

An increase of sugar intake during pregnancy is unnecessary. It is a general principle that an excessive amount of sugar should be avoided in the diet. Some sugar substitutes, especially cyclamate, are known to cause congenital abnormalities in animals when administered in high dosage, and although there is no definite evidence of this in the human they should be avoided. Recent legislation has been helpful in removing the cyclamates from the market so that sugar substitutes now available are quite safe.

Iron and supplementary elements

Iron is essential for the formation of haemoglobin, which is one of the main constituents of the red blood cell and carries oxygen around the body. A deficiency of iron causes anaemia and one of the most important aspects of antenatal care is the prevention of anaemia in the mother. Iron is to be found in nearly all meat, especially liver and kidneys, as well as in eggs, green vegetables such as spinach, cabbage, brussels sprouts and broccoli. Small quantities are present in root vegetables as well as in fish.

Calcium is one of the most important elements for the growth of the fetus and if the mother has insufficient calcium she may suffer from osteomalacia where the fetus takes calcium from her bones and they become softened and bent. This is occasionally seen in some developing countries where a woman has had many children. The loss of calcium from the mother during pregnancy has nothing to do with dental caries or bad teeth. Calcium is found in cheese, milk and cream. It is also present in fish, nuts, eggs and green vegetables such as broccoli and spinach.

The trace elements—phosphorus, copper, iodine, manganese, magnesium and cobalt—are essential for the formation of blood cells and many other tissues in the body. Only minute quantities are required by the body for its satisfactory function. A complete absence of them, however, will lead to gross deficiencies. The majority of these elements are found in small amounts in most of the proprietary iron preparations that are available.

Phosphorus is present in seafoods, cheese, eggs, milk, meat, onions and wholemeal bread.

Copper is present in most meat, liver, cheese and beans.

Iodine is present in nearly all fish foods and fish extracts. It is also possible to buy iodized salt which is sold in those areas where there is a natural shortage of iodine which can lead to the formation of goitre.

Manganese is found in most vegetables, especially peas, beans, wheat products, green vegetables and also in animal liver.

Magnesium is present in peas, beans, nuts and grain foods.

Folic acid is now accepted as a routine supplement during pregnancy although it is found in green leaf vegetables, yeast, liver and kidneys. A deficiency of folic acid causes megaloblastic anaemia, a particular type of anaemia which only affects pregnant women. Between 5 and 10 per cent of all pregnant women suffer from it, especially those who have repeated pregnancies at very short intervals and those who are expecting twins or triplets.

Folic acid may be administered as a separate tablet but is usually combined with the ordinary iron in one tablet. You will be told how many tablets you should take each day and these will provide you with all the iron and folic acid you require. Recent research suggests that folic acid supplements decrease the incidence of neural tube defects such as spina bifida (see Chapter 36).

Pica (abnormal food desires)

Some women develop abnormal and very peculiar likings for strange food during pregnancy. These are slightly different from the sort of food craze that affects everyone at times and to which most women are subject intermittently throughout their pregnancy. The result is a real craving for a particular type of food which they would not normally eat. These cravings are usually associated with materials that contain iron. Such food cravings are very uncommon today, but used to be very frequent in the past. There are many documented instances of women eating soil and coal, which in retrospect are interpreted as a subconscious desire to obtain iron.

Pica today is a rare phenomenon and is not to be confused with a particular liking for certain foods which women develop during pregnancy. Unfortunately, the likings are usually for carbohydrate foods and are therefore followed by undue weight gain. They can be controlled. On the other hand pica is almost completely uncontrollable and it is only with extreme difficulty that the woman can be weaned away from her abnormal desire. The primary treatment for such conditions is, of course, to correct any anaemia or vitamin deficiency.

14 Drugs in Pregnancy

Drugs which cross the placenta

All the material that the fetus requires for its growth and survival must be supplied to it from the mother by way of the placenta. Everything is passed in a comparatively simple chemical form for the fetus to manufacture into complex proteins and other substances. Similarly all the excreted products from the fetus are passed back to the mother across the placenta as simple chemical compounds. The most important chemical passed to the fetus is oxygen. The red blood cells of the fetus contain a haemoglobin, slightly different to that present in ordinary adult cells, which has the ability to absorb oxygen readily from the maternal blood and transfer it to its own tissues easily. Similarly all the fats, proteins and carbohydrates which the fetus requires for its growth must come from the mother. It follows then that any condition which affects the health of the placenta ('placental insufficiency'), or the passage of chemicals to the fetus (for example poor nutrition in the mother), will affect the health of the fetus. It is for this reason that a mother may be given extra oxygen to breathe if her fetus is distressed or short of oxygen.

Most drugs are simple chemicals which upon being introduced into the mother will pass from her circulation to that of the fetus because of a lower concentration on the fetal side of the placenta. Some of these may be beneficial to the fetus while others may cause harm, and those that are harmful are usually only capable of causing damage or trouble at a specific time during pregnancy. Although many different drugs may be taken by women, the ability to cross the placenta depends on the exact size of the drug molecule. Those chemicals with small molecules will pass easily into the circulation of the baby whereas those with large molecules will not.

Commonly used drugs such as aspirin, codeine and barbiturates (sleeping pills) do cross to the baby but rarely cause any harm. Most antibiotics cross the placental barrier and are present in the fetal circulation very shortly after administration to the mother, and in fact some of these are actually used to treat the fetus either during pregnancy or during labour when some obstetricians consider that the administration of antibiotics is advisable after a woman has had ruptured membranes for 24 hours. During recent years there have been some tragedies when the administration of drugs to the mother has led to mild, or even severe, congenital abnormalities in the fetus. The Thalidomide tragedy occurred some years ago when a supposedly safe and mild sedative was given to women in early pregnancy. Over 5,000 children throughout the world were born with limb defects, in some cases no limbs at all. Drugs which affect the fetus during its formative time, generally during the first 12 weeks, are said to be teratogenic. Today any new drug marketed into Britain has to have official approval of a special committee established to ensure that no such similar tragedy should occur. Very rigid regulations have to be adhered to before drugs can be sold to the public, particularly those that might be administered to women during pregnancy, and all new drugs are tested specifically in animals in order to assess their action upon the growing fetus.

Drugs have to be used correctly. They are safe in their correct dose but potentially dangerous or even lethal if that dose is exceeded or given at the wrong time or in the wrong manner. Furthermore, the effect on the fetus may depend on the stage of pregnancy at which the drug is given. A simple example demonstrates this. Should you have the misfortune to injure yourself and perhaps break a leg in the earlier part of your pregnancy you may be given a very large dose of pethidine or morphine in order to relieve the pain until your leg can be treated. Such a large dose of pethidine or morphine will certainly do your baby no harm. If, on the other hand, you are given a similar dose of pethidine or morphine about half an hour before your baby is to be delivered, then its breathing might easily be depressed when it is born, to such an extent that it has considerable trouble in establishing satisfactory respiration.

Should any drugs be taken?

In recent years, with the growing awareness that some diseases and illnesses in man have been substantially caused by toxic substances in the environment or the medical administration of drugs, some people have questioned the safety of any drugs given to the pregnant woman—including even iron tablets. Indeed, many of the minor alterations in a woman's body which lead to discomfort and complaint can be treated by a change in routine, rather than by drugs. Nausea or heartburn may respond to a change in diet, and eating small dry meals frequently. Constipation may improve with a diet containing more fibre. Inability to sleep may respond to a cup of warm milk, listening to music or reading a book before trying to sleep.

On the other hand, pregnancy may lead to major alterations in the body, or give rise to complications where drugs become mandatory to improve both the mother's and her baby's well-being. In rare instances, this may even include the life of mother and child. A simple and common example of this is iron-deficiency anaemia. The anaemic woman will feel tired and exhausted and not enjoy her pregnancy as well as she might.

Her body will be poorly prepared for the incredible physiological changes which occur during labour and the early puerperium She is more susceptible to infections during pregnancy, especially of the urinary tract. Her baby is more likely to be small and growth-retarded, and to be born prematurely. It may become distressed very easily during labour, and require special nursing care after it is born. The anaemic mother may become shocked very easily if she loses a lot of blood during delivery, and is more susceptible to infection in the puerperium, with all its dangers of thrombosis and even death. Hence, a whole chain of tragic events may occur if a simple anaemia is not detected and treated properly early in pregnancy.

Sometimes life-threatening situations may arise where drugs alone will save the mother and baby. For example, the diabetic with poor control of her illness may need large doses of insulin. The eclamptic woman, although rarely seen nowadays, urgently needs drugs to lower her blood pressure and to stop the fits.

These examples are given to put drugs into their right perspective. Given judiciously and only when medically necessary, their side effects will not be apparent or will be minimized. Of course there are some drugs given which may have side effects on the baby. In such cases, women are usually on long-term drug therapy for some medical disorder, for example diabetes, thyroid disease, high blood pressure, artificial heart valve or epilepsy. Both the doctor and the fully informed woman must weigh up the risks to the fetus of these drugs, as well as the risk to the woman's life of continuing pregnancy without their benefit. Such decisions can only be made by all the specialists involved in the woman's case.

Groups of drugs

The best way to discuss various drugs may be to describe their individual actions and the types of drugs that may be prescribed, and then to consider the different stages of pregnancy at which harm may occur.

Alkalis are taken for the relief of indigestion and heartburn, and appear harmless if taken in the prescribed dose. In large amounts they may decrease the amount of iron being absorbed and cause anaemia. Aluminium hydroxide does not have a laxative effect which other antacids may have. Magnesium trisilicate has a high sodium content and should not be given to women with heart disease, oedema or pre-eclampsia.

Antihistamines are mainly used to treat nausea and early morning sickness. Simple measures such as avoiding greasy foods and small frequent meals of dry foods should be tried before taking drugs. The risks to the fetus are not proven but only mild drugs such as promethazine (Avomine) should be used. In hyperemesis gravidarum (see page 182) stronger drugs may be given by injection.

Purgatives should, ideally, never be required. In many cases the constipation of pregnancy is a worsening of constipation in the non-pregnant state. It is important that women be educated to eat more fibre, be active, drink sufficient fluids and re-train bowel function so that the urge to stool is felt. If purgatives are necessary, the simplest possible drugs should be used first.

1 Stool bulk-forming drugs such as bran, Normacol and many others increase faecal mass, which increases the normal bowel movement.

2 Stimulant laxatives such as castor oil, Dorbanex, syrup of figs and senna derivatives increase bowel motility and may cause severe cramps if taken in excess. Plenty of fluids should also be taken.

3 Faecal softeners such as liquid paraffin lubricate and soften the faecal mass. Paraffin leaks through the anus and stains the underwear and may interfere with the absorption of certain vitamins (A, D and K).

4 Saline laxatives such as Milk of Magnesia and Epsom salts draw fluid into the bowel and therefore lots of fluids should be drunk.

Analgesics such as aspirin, codeine and paracetamol are taken for the relief of simple aches and pains or for the relief of headache and may be taken in early pregnancy quite safely. Codeine should not be taken regularly as it may be addictive (see below). Paracetamol in large doses can cause liver damage. Aspirin should not be used in large amounts towards the end of pregnancy as it interferes with the production of prostaglandins in the uterus (see Chapter 25). These small hormones are probably involved in the initiation and continuation of labour, and large amounts of aspirin may delay the onset and progress of labour. Aspirin can also cause clotting problems in the new-born baby. Drugs to treat migraine should not be taken if they contain ergotamine or its derivatives, as this causes the uterus to contract and is given to women to prevent haemorrhage immediately after the baby is born.

Anti-inflammatory drugs such as aspirin and indomethacin (Indocid) are given for the treatment of rheumatoid arthritis and chronic joint pain. They all act by inhibiting prostaglandins, and Indocid suppositories are sometimes given to women in premature labour to try to inhibit contractions.

Antibiotics should only be prescribed for a good medical reason.

1 Penicillins such as ampicillin are often prescribed for a urinary tract infection in pregnancy and appear to be safe at all stages.

2 Tetracyclines are the only antibiotic known to be teratogenic if taken in early pregnancy and can cause cataracts and bone abnormalities. Given later in pregnancy, they are stored in the teeth and bones of the fetus and cause ugly yellow staining of the deciduous ('milk') teeth if given after the 14th week, and of the permanent teeth any time after the 28th week.

3 Sulphonamides are often used to treat urinary tract infections and are safe in early pregnancy. They should be avoided in late pregnancy as they can precipitate jaundice in the new-born.

4 Streptomycin and other anti-tuberculosis drugs must be used with care as some are teratogenic and streptomycin can cause damage to the fetal ear, resulting in nerve deafness.

5 Penicillin allergy. Women who are allergic to penicillin may be given cephalosporins (e.g. Velosef), nalidixic acid (Negram) or nitrofurantoin (Furadantin) for urinary tract infections.

Tranquillizers. Mild drugs are often prescribed for anxiety although clearly the cause of the problem should be sought. These drugs are appropriate as a short course for a limited period of time. Barbiturates have been largely replaced by the benzodiazepine group of drugs which includes Valium, Librium and Mogadon. All are addictive with prolonged usage. Diazepam (Valium) taken before labour can cause the baby to have respiratory depression and problems with feeding and maintaining a normal body temperature.

Sedatives are sleeping pills. Barbiturates are addictive and milder substances such as nitrazepam (Mogadon) or chloral are safer. All will cause an abnormal sleep pattern with prolonged usage and rebound sleeplessness and rarely withdrawal symptoms when stopped.

Diuretics. There is some evidence that these are useful in reducing the oedema of pregnancy or pre-eclampsia, especially in late pregnancy. Large doses can lead to bleeding problems in the new-born.

Special drugs

Under the heading of special drugs are those drugs taken by a woman for some underlying disease or condition either daily or intermittently according to the demands of her illness. You should discuss the whole question of pregnancy with your doctor beforehand, even though most of these drugs may be taken safely during pregnancy.

Steroids should be avoided during pregnancy because of the slight risk of cleft palate in the fetus. When given chronically they may lead to suppression of the baby's adrenal glands and steroid production, so that the baby must receive cortisone treatment. However, some women will need to be on steroids, e.g. those with severe asthma or rheumatoid arthritis. Skin creams for eczema which contain cortisone derivatives should not be used for prolonged periods, as they are absorbed through the skin.

Thyroid drugs. Pregnant women with an over-active thyroid gland are given anti-thyroid drugs because surgical operation is hazardous during pregnancy. Drugs such as Carbimazole cross the placenta and can cause the baby to be born with insufficient thyroid hormone. They are therefore stopped towards the end of pregnancy and thyroid supplements given instead. Women suffering from an under-active thyroid gland rarely conceive and have a high incidence of spontaneous abortion and still-birth. The baby may have an under-active thyroid as well (cretinism). These women are put on thyroid replacement with thyroxine.

Diabetes during pregnancy is discussed in Chapter 21. Women who suffer from diabetes usually know a great deal about their disease and its control because they are members of a diabetic association. It requires very careful management during pregnancy. A very high blood sugar or an overdose of insulin can prove harmful to the fetus just as it can be to the pregnant woman herself. The rigid control of blood sugar levels during pregnancy is absolutely essential because it is well known that the unstable diabetic woman has a slightly higher incidence of congenital abnormality in her child than the non-diabetic woman. It is also known that the diabetic woman whose blood sugar is carefully controlled and who does not allow her blood sugar to fluctuate into the wild limits of abnormality does not have a higher incidence of congenital abnormality amongst her children, neither does she suffer from all the other problems that beset the pregnancy of the vulnerable diabetic. Insulin is always used in pregnancy because the oral hypoglycaemic agents cross the placenta and lower the blood sugar in the baby.

Cytotoxic drugs are used in the treatment of some types of cancer and malignant disease of the bone marrow, and because of the damaging effect they exert upon dividing cells, they are absolutely forbidden at any stage during pregnancy. These include methotrexate which may be given to some women with severe psoriasis, and cyclophosphamide or azathioprine which may be given to some women with severe auto-immune diseases or renal disease, including transplants.

Anti-convulsants all cause folic acid depletion and therefore supplements are given during pregnancy. Phenytoin (Epanutin) and primidone are teratogenic in animal studies. However the risk of uncontrolled epileptic fits may be far greater than the slight risk of congenital abnormality.

Anti-coagulants such as warfarin are teratogenic and may cause facial and bone deformities, cataracts and mental retardation if taken early in pregnancy. In mid-pregnancy they are comparatively safe but later, because they cross the placenta, they may cause bleeding problems in the fetus.

Injectable drugs such as heparin do not cross the placenta and therefore are used at the end of pregnancy.

Psychotropic drugs may be taken by some women with psychiatric disorders and include tranquillizers such as chlorpromazine (Largactil) and haloperidol (Serenace), as well as anti-depressants called monoamine oxidase inhibitors. All such women should be under specialist psychiatric care. There is some evidence that Largactil may cause eye damage to the fetus and the new-born baby may be floppy and have trouble in maintaining his body temperature.

Addictive drugs

Some of these drugs such as alcohol and nicotine are used in a socially acceptable way, although there is evidence that even small amounts may have a harmful effect on the fetus, and the woman trying to conceive should stop taking them before conception. Other drugs such as heroin are only used by addicts and these women should be encouraged to seek professional help.

Cannabis and LSD. Although little is known about the effects of these drugs on the fetus, it appears that both may be teratogenic (LSD causes chromosome damage) and both may cause growth retardation of the fetus.

Opiates. Babies who are born to heroin addicts, or mothers on methadone replacement, become addicted *in utero* and suffer withdrawal symptoms with irritability, shaking, vomiting and diarrhoea, sweating, sneezing, and feeding problems. They tend to be growth-retarded and may die from their addiction.

Alcohol. Recent research from the United States suggests that up to 25 per cent of pregnant women who may drink as little as 1 oz of alcohol twice a week are more likely to have a spontaneous abortion than women who do not drink. However, many women continue to drink moderately without any problem during pregnancy, although some develop an aversion to it. Alcohol abuse results in an increase in mid-trimester abortion and premature labour (even though alcohol can be used intravenously as a drug to stop premature labour). Alcohol in excess is teratogenic and babies born with the so-called 'fetal alcohol syndrome' are growth-retarded with characteristic facial deformities, cardiac malformations and mental retardation. At least 40 such children have been identified in the West Scotland region in the past ten years.

Nicotine. Women should not smoke during pregnancy. The fetus is affected by nicotine, carbon monoxide and other substances in cigarettes, just as in adult life. Ultrasound shows that the fetal breathing pattern is disturbed and the heart rate increases even if the mother is not smoking herself but merely sitting in a smoke-filled room ('passive smoking'). Constriction of the placental vessels results in fetal growth retardation and this depends on the number of cigarettes smoked each day. Smoking has been associated with premature delivery and rupture of membranes, a doubled risk of early spontaneous abortion, ante- and post-partum haemorrhage, congenital abnormality, still-birth and a higher risk of neo-natal death.

There are many things about a baby that cannot be assessed, such as its liver function, its kidney function, its heart condition or its intellect. Its weight, however, can be measured. Many people have an unhappy feeling that when medical science has advanced sufficiently to measure the physiological and mental powers of the new-born infant it might well be found that the babies of women who smoke do in fact suffer from deficiencies other than just a simple reduction in size. There is evidence today that smoking after the 16th week of pregnancy causes mental and physical retardation in later childhood.

Hormones

Hormones are often given in early pregnancy for one of two reasons. Firstly, to try to confirm the diagnosis of pregnancy: a small amount of oestrogen and progesterone is given for one, two or even three days and, if the woman is not pregnant, then a period will follow. If she is pregnant there will be no bleeding. Such hormones are not recommended as it is controversial whether they may be teratogenic. This also applies to women who conceive whilst taking the oral contraceptive pill (see Chapter 43). Secondly, hormone is given either by mouth or by injection over a fairly prolonged period to treat a threatened abortion or to treat women who have previously miscarried or who are shown to be deficient in progesterone. This can be diagnosed by taking a scraping of cells from the vagina and looking at their hormonal status under the microscope. There is no evidence that hormones given for any reason other than this uncommon one, called corpus luteum deficiency, have any benefit in maintaining a pregnancy. In fact, if a woman is going to abort, giving a hormone simply delays the diagnosis by preventing the bleeding which alerts the woman that something is wrong.

Oestrogen in large doses was given to women in the United States to prevent spontaneous abortion, and we now know years later that female infants born to those mothers run the tragic risk of acquiring a rare form of vaginal cancer. Some older preparations of progesterone can cause virilization (development of masculine characteristics) of a female child, because they are broken down to male hormones in the body. These are no longer given, and the hormone preparations that are presently in use are quite safe.

Anaesthesia

Local anaesthetics in the prescribed dose may be administered during pregnancy without any harm coming to the pregnant woman or to her baby. This is particularly applicable to dental anaesthesia.

General anaesthetics and operations are best avoided during pregnancy if possible, but may sometimes be necessary, e.g. for appendicitis or the removal of an ovarian cyst. After the first trimester this appears to be safe with adequate oxygen supplied to the baby as well as the mother during the operation. However, nitrous oxide inhaled over a long period may be teratogenic in early pregnancy, and women who work in operating theatres have a higher risk of aborting spontaneously. At the other end of pregnancy, the baby born by Caesarean section under general anaesthetic may have more trouble initiating breathing than the baby born under epidural anaesthetic (see Chapter 24).

Drugs normally administered during pregnancy

Iron and simple iron preparations are essential for the mother's welfare and the prevention of anaemia during pregnancy. The majority of iron tablets available for pregnant women have been specifically prepared for the purpose and also contain the various trace elements required such as copper, manganese, magnesium and cobalt. Even iron, however, should not be given to women who suffer from a very rare disease called thalassaemia until fairly extensive blood tests have been carried out. Thalassaemia is extremely rare in Great Britain and the routine tests performed on a woman's blood at the very commencement of pregnancy automatically ensure that this disease is diagnosed. Do not worry about taking your iron pills.

Vitamin supplements have now become a part of normal antenatal care. They are perfectly safe and should be taken as prescribed.

Calcium supplements are frequently prescribed during pregnancy especially to those people who suffer from muscular cramps. In many countries calcium supplements are given as a routine together with iron and vitamin preparations. It is not true that excess calcium will cause the baby's bones to become brittle or its skull to be unduly hard so that delivery is difficult.

Fluoride. The role of fluoride in preventing dental decay is generally accepted and some dentists do support the routine administration of fluoride to women during pregnancy on the principle that their children will therefore have less dental decay.

Drugs at different stages of pregnancy

The first trimester is the first 14 weeks of pregnancy and it is during this stage that drugs or other factors may lead to the formation of congenital abnormalities in the rapidly developing fetus. Drugs administered after the end of the 12th week of pregnancy should not result in any developmental abnormality of the baby because by that time all its organs are properly formed and cannot, therefore, be damaged. Teratogenic drugs should not be given at any stage of pregnancy. These include Thalidomide, phenytoin, anti-thyroid drugs, anti-cancer agents, some sex hormones, alcohol, tetracycline and some anaesthetic agents.

The second trimester is from the 14th to the 28th week of pregnancy and is the stage of the main physiological growth of the fetus as well as the development of its enzyme systems and other highly complex endocrinological processes. Abnormalities in the development of these processes would not be immediately obvious at birth but discoloration of the teeth by the administration of tetracycline, damage to nerves of the ear by the administration of streptomycin or hidden damage to the baby by overdose of insulin can all occur during this stage of pregnancy.

The third trimester is from the 28th week until delivery. It is during this time that thyroid drugs may cause abnormal growth of the thyroid gland and other drugs such as anticoagulants may adversely affect the baby. Cigarette smoking is thought to exert its main effect after the 16th week of pregnancy. Sulphonamides taken late in pregnancy may prevent the new-born baby's liver from dealing quickly with jaundice. Valium in moderate doses for some weeks before delivery may make the baby sleepy, slow to cry and poor to feed after delivery. Methadone and heroin exert their main addictive effects on the baby at this stage, and large doses of aspirin and other anti-inflammatory drugs may prolong pregnancy.

Labour. The administration of hypnotic, analgesic and anaesthetic drugs during labour is very carefully controlled because nearly all, if not all, of these drugs do in fact cross the placenta to the fetus. A woman who is sedated too heavily during labour may give birth to a baby so heavily sedated that it may be slow to breathe spontaneously. Drugs given to control blood pressure may have transient effects on the baby's heart rate and ability to metabolize glucose, and Syntocinon may cause jaundice in the new-born.

Drugs and breast feeding

Nearly all drugs given to the mother will find their way into breast milk but usually in such small amounts as not to affect the baby. Laxatives, especially senna derivatives, may cause colic and diarrhoea in the new-born. Antibiotics such as tetracycline and streptomycin should be avoided, as should sulpha-containing drugs. Anti-thyroid drugs may cause a goitre in the baby. Steroids should be avoided, as should all sedatives or tranquillizers such as barbiturates or Valium which will cause drowsiness and sometimes feeding problems. Even alcohol, if ingested in large amounts, can cause intoxication in the baby. Anticoagulants and large doses of aspirin can cause bleeding problems in the infant. Women who are advised not to breast-feed for a medical reason, or whose baby has died, can be given a safe drug called bromocriptine to stop the production of milk, and relieve the discomfort in the breasts.

15 Care of the Breasts

On your first visit to the antenatal clinic you will probably be asked if you wish to breast-feed your baby. If you have not yet decided or are in doubt you should discuss it with the midwife. You don't have to decide immediately but the sooner the better because the preparation for breast-feeding should begin in early pregnancy.

You will be instructed in the advantages of breast-feeding and if you are going to feed your baby yourself your intention to do so will be encouraged. You must also realize, even at this stage, that if you do not wish to breast-feed, or some unforeseen circumstance leads to failure of breast-feeding, proper artificial feeding, despite its additional labour, is both safe and effective.

The routine examination of the mother's breasts at the first antenatal clinic includes an assessment of the suitability of the nipples for breast-feeding. The breasts and nipples are re-examined at regular intervals. If by the sixth month of pregnancy the nipples are retracted (turned inwards) then shells should be worn daily until the nipples become everted.

An adequate diet during pregnancy is fundamental as it has a direct influence on normal healthy development of the unborn child and is an important factor in successful breast-feeding.

The size of the breasts before pregnancy has no influence on the mother's ability to breast-feed successfully.

Cleanliness of the breasts

Antenatal care aims at promoting and maintaining cleanliness of the breasts, particularly the nipples. The breasts and nipples should be carefully washed and dried each day, particular attention being paid to the undersurface of the breasts and to removing any crusted secretions on the nipples.

Expression of colostrum

If the onset of breastfeeding has been difficult in a previous pregnancy, and sometimes in a first pregnancy, it is helpful to express colostrum which is similar to milk before the baby is due. The midwife will instruct on expression of colostrum by the pregnant woman herself. The hands and breasts are lubricated with baby oil. The fingers and palms grasp the breast and stroke gently in a downward direction towards the nipple for a few moments. The finger and thumb are then placed on the outer margin of the pigmented area surrounding the nipple and with a squeezing movement the colostrum is expelled from the breast.

Some women may only produce colostrum after the baby is born. Nevertheless, learning how to handle the breasts before the birth is useful, as many women may need at times to express milk once lactation has begun.

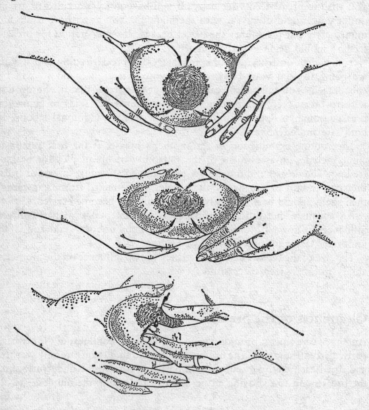

Fig. 21 Expression of colostrum

Brassiere

The weight of the enlarged breasts tends to pull them down so that the tissue attaching the breasts to the chest wall and the skin over the upper part of the breasts become stretched Stretching of the supporting tissues causes the breasts to sag and must be prevented during pregnancy by wearing a good supporting brassiere. Enlargement of the breasts may increase the bust measurement by as much as 8 to 10 cm. Well-supported breasts will not lose their shape but it is surprising how quickly breasts will sag if they are not adequately supported. This is, of course, particularly applicable to the few days immediately after delivery. It is true that, following pregnancy, delivery and breast-feeding the breasts will never regain the same consistency that they had before pregnancy commenced, but if they are properly supported and looked after there is no reason why they should change their shape or droop.

The nipple

Different advice is frequently given about care of the breasts in pregnancy and this advice changes not only from year to year but also from town to town and country to country. It is often incorrectly stated that the nipples should be bathed in alcohol in order to 'harden the skin' or scrubbed with a soft brush. Nipples of normal shape and size require no care other than the daily use of soap and water, and perhaps massage of the nipples and the surrounding skin with a bland cream such as lanolin once each day to make the skin soft and pliable, and gentle moulding and drawing out of the nipples between the thumb and index finger. Dry skin is thus avoided. This procedure can conveniently become part of the daily bath routine.

Inverted nipple

Inversion of the nipple is usually a congenital condition in which the nipple fails to protrude at all, or remains flat or inverted when stimulated. It is obvious that a child cannot feed from a breast unless the nipple protrudes so that it can be placed completely within the child's mouth. Inversion can be corrected or cured by manipulation and by wearing Woolwich breast shells. These should be worn underneath a closely fitting brassiere with good supporting straps so that the nipple protrudes through the aperture on the flat surface of one side of the shell. The shell consists of two plastic halves screwed together and its particular shape together with the woman's continual movement exert a gradual, constant, evenly distributed pressure on tissues and structures immediately around the nipple, which will eventually cause normal protrusion of the nipple. The time during pregnancy at which a woman should begin wearing breast shells varies with the severity of the inversion of the nipple. Most authorities recommend that they should be worn during the last six to eight weeks of pregnancy, initially for only one or two hours a day, preferably during the afternoon. After about one week the shells may be worn for progressively longer periods each day until after three or four weeks they are being worn throughout the day. There is no need to wear the shells at night.

In the last three or four weeks of pregnancy some secretion may occur from the nipple. This is completely normal and providing the shells are worn with the air-hole uppermost the secretion will be collected in the shell itself.

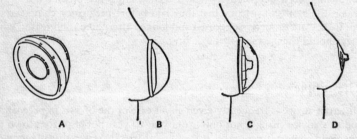

Fig 22   Breast shells
A   breast shell
B   breast shell on retracted nipple
C   nipple protracting into shell
D   nipple fully protracted after wearing breast shells

Care must be taken that the shells are not worn for an excessive length of time each day and this must be judged by the individual. If they are worn for too long the skin around the nipple becomes sore and tender. The shells should be washed and dried each day after taking them apart to empty the colostrum. The skin of the breast that is in contact with the plastic should be lightly powdered to avoid irritation due to perspiration.

16 Maternity Benefits

The social services in Great Britain provide certain benefits for a woman during her pregnancy. The rules and regulations governing these benefits are continually changing, especially the financial benefits which are seldom constant for more than a year at a time.

The maternity benefits as set out in this chapter are those in force at the time of writing and will almost certainly have been changed by the time you come to read it. For up-to-date information you should write to the Department of Health and Social Security or enquire at your local post office or local social security office for the appropriate pamphlets (MV11 and NI17A) dealing with free welfare foods and maternity benefits.

Maternity grant

If you satisfy the rules for maternity grant you will be sent a Girocheque for £25.

If the baby is stillborn the grant will be paid provided the pregnancy lasted for 28 weeks or longer.

If you have twins or triplets, etc., you can get a grant for each child who lives for more than 12 hours (although if all died, one grant would still be paid).

How to claim. You claim your maternity grant by filling in form BM4. You can get the form from your local social security office or maternity or child health clinic.

When to claim. You can claim at any time from the 14th week before your baby is expected until 3 months after your baby is born.

If you do not claim until more than 3 months after the birth, you will not get the grant unless you can show you had good reason for not claiming earlier.

The grant can't be paid at all if you make your claim more than 12 months after the birth.

The new rules

You qualify for the grant if you have lived in Great Britain for a total of more than 182 days (26 weeks) in the 52 weeks before the week in which your baby is expected. If you claim after the birth this rule must be satisfied before the date of the birth.

If you normally live in Great Britain but you cannot satisfy the rule because you've been temporarily abroad, you can count towards the total any days in those 52 weeks when you were abroad if you comply with certain conditions (see leaflet NI17A).

If you have been abroad in a European Community country or a country with which the United Kingdom has a reciprocal agreement which covers maternity grant, you may be able to get the grant even though you do not satisfy the above rules.

If you claim before the birth, you must be in Great Britain when you make your claim.

If your baby is born abroad

If you are going to have a baby in a country which has a reciprocal agreement on social security with the United Kingdom (other than Israel) or in one of the other countries of the European Community, claim your maternity grant at the normal time.

If your baby is born abroad, you will get the grant if you can meet the normal rules (the more than 182 days in 52 weeks rule) and one of the following:

1 you are entitled to child benefit for the week following the birth;
2 you are confined during a temporary absence from Great Britain which was not intended to last more than 4 weeks;
3 you were a serving member of HM Forces up to 13 weeks before your baby was born;
4 either you or your husband have paid contributions (or have credits) on earnings of at least 50 times the lower earnings limit in the last complete tax year ending more than 3 months before the birth. If you meet this rule on your husband's National Insurance record you must be living with him at the time of the baby's birth or, if you are a widow, you must have been living with him when he died.

Maternity allowance

The weekly maternity allowance can be paid only on your own contributions. As your contributions do not count for benefit until some time after you have paid them, you could still qualify for the allowance on contributions you paid some while ago. So check carefully the contribution conditions.

Only full contributions count, not the reduced-rate ones that some married women and widows can pay

You can claim maternity allowance each time you have a baby if you have enough contributions paid or credited in the right tax year. You may qualify even if you have not worked since your last baby was born. You can qualify for the allowance from the start of the 11th week before the week in which your baby is expected (but not while you are doing paid work). Unless your baby is born later than expected, the allowance will be paid until the end of the 6th week after the expected week of confinement. In this way, the allowance can last for up to 18 weeks. If your baby is late, payment of the allowance may be extended.

If you do not claim until after the baby is born, the allowance is normally payable for the week of the birth and the 6 following weeks. Maternity allowance can be paid with maternity pay from your employer. But the maternity allowance cannot be paid at the same time as you are getting any other weekly National Insurance benefit (e.g. sickness or unemployment benefit, or widow's benefit), an unemployability supplement of any kind or a training allowance from public funds. If you are entitled to more than one benefit at the same time you will normally get an amount equal to the greater, or greatest, of them.

How to claim. You claim the allowance by filling in both sections of form BM4. You get the form from your social security office or maternity or child health clinic.

When to claim. Claim as soon as you can after the beginning of the 14th week before your baby is expected, even if you are still working. If you claim later than the 8th week you may lose the allowance for some of the weeks before the one in which you make your claim.

If you want to claim for someone who is dependent on you, tick the appropriate box on page 2 of form BM4 and you will be sent a claim form to fill in. Do not delay claiming or you may lose the extra benefit for any period earlier than one month before you claim the increase.

How the allowance is paid. If you qualify, you will get a book of weekly orders containing the allowance to which you are entitled. If you are entitled to extra benefit for a dependant, this will be included. See leaflet NI196 for the weekly rate.

The National Insurance contribution rules

To get maternity allowance you must meet two contribution rules:

First contribution rule. In any one tax year since you started work, you must have paid a minimum amount of employed or self-employed contributions. This minimum is equal to the amount of contributions that would be payable over 25 weeks by someone with weekly earnings at the lower earnings limit.

You must meet this rule before the Sunday of the 11th week before the week in which your baby is expected (or the Sunday of the 11th week before the week in which the baby is born if you claim afterwards).

The first rule is met if you paid 26 flat-rate Class 1 contributions before 6 April 1975.

The rule can also be met if you paid Class 1 contributions on earnings totalling at least 25 × the lower earnings limit, even though your employment lasted for less than 25 weeks.

Second contribution rule. In the relevant tax year you must have paid or been credited with Class 1 or 2 contributions equal to the amount payable on earnings at the lower earnings limit for 50 weeks.

In the 1982–83 tax year, for example, a woman earning £29.50 a week would need to have paid contributions on earnings of at least £1,475 (50 × 29.50) to satisfy the second condition; if she were earning more than £29.50 per week she would have paid enough in less than 50 weeks.

If you meet the first contribution rule but do not fully meet the second, you may be able to get benefit at half or three quarters of the standard rate. If you have received sickness, invalidity or unemployment benefit for a day within 8 weeks of the relevant time, you are likely to be entitled to maternity allowance at the same rate.

Credited contributions

Credited contributions can help you to meet the second contribution rule. Credits are equal in value to contributions paid on earnings at the weekly lower earnings limit. Credits awarded in the relevant tax year for weeks when you were undertaking training approved by the DHSS or claiming unemployment or sickness benefit or maternity allowance may count towards the second contribution rule in certain circumstances.

You may also be entitled to special credits to help you to meet the second contribution rule if you are or were a short time ago (see leaflet NI17A):

1 a school-leaver or other new contributor;
2 a student, trainee or apprentice;
3 a divorced woman;
4 a widow.

If you think credits may help your claim, tell the social security office when sending in your claim form.

Credits while you are getting maternity allowance. You will normally be entitled to be credited with a contribution for each complete week for which you receive maternity allowance.

Extra allowances if your baby arrives late

Your allowance will be paid until 6 weeks after your baby is born. Write and tell the social security office if your baby is late and enclose either the certificate of confinement supplied by your doctor or midwife or the baby's birth certificate.

If your baby has not been born by the date of the last order in your order book, tell the social security office (not later than 6 weeks after that date) that you are still expecting your baby.

Claiming after your baby is born

You will not get the allowance for the full period of 18 weeks unless your baby has been born more than 11 weeks early, or you can give some other good reason why you have not claimed before. If you claim within 3 weeks after the baby is born, the allowance is paid for 7 weeks starting with the week of the birth. If you claim later than this, you may lose even more benefit.

If you have delayed your claim until after the birth and your baby arrived earlier than expected, ask the midwife or doctor to give you a certificate of confinement, giving on it the date on which the baby had been expected. You may then get the allowance up to the end of the 6th week after the week in which the baby was expected.

Increased benefit for your dependants

An increase of your allowance may be paid for a dependent child or children, if you are a single parent or your husband is earning no more than £16 (1983 figure) a week. Increases may also be payable for one adult dependant (a husband earning less than £16 or a woman who looks after your children). Fuller information can be found in the leaflet.

If your maternity allowance is paid at a reduced rate because you cannot fully meet the contribution conditions, any increase for an adult dependant (but not for a child) will be paid at a lower rate. An increase for a dependant may also be reduced or not paid at all if other payments are being made for that dependant.

Invalidity benefit

After getting maternity allowance or sickness benefit for 168 days, you can get invalidity benefit. See leaflet NI16A.

If you are or have been abroad

There are reciprocal agreements affecting maternity benefit between the UK and some other countries (Austria, Cyprus, Finland, Guernsey, Israel,

Jersey, Norway, Portugal, Spain, Sweden, Turkey and Yugoslavia) and there are also arrangements with the other countries of the European Community (Belgium, Denmark, Federal Republic of Germany, France, Gibraltar, Irish Republic, Italy, Luxembourg, the Netherlands and Greece). This may help you to qualify for maternity allowance if you (or your husband) have paid contributions in, or your baby is born in, one of those countries, or enable you to get the benefit while you are there or on your return to the UK. For information about these agreements, write, stating the country concerned, to the Department of Health and Social Security, Overseas Branch, Newcastle upon Tyne NE98 1YX.

Further information

If you need further advice or help in completing the forms, contact your social security office.

Expectant mothers are entitled to free prescriptions and free dental treatment and new mothers to free prescriptions for 12 months after the birth. Women whose families are entitled to the family income supplement or supplementary benefit also qualify for a range of other free services, including free milk and vitamins. Details can be found in leaflets P11, D11, G11, H11 and MV11 from post offices and social security offices. H11 (help with fares to hospital) can also be obtained from hospitals.

Employment rights for the expectant mother

If you are expecting a baby and are in full- or part-time employment, recent employment legislation gives you certain rights such as time off to receive antenatal care or to return to your job after the birth. These rights are generally available to all women employees, but they are all subject to conditions and limitations, so it is essential to read the Department of Employment's booklet PL710.

Some women are not covered by the provisions of this legislation, for instance, women who work freelance or abroad or who are members of the police force or armed forces.

If you are expecting a baby and working, you should obtain leaflet PL710 from a Jobcentre, employment office or unemployment benefit office and read it carefully. You should also check your contract of employment or your trade union's agreement with your employers to see what additional rights you may have.

Time off for antenatal care

You are entitled to have time off work, with pay, to receive antenatal care. However, you must make an appointment first and then ask permission of your employer to keep that appointment. The employer has the right to ask to see your appointment card and a certificate from a doctor, midwife or health visitor to say that you are pregnant.

Unfair dismissal

If your employer sacks you because you are pregnant or because of a reason connected with your pregnancy, you may be able to complain to a tribunal of unfair dismissal. Your rights depend on how long you have worked for your employer, whether the firm is big or small and how many hours you work each week.

Some dismissals by reason of pregnancy may be considered as 'fair' in terms of the legislation, for instance, if it is illegal for pregnant women to do certain jobs or if it is impossible for a woman to do her job adequately while she is pregnant. However, the dismissal becomes unfair if the employer does not offer suitable alternative work.

Someone who is dismissed 'fairly' and not re-engaged in suitable alternative work is still entitled to maternity pay from the employer and has the right to return to her original job after her maternity absence, provided she fulfils certain conditions.

Maternity pay

If you satisfy the necessary conditions, your employer should give you maternity pay for six weeks. If you leave work at or after the 11th week before your expected date of confinement, you should receive nine tenths of your normal week's pay, less the amount of the maternity allowance. Your employer can claim this money back from a government fund. If your employer refuses to give you maternity pay to which you are entitled, you can ask the Department of Employment to pay you direct from the fund. Full details are in booklet PL710.

Some contracts of employment provide for full salary (less the maternity allowance) to be paid to the employee for longer periods than those laid down by the legislation, so it is wise to read your contract of employment, staff regulations or trade union agreement carefully.

The right to return to work

A woman has the right to return to her former job at any time before the end of the period of 29 weeks beginning with the week in which her child was born and to be treated in exactly the same way as if she had not been absent. However, she must meet all the conditions laid down.

She must have worked continuously for at least two years with the same employer (five years if she works for 8 to 16 hours a week only) and she must continue to work until the beginning of the 11th week before the expected week of her confinement. She must also, if it is reasonably practicable, tell her employer in writing that:

1 she will be (or is) absent from work to have a baby; and
2 she intends to return to work for her employer after her absence; and
3 the expected week of confinement (or if the confinement has occurred, the date of confinement).

Her employer may ask to see a certificate of the expected week of confinement signed by a doctor or midwife.

The employer is entitled to write to the employee 49 days after the date given as the beginning of the expected week of confinement to ask the employee to confirm in writing that she intends to return. The employee must reply within 14 days or as soon as is practicable, otherwise she will lose the right to return.

The employee must also inform the employer in writing of the date she proposes to return at least 21 days before that date. She is free to decide on that date, provided it is before the end of the period of 29 weeks beginning with the week in which her child is born. The date can be changed for medical or for personal reasons (but only once in the latter case).

It is most important that the woman who wishes to return to work notifies her employer of her intentions at the correct times and gives him all the necessary information. Booklet PL710 has a useful appendix of sample letters for both employee and employer to use; these letters include all the details required.

There are cases where a woman does not get her job back. Her job may have become redundant during her absence or her employer may find it impracticable to have her back. If she is employed by a firm with fewer than 5 employees, the firm does not have to take her back. All these situations are explained in booklet PL710.

If, when she has carefully read the booklet, a woman feels that her rights have been ignored, she should go to a Jobcentre, employment office or unemployment benefit office and ask for leaflet ITL1 and a form of application to an industrial tribunal. A conciliation officer of the Advisory, Conciliation and Arbitration Service will probably try to get both sides to reach a settlement without going before a tribunal. It is also possible to get advice from a conciliation officer without making a formal application to a tribunal first.

17 The Health of the Fetus

The baby is completely formed by the end of the 12th week of pregnancy and it is usually during these first 12 weeks that the baby can be severely damaged. After about the 16th week when the afterbirth, or placenta, is fully developed and completely functioning it is extremely difficult to harm the fetus because it is then purely growing and maturing.

All drugs should be avoided if possible during the first 12 weeks of pregnancy and certainly no drugs should be taken without the doctor's advice. Simple drugs such as aspirin for headache, alkali for indigestion, and also mild purgatives if necessary, will cause no harm (see Chapter 14).

Diseases which may affect the fetus

There are many conditions which occur both before and during pregnancy which may adversely affect the health of the fetus. These may be divided into two sections: infections which occur in the mother and are transmitted across the placenta to the fetus (direct infection of the fetus from the vagina while still within the uterus is virtually unknown); general or localized diseases of the mother, which, for some reason or another, will adversely affect the baby.

Infections

The main infections which may seriously affect the fetus are rubella and syphilis. Rubella has been discussed extensively in Chapter 11. It affects the baby mainly during the first 12 weeks of pregnancy. The infection is transmitted from the mother across the placenta to the fetus and may damage the eyes, the ears, the heart or other organs as they are developing. Maternal infection by rubella after the 12th week of pregnancy may not cause congenital abnormality for by this time all the organs are fully developed but the virus may interfere with maturation and cause a hearing defect.

There is evidence that all virus infections may adversely affect the developing fetus and although the incidence of congenital abnormality as a result of rubella is far greater than from other virus infections such as Asian flu and mumps, these are nevertheless associated with an increased incidence of congenital abnormality.

Syphilis is caused by an organism called treponema pallidum which can only cross the placental barrier after the 20th week of pregnancy. It may severely affect the fetus and lead to its death within the uterus, or, if the baby lives, he will most certainly be delivered with congenital syphilis. The diagnosis of syphilis at the beginning of pregnancy is of the utmost importance because if it is satisfactorily treated before the 20th week the baby will not be affected.

Toxoplasmosis is an extremely common parasitic disease in the human affecting approximately 30 per cent of people by the age of 30. Although this is a relatively common disease, very little is known about it or its mode of spread. In the very few instances when a woman develops active toxoplasmosis during the first 12 weeks of pregnancy she does run a small risk that her baby might have his eyesight or other organs affected. Toxoplasmosis is rather like rubella in that a previous attack confers life-long immunity and the only time at which a baby can be affected is when an initial and acute attack occurs in the mother within the first 12 weeks of pregnancy. Despite the very common incidence of toxoplasmosis the number of people who develop toxoplasmosis during early pregnancy is very small indeed and the number of instances of congenital toxoplasmosis is also small. The parasite may be picked up from cat faeces.

There are a number of unusual diseases which may also affect the fetus in the uterus, one of which is severe malaria. Apart from the above mentioned diseases, other infections of the fetus within the uterus are extremely rare.

General diseases affecting the mother

It is certainly true to say that the fetus within the uterus behaves as a parasite and extracts from the mother as much as it requires for its own growth and nutrition. Certain conditions in the mother, however, do adversely affect her ability to supply the child with its nutritional requirements, or alternatively will lead to the formation of a small placenta so that the fetus cannot grow as rapidly as it might otherwise.

Severe anaemia and deficiency states in the mother may adversely affect her ability to transfer oxygen and other nutritional substances to the baby which may then be retarded in its growth. There are certain factors which seem to prevent the development of a proper placenta and therefore adversely affect the fetus. These include chronic kidney disease, a persistently raised blood pressure and pre-eclampsia. There are also other, as yet unknown, factors which predispose to the development of a small placenta and which may lead to a baby being delivered prematurely or being dysmature. (A dysmature baby is a baby who is small but otherwise perfectly normal.)

Diabetes may also adversely affect the baby.

A very high temperature can sometimes cause the onset of premature labour.

Traumatic injury to the baby *in utero*

It is almost impossible to cause physical injury to a baby within the uterus as a result of a direct blow or accident as he is extremely well cushioned. The uterus itself is carefully protected even in a thin woman not only by the maternal spine and pelvis but also by the anterior abdominal wall. The uterus is soft and flexible and the baby lies within a fluid sac inside it. The amniotic fluid in which the baby floats protects him from being harmed by a direct blow. It would take the most violent and severe of blows with a sharp instrument to damage the baby in the uterus. Many women have fallen down stairs and off stepladders without doing their pregnancies or babies any harm despite quite extensive injuries to themselves.

The immunity of the fetus

Virus infections of the new-born baby are uncommon. During his time in the uterus and for 6 weeks after delivery the baby has no active immunity to any disease to which he may be exposed because he cannot manufacture antibodies. The diseases which may affect the fetus are discussed above and it will be noted that, with the exception of the viruses, only a few micro-organisms including those of syphilis and toxoplasmosis are capable of crossing the placental barrier to infect the fetus, so that the fetus does not need to develop antibodies against any of the common bacterial diseases. This deficiency is compensated to a certain extent by the passage of antibodies from the mother across the placenta to the fetus. The new-born infant, therefore, possesses antibodies in his blood of approximately the same strength and to the same diseases as those which are present in the mother's blood. This is known as a passive immunity and after a time, which varies from 6 to 12 weeks, these antibodies gradually disappear from the baby's blood, and he then becomes susceptible to all these diseases.

Immunity to two most important diseases is not passed from the mother to her baby. One is tuberculosis, to which the new-born infant is particularly susceptible even if the mother has active disease and therefore a high level of antibodies, and the other is whooping cough. A new-born baby must be protected from all infectious diseases and especially these two.

A certain amount of immunity is supposed to be conferred as a result of breast-feeding. Breast-milk certainly contains antibodies to various diseases but it is uncertain how much immunity they confer on the baby.

Diseases contracted by the fetus during birth

There are certain viral and bacterial diseases which may be contracted by the fetus during labour and the passage through the birth canal.

Gonorrhoea is a venereally transmitted disease which may not be symptomatic in the mother. However, the baby's eyes may become infected during birth and blindness result unless treated with penicillin or other antibiotics.

Monilia (see Chapter 12) may cause 'thrush' to develop in the baby's mouth and on the skin. This is treated with the same fungicidal preparations as in the mouth. It is for this reason that all women with vaginal discharge and irritation should tell their doctor.

Genital herpes virus (related to the virus which causes 'cold sores' on the face) may cause recurrent attacks in an affected woman. Any woman who becomes pregnant should tell her doctor if she has had herpes in the past. In the last few weeks of pregnancy swabs are taken from the vagina to ensure that the virus is not actively present. If it is, then the woman will be advised to have a Caesarean section, for there is a 50 per cent chance that the baby will die if it contracts the viral disease during the process of vaginal delivery. Women who are carriers of hepatitis B may also infect their babies during birth and a blood test can be done within the first few months of life to see if the baby is a carrier.

18 Complications of Pregnancy

This book presents the facts concerning pregnancy and is intended to make pregnant women aware of what is happening to them It is also intended to inform them about the many changes associated with pregnancy so that they are aware of some of the warning signs of dangers which may be involved. Pregnant women are highly susceptible to suggestion and it is very difficult to warn them about complications without creating doubts or making them afraid. Antenatal care today prevents many complications and can deal satisfactorily with most of those that do arise, and as long as pregnant women attend the antenatal clinic regularly and heed any warning symptoms they need not worry about their progress.

A normal pregnancy requires very little more than a certain amount of homage, and it is reasonable to expect a woman to take more care of herself when she is pregnant. She should have more rest; she should not take drugs and should not expose herself to undue dangers or to the risk of infections which might possibly harm her unborn infant. The pregnant woman can behave almost normally in the early part of pregnancy apart from these cautions, since the fetus is extremely well protected within the uterus. She need not restrict her activities in any way, unless she usually undertakes a lot of physical activity, in which case she should ask her doctor about continuing. The ability of a pregnancy to continue quite normally despite the most outrageous insults is shown by the number of women who attempt to get rid of unwanted pregnancies and find that all their efforts are completely unsuccessful.

Bleeding in early pregnancy

When a pregnancy occurs the first period that should come after the implantation of the ovum is normally suppressed, so that there is no bleeding. Subsequently all the periods that would normally occur are likewise suppressed throughout the pregnancy. This is because a greater amount of the hormone progesterone is being produced. It occasionally happens, however, that the level of progesterone is not sufficiently high and a certain amount of bleeding occurs when the period would be expected. This usually goes under the heading of a 'partially suppressed period'. Bleeding at this time is usually comparatively slight and may last for only a few minutes, a few hours or perhaps for one or two days. The loss is much less than usual and the colour is darker. There is no pain.

It is not generally recognized that a woman can have partially suppressed periods while she is pregnant and it is therefore understandable that although she may feel some of the symptoms of pregnancy she may not realize that she is pregnant, and it is only in retrospect that she will appreciate that the period was both shorter in duration and less in quantity than normal.

Occasionally a small amount of bleeding may occur at the time of the second or even the third period and there are instances in which women have continued to have virtually normal periods for six or more months of what was an otherwise normal pregnancy.

Bleeding at the time of an expected period in early pregnancy may cause some confusion concerning the exact date of conception and therefore the expected date of delivery. If, during your first visit to the doctor or the antenatal clinic, your uterus is found to be slightly more advanced in size than the dates suggest, you may be asked for exact details of your last period in case this was partially suppressed.

The true significance of bleeding at the time of a suppressed period in early pregnancy is not clear, for while in the majority of instances it does not seem to affect the pregnancy it does indicate that the pregnancy is unstable and it is certainly true that miscarriage is more likely in a woman who has had a partially suppressed period than in one who has not. Caution therefore being the watchword, doctors consider it wise for a woman who has bled at the time of her first period to avoid intercourse and rest quietly in bed for a few days when her next period would be expected.

The bleeding at the time of a suppressed period is bleeding from the mother's uterus, not from the pregnancy or the baby. The baby is not adversely affected by it and if the pregnancy continues to progress satisfactorily the baby will develop normally.

Internal sanitary tampons should never be used during pregnancy.

Cervical erosion

Bleeding in the early stages of pregnancy may also come from abnormalities or diseases of the cervix.

Cervical erosion is a particular type of very superficial ulceration that occurs on the neck of the womb either before or very often during early pregnancy. It may occasionally become infected and give rise to a rather profuse yellowish, and sometimes irritating, vaginal discharge. A cervical erosion may bleed but this is usually very slight and may only be a stain. Bleeding may sometimes be provoked by intercourse at any stage of pregnancy However, a cervical erosion does not usually bleed, even after intercourse, unless it has become infected. It 's not treated during pregnancy although when it becomes infected local treatment with cream or pessaries is usual.

Abortion

Bleeding from the vagina is abnormal at any stage of pregnancy and may be due to many causes. Some are of little or no significance while others are potentially more dangerous. There is no way a pregnant woman can know if any bleeding from which she is suffering during pregnancy is significant or not, and she must, therefore, report it immediately to her doctor. Similarly she must report an excessive vaginal discharge or any acute abdominal pain.

An abortion by definition is the discarding by the uterus of the products of conception before the 28th week of pregnancy. There is no difference between an abortion and a miscarriage despite the frequently held view that an abortion is something that is induced and a miscarriage is something which occurs spontaneously. The two terms are synonymous and are so used here.

A threatened abortion is bleeding from the vagina during the first 28 weeks of pregnancy and is not accompanied by any pain.

Inevitable abortion. A threatened abortion becomes an inevitable abortion when the woman experiences pain due to uterine contractions or when, on examination, the cervix, or neck of the uterus, is found to be opening so that abortion must inevitably occur sooner or later.

A complete abortion has occurred when all the products of conception have been passed from the uterus.

An incomplete abortion is a condition in which part of the products of conception have been passed but some remain within the uterus.

A missed abortion is said to occur when the pregnancy has died within the uterus but the uterus has failed to expel it. The dead pregnancy will be aborted sooner or later.

Recurrent abortion is miscarriage on three or more occasions. The cause may vary on each occasion so the abortion may occur at different stages during different pregnancies.

Habitual abortion is the term usually reserved for miscarriage on three or more occasions at approximately the same stage of pregnancy and therefore assumed to be for the same reason each time.

Threatened abortion

Any bleeding which occurs at any stage during the first 28 weeks of pregnancy must be considered a threatened abortion until proved otherwise. If a woman notices any such bleeding she should go to bed immediately and stay there until she has been seen or advised by her doctor. The bleeding may be very slight in amount and may or may not be mixed with mucus. On the other hand it may be comparatively severe and even as heavy as a normal period. Occasionally there may be a dull aching discomfort in the lower abdomen. A small amount of backache, especially in the lower part of the back, may occur both before and with the bleeding. The abdominal discomfort and the backache usually pass with rest in bed. It frequently happens that a woman is first conscious of the bleeding when she passes urine. This does not mean that micturition has made the uterus bleed, but that the uterus has been bleeding slowly into the vagina for some time before micturition and on straining slightly blood appears from the vagina as urine is passed.

There are many causes of threatened abortion, some of which are known and many of which are not. Possibly the commonest cause is hormone imbalance so that the bleeding occurs at the time when the woman would be having a period and is called a 'partially suppressed period'. If the amount of circulating hormone is insufficient to maintain a pregnancy this will first become apparent when it fails to suppress completely the next menstrual period. Such bleeding may be slight in amount or, if the hormone levels are really low, it may become much more severe and may end in actual abortion.

A threatened abortion most commonly occurs at the time of the first, second or third suppressed period, that is at 4, 8 or 12 weeks of pregnancy. It also occurs at about the 14th week of pregnancy because it is at this stage that the placenta, which may be inefficient, takes over the production of hormone from the corpus luteum of the ovary.

The correct treatment for threatened abortion is immediate bed-rest. This means complete rest: going to bed, staying there and resting as quietly as possible. The woman may be allowed up for toilet purposes but for no other reason.

When a threatened abortion first begins the loss is usually bright red or pink which means that the blood is coming almost directly from the uterus. When it stops bleeding the colour of the loss from the vagina changes from bright to dark red and then brown. Normally bed-rest is continued until three days after the brown discharge has ceased.

Internal sanitary protection must not be used at any time during pregnancy unless specifically requested by your doctor. Sanitary towels must be used and changed frequently. They should be saved for your doctor to examine.

Complete bed-rest may, of course, be impracticable for someone who has no help in the house or for someone who has to look after small children, but it is nevertheless the ideal and the maximum rest possible must be taken. A mild amount of sedation or tranquillizer is frequently administered to women when they threaten to miscarry because not only are they upset but it also helps them to rest quietly. Threatened abortion used to be treated by giving some sort of progesterone tablets or injections but this treatment has many disadvantages and no advantages so it is no longer recommended.

It is impossible to know how many threatened abortions settle down and how many proceed to actual miscarriage. A threatened abortion does indicate a certain instability of the pregnancy and care should be taken to rest quietly at the time when the next period would normally be. The pregnant woman's activities should also be appropriately restricted for at least the first 14 weeks of her pregnancy. Sexual intercourse should not occur until the baby has been felt moving and in any event not until her doctor advises.

Inevitable abortion

Inevitable abortion is associated with pain in the lower abdomen which feels rather like the cramp of a period pain. The initial bleeding usually increases in amount and becomes brighter in colour. The woman should go to bed immediately and notify her doctor who will decide if admission to hospital is advisable. The amount of discomfort or pain depends on the stage of the pregnancy. The pain is actually caused by the uterus contracting so that it will eventually expel the pregnancy.

There is little that can constructively be done to treat an inevitable abortion and this is usually bed-rest and the administration of a sedative drug together with something to relieve the pain or discomfort if necessary.

Complete abortion

An abortion begins as a threatened abortion and proceeds to become inevitable after which the contents of the uterus will be completely expelled or only partially expelled (incomplete abortion). Complete abortion is said to occur when all the products of conception have been passed so that the uterus no longer contains any of the products of conception. A complete abortion may take only one hour from the onset of bleeding and may be accompanied by comparatively little pain. Alternatively the process may take many hours and be associated with severe lower abdominal pain and profuse bleeding. If abortion is rapid it may be completed before the doctor arrives, or if slow, admission to hospital may have been arranged while the abortion was either threatened or inevitable.

When the abortion is complete all discomfort and pain ceases and the amount of bleeding rapidly diminishes. The abortion itself is passed as a clot of liver-like material which should if possible be saved for the doctor to examine and confirm that all the products of conception have been passed. The main treatment is rest in bed for one or two days and then a gradual return to normal activity over the next four or five days.

Incomplete abortion

An incomplete abortion is a condition in which part of the products of conception have been expelled but some remain because they are adherent within the uterus. This is the only type of abortion that really causes problems, since the part of the pregnancy remaining predisposes the woman to the two major complications of abortion, which are haemorrhage and sepsis. Incomplete abortion can be the result of either an induced abortion or a spontaneous miscarriage. The diagnosis is usually made when bleeding continues from the uterus after some of the pregnancy has been passed. If a woman thinks she is suffering from an incomplete abortion she should get in touch with her doctor or with the nearest hospital as soon as possible.

The first measure in treating an incomplete abortion is to stop the bleeding from the uterus. This is done temporarily by giving an injection of a drug such as ergometrine or syntometrine which may cause uterine cramp to return together with lower abdominal pain, but the contracted uterus will cease to bleed. The woman is then transferred to hospital where the retained products of conception are removed from within the uterus by curettage, or scraping, while she is under a general anaesthetic. Once the products of conception have been completely removed the uterus will stop bleeding and there will be no danger of infection.

It cannot be emphasized too strongly that any woman who has had an abortion and finds herself bleeding heavily should seek help from her doctor or from the nearest hospital as soon as possible.

Missed abortion

When a pregnancy has died within the uterus but the uterus has failed to expel it a missed abortion has occurred. It will inevitably be aborted spontaneously sooner or later. A missed abortion can be a most disturbing and difficult problem. The story usually goes something like this. A woman is pregnant and she has all the signs and symptoms of early pregnancy but at about the 8th week she has a small amount of either bright or dark vaginal bleeding. She goes to bed, rests, the bleeding stops and she assumes that her pregnancy is continuing normally. Eventually however, because it is dead, hormones are no longer manufactured and she may slowly become aware of what is happening because the nausea, sickness and breast activity will cease and she will no longer 'feel pregnant'. A few days later a further small amount of brown or red bleeding may occur and this type of loss may continue intermittently for several weeks. There is no pain and the uterus does not contract or do anything to expel the dead pregnancy.

It is impossible to distinguish an early missed abortion from a threatened abortion but later the doctor will notice the absence of the signs of pregnancy and also that the uterus is small for the expected duration of pregnancy. A missed abortion is a very distressing condition and naturally the woman may wish to go into hospital as soon as possible to have it removed by operation.

Where an ultrasonic scan can be performed, it will show the absence of a fetal heart beat and a failure of the fetus to grow properly and so make an accurate diagnosis. The woman will be admitted to hospital in order to have a curettage under general anaesthetic. In this way the uterus is emptied and will return to normal within one or two weeks.

Recurrent abortion

Recurrent abortion is miscarriage on three or more occasions. The cause may vary on each occasion so the abortion may occur at different stages during different pregnancies. The causes of recurrent abortion are usually multiple so that one abortion cannot be related to another. Some may be the result of hormone deficiency, others the result of abnormal development of the pregnancy, and these may be related to abnormalities of the uterus or illness of the mother.

The prevention of recurrent abortion does, of course, depend upon discovering the cause. Fairly extensive investigations may be necessary to do this, but once the cause, or causes, has been determined, preventive measures or particular treatments can be undertaken to prevent a recurrence during a subsequent pregnancy. The husband will probably be examined and a seminal analysis performed. A higher than usual percentage of abnormal or dead sperms is sometimes considered a frequent cause of abortion.

Habitual abortion

Miscarriage on three or more occasions at approximately the same stage of pregnancy is assumed to be caused by the same factor each time, and is termed habitual abortion. It is impossible to define here the cause of habitual abortion, which may vary from congenital abnormality of the uterus to incompetence of the cervix. Extensive investigations may be necessary to discover why habitual abortion is happening and even then it may be very difficult to arrive at a definite diagnosis. The prevention and treatment of this type of abortion naturally depend upon its cause. Investigations may have defined the reason for the previous habitual abortions and factors such as fibroids can be treated before the next pregnancy.

If the cause is known and pregnancy has already been established the woman will be treated to prevent further miscarriage.

Dangers of abortion

There are two main dangers involved in any abortion. The first is haemorrhage and the second sepsis. Both induced and spontaneous abortion may result in the retention within the uterus of a small amount of the chorionic villi (incomplete abortion) whose very presence allows the uterus to continue bleeding and also predisposes it to infection.

Haemorrhage occurring in an abortion can be temporarily controlled by giving ergometrine or syntometrine to make the uterus contract. The remaining products of conception are then removed by curettage. If a woman has had an induced abortion and finds herself bleeding excessively she should seek medical help immediately because if some of the pregnancy still remains in the uterus the bleeding will continue until it has been removed.

Infection only occurs when a portion of the pregnancy is still retained within the uterus or as a result of induced abortion. The main symptoms of infection are pain and temperature, and any woman who has lower abdominal pain together with a temperature shortly after an abortion or miscarriage should seek medical aid immediately. Infection during or following an abortion can be serious if not treated promptly.

Gap before next pregnancy

Once a woman has miscarried, how long should she wait before she again becomes pregnant? The answer must be an individual one and will vary according to her age, health, circumstances and the reasons for the miscarriage. Sexual intercourse itself may be resumed as soon as vaginal bleeding has ceased. The better success rate for pregnancies of women waiting three months after a miscarriage before getting pregnant is now well established; thus, while a short wait may be desirable for various reasons, there is more than an element of truth in the saying that a uterus will not accept another pregnancy until it is fit and well enough to do so.

Some special treatment may have to be performed to prevent abortion recurring in which instance the space before another pregnancy will be advised by the doctor. There is no sense in waiting for longer than three months, time is always precious.

Blighted ovum

A pregnancy where the fetus does not develop properly is termed a blighted ovum. The fetus may fail to develop at all. Strange as it may seem, a fetus is not an essential part of an early pregnancy although it is appreciated that the reason for the pregnancy is the production of a fetus. Occasionally the mass of cells in the centre of the pregnancy that is destined to differentiate and develop into the fetus fails completely to get going. The whole pregnancy starts to develop normally; the chorionic villi grow on the outer side of the blastocyst and they implant in the wall of the uterus; the chorionic villi produce chorionic gonadotrophin, which stimulates the pituitary to release luteinizing hormone, which in turn provokes the corpus luteum in the ovary to produce large amounts of progesterone. Thus pregnancy is established.

At about this stage a group of cells known as the inner cell mass normally start dividing and differentiating into the different organs of the baby, but the presence of a developing fetus is not essential for the early part of pregnancy. At about the 6th week, however, the fetus should be developing its circulation and it is shortly after this, at about the 8th week of pregnancy, that the first signs that all is not well may appear since the chorionic villi must establish a circulation with the fetus so that they can form the placenta. There may be a small amount of bleeding and, as a result of a very gradual reduction in hormone levels, the woman may be aware of a slight reduction in the symptoms of pregnancy. If a circulation between the fetus and the chorionic villi is not established by about the 10th week of pregnancy, continuous or intermittent bleeding may begin, and will be followed eventually by pain and complete abortion of the pregnancy from the cavity of the uterus. Such a pregnancy contains a small amniotic sac but no fetus within its cavity.

The exact reason for a blighted ovum is not known but it is generally considered to be caused by fertilization of a normal ovum by an abnormal sperm. It is impossible to prove this theory but in the majority of instances where a blighted ovum is known to have occurred, the husband's seminal count is usually deficient and contains more abnormal sperms than usual.

It is not known exactly how many abortions are due to blighted ova. It is however a commonly accepted view that approximately 1 in 5 of all human pregnancies are grossly abnormal and therefore miscarry spontaneously at about the time of the first period or they are blighted ova and miscarry at about the 8th or 10th week. Some authorities consider that blighted ova constitute 1 in 10 of all human pregnancies. If the theories about a blighted ovum are correct, then once it has been diagnosed the husband should be examined and any abnormality in his seminal analysis corrected. However, it is an unfortunate fact that some couples are destined to produce more than their fair share of blighted ova when no abnormality can be found in either partner. In such instances there is no constructive treatment to prevent a recurrence in a subsequent pregnancy. Only rather thankless reassurance can be given that sooner or later a normal pregnancy is bound to occur and that, when it does, it will continue normally into the production of a normal infant.

A blighted ovum can be diagnosed as early as the 6th week by ultrasonic scan because the early developing fetus will not be visible. By the 7th week the ultrasonic scan will fail to demonstrate a normal fetal heart, the presence of which must automatically exclude a diagnosis of a blighted ovum.

Treatment for a blighted ovum is by dilatation and curettage, once the diagnosis has been confirmed by ultrasonic scan. The diagnosis and the treatment may be very difficult for some women to accept, especially if there is a history of infertility. Women often blame their doctors, very unfairly, for treating them as though they had a normal pregnancy when their pregnancy 'was bound to fail'. If a woman who is 6 or 7 weeks pregnant starts to bleed from the vagina she will call her doctor who will diagnose a threatened miscarriage, the treatment for which is always conservative, namely bed-rest and sedation. Even if the doctor has extensive tests done on the blood, the urine and the vaginal secretion, he will only be able to confirm the diagnosis by ultrasonic scan. A blighted ovum is destined to fail eventually despite anything he can do.

Incompetent cervix

An incompetent cervix will cause miscarriage at about the 20th week of pregnancy.

The canal of the cervix is about 2.5 cm in length narrowing at its lower end where it joins the vagina (the external cervical os) and at its upper end where it joins the body of the uterus (the internal cervical os). During pregnancy, while the uterus is enlarging the cervix must remain closed otherwise the fetus would fall through into the vagina. There are many circular muscle fibres surrounding the cervix, especially the internal cervical os, which normally keep it tightly closed throughout pregnancy despite the continuous recurrence of Braxton Hicks' contractions.

The muscle surrounding the internal os may have been damaged so that it is incapable of keeping the cervix closed during pregnancy. The internal cervical os will then start to open soon after the 14th week, and by about the 20th week of pregnancy the cervix will be about 1 in. dilated. At this stage the membranes, or bag of waters, will bulge through the cervix into the vagina and will eventually break. There will be a sudden loss of a large quantity of water from the uterus and the vagina followed by miscarriage which usually occurs fairly quickly with comparatively little discomfort

The main causes of incompetent cervix are:

Injury During a particularly difficult or rapid labour, or where a baby is unduly large, the muscle fibres of the internal cervical os may occasionally be damaged and the next pregnancy miscarries at about the 20th week

Operative When the cervix is injured at an operation for the treatment of painful periods, or to perform an abortion, the circular muscle fibres around the internal cervical os may be damaged sufficiently to render the cervix incompetent in the next pregnancy.

Very few women suffer from an incompetent cervix where there is no history of previous operation or pregnancy.

Fortunately an incompetent cervix is a comparatively rare condition. The diagnosis cannot be made until after the first miscarriage when the history alone is sufficiently definite and classical for the cause to be established. If there is any doubt a special X-ray of the uterus is diagnostic. The treatment usually recommended is the insertion of a special stitch (Shirodkar suture) around the cervix either before or during pregnancy. The preference in Great Britain is usually to insert the suture during pregnancy and this is done under anaesthetic, generally at the 14th week or shortly afterwards, at which time the pregnancy is known to be in its most stable condition.

The Shirodkar suture is made of nylon or a similar material which is placed around the cervix like a purse-string to prevent it from opening. It is a comparatively simple procedure. This treatment has a very high success rate and over 75 per cent of the pregnancies proceed to term. The stitch is removed at about the 38th week (or before, if the woman goes into labour at an earlier date) and the onset of natural labour may begin quite soon afterwards or not until term.

Ectopic pregnancy

Ectopic pregnancy is described in Chapter 19 but is mentioned here because it may be a cause of bleeding in early pregnancy and may sometimes be confused with a true abortion. An ectopic pregnancy is a pregnancy that is situated outside the cavity of the uterus and most frequently occurs in the Fallopian tube. The first symptom is pain, becoming severe, followed by bleeding, whereas in abortion bleeding invariably precedes any pain or discomfort.

Hydatidiform mole

Hydatidiform mole is a strange abnormality of pregnancy in which the placental tissue alone develops in much the same way as it does in a blighted ovum In hydatidiform mole, however, the chorionic villi continue to develop and multiply so that instead of producing a smaller amount of chorionic gonadotrophin they produce an excessive quantity and thus guarantee that the 'pregnancy' continues. A pregnancy test will be positive even when the urine is diluted more than 200 times which gives some indication of the amount of hormone being produced by the hydatidiform mole. The chorionic villi gradually become distended and cystic so that the whole uterus is filled with a mass of tissue which resembles a bunch of small grapes.

Hydatidiform mole is a rare complication of pregnancy in Britain. All the signs and symptoms of early pregnancy are present and may frequently be rather excessive. It may be first suspected at about the 14th or 16th week of pregnancy when the uterus is much larger than it should be. This rapid enlargement may also cause intermittent vaginal bleeding. The diagnosis may be very difficult, especially in the early stages of pregnancy although the continuous intermittent loss of a small amount of bright or darkish blood may arouse suspicion. No fetal movements will be felt and a fetal heart will not be heard. The findings on ultrasonic scan are diagnostic and this should be performed as soon as possible if a hydatidiform mole is suspected. The diagnosis may also be confirmed by repeated findings of a positive pregnancy test when the urine is diluted more than 200 times.

A hydatidiform mole must be removed from the uterus and this is usually done by dilatation of the cervix followed by curettage or aspiration while the woman is anaesthetized. Alternatively she may be given Syntocinon, or a similar hormone, such as prostaglandin, to make the uterus contract sufficiently to expel its contents after which curettage is performed to ensure that the uterus is completely empty. Following this she is regularly followed up with urine and blood samples for about 2 years to ensure that there is no further growth of tissue. She may then go ahead with another pregnancy.

Antepartum haemorrhage

Before the 28th week of pregnancy any bleeding is, by definition, a threat to miscarry or abort and is known as a threatened abortion. After the 28th week, however, when the child is viable, such bleeding is known as antepartum haemorrhage.

Bright red blood coming from the vagina after the 28th week of pregnancy should be reported to the doctor or midwife immediately regardless of the hour of day or night at which it is first noticed. It can easily be distinguished from the small quantity of pinkish or brownish mucus which a woman often passes at the onset of labour. The passage of such a pink mucous plug should not cause any alarm, but if this occurs before the 36th week of pregnancy the doctor should be notified.

An antepartum haemorrhage may fall into one of three main categories:

Placenta praevia is a condition in which the placenta, instead of being attached to the upper part of the uterus, is attached to the lower part in the region of the lower uterine segment or the cervix

Accidental antepartum haemorrhage (abruptio placentae) is a comparatively rare condition in which the placenta is normally implanted in the upper part of the uterus but detaches from it prematurely and results in vaginal bleeding.

Incidental antepartum haemorrhage is haemorrhage which occurs from the genital tract but not from the site of the placenta or its implantation. Such haemorrhage may result from injury, infection, ulcers on the neck of the womb, polyps or, most commonly, the onset of labour.

Placenta praevia

The placenta is normally situated in the upper part of the uterus and usually on the posterior wall. Occasionally, probably due to a fault of implantation of the ovum, it is situated in the lower part of the uterus and is known as placenta praevia. A placenta implanted in the lower uterine segment will be below the baby's head. Changes occur in the lower part of the uterus and the cervix during the last two months of pregnancy in preparation for labour. These are mainly stretching of the lower segment with a gradual softening and shortening of the cervix. The placenta is then

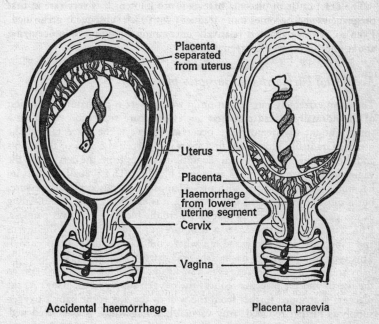

Accidental haemorrhage   Placenta praevia

Fig. 23 Antepartum haemorrhage

ınevitably separated to some extent from the uterus. Separation of the placenta always results in bleeding. It is important to remember that the bleeding which occurs in placenta praevia is the mother's blood and not blood from the baby's circulation. A baby is never harmed or injured in any way by what may occasionally seem to be quite a lot of bleeding.

Any bleeding after the 28th week of pregnancy should be reported to the doctor. Bleeding which occurs during the last two months of pregnancy is especially significant and the woman is nearly always admitted to hospital until a diagnosis of placenta praevia has been proved or disproved by ultrasonic scan. If a diagnosis of placenta praevia is proved then she will probably have to remain in hospital until delivery. A placenta that is situated over the lower uterine segment will almost certainly cause more bleeding before the onset of labour and will certainly bleed again when labour starts. If the woman is under proper supervision in hospital any further haemorrhage can be investigated immediately and appropriate steps taken to ensure safe delivery without danger to the mother or her child. In severe degrees of placenta praevia it may be necessary to perform Caesarean section. In mild degrees of placenta praevia normal labour is allowed to proceed but the membranes may be artificially ruptured shortly after the onset of labour.

The exact cause of placenta praevia is not known. It is very rare in first pregnancies and becomes more frequent with each subsequent pregnancy. Even so, it still remains a relatively uncommon condition only occurring about once in every 100 pregnancies.

Accidental haemorrhage (abruptio placentae)

This is an extremely rare condition in which there is premature separation of the normally placed placenta. Such premature separation results in a small amount of haemorrhage occurring between the placenta and the uterus. Gradually blood will find its way between the wall of the uterus and the membranes of the fetal sac until it escapes from the cervix into the vagina and is then recognized as vaginal bleeding. This type of antepartum haemorrhage is associated with pre-eclampsia or a raised blood pressure, but it must be emphasized that, even so, it is extremely rare. The bleeding causes pain, unlike placenta praevia where the bleeding is always painless. Pain, tenderness and soreness will be present over the area of the uterus and especially over the exact site where the haemorrhage has occurred. This type of antepartum haemorrhage is extremely dangerous to both the baby and the mother because even a small amount of haemorrhage between the uterus and the placenta reduces the oxygen supply to the baby. As the placenta is stripped further from the wall of the uterus the baby's oxygen supply is further reduced. Any vaginal bleeding which is associated with continuous abdominal pain should be immediately reported to the doctor or midwife, who will almost certainly arrange for urgent admission to hospital. Treatment usually includes sedation to control the pain and high blood pressure, blood transfusion and rapid delivery by Caesarean section if labour does not begin quickly and proceed rapidly.

Recurrences of either placenta praevia or abruptio placentae in subsequent pregnancies are very rare. Approximately half the total number of patients who suffer from abruptio placentae have had six or more children.

The placenta can be dislodged as a result of a violent blow on the uterus. This, however, is an extremely rare injury virtually unseen today. It is almost impossible to injure the uterus, placenta or the fetus as a result of falling down; even falling down stairs seldom results in any damage to the uterus or its contents.

Incidental haemorrhage

Incidental haemorrhage may be due to a variety of causes, but essentially it means that there is vaginal bleeding which is coming from a site other than the placenta. The commonest bleeding during pregnancy is the small amount of blood, or 'show', which nearly always accompanies the onset of labour. Bleeding may also come from an erosion on the cervix, or cervical tumours. Such erosions are very common in pregnancy and in fact occur in about 75 per cent of all pregnant women. Vaginal infections are also common in pregnancy and are liable to bleed. Injuries to the vagina will also cause bleeding, but these are extremely unusual in pregnancy and usually result from attempts to procure an abortion. Injury resulting from intercourse in pregnancy is extremely rare.

Severe sickness in pregnancy

Severe sickness in pregnancy, otherwise known as hyperemesis gravidarum, is much less common than it used to be. Nausea is a very common symptom in early pregnancy, frequently associated with a certain amount of vomiting. If vomiting becomes excessive then the pregnant woman will show signs of starvation by the presence of acetone in her urine (and it is for this reason that each woman's urine is tested at the antenatal clinic for acetone as well as for sugar and protein). The sickness which occurs normally in early pregnancy and perhaps again in later pregnancy is discussed in Chapter 12 together with its management and normal treatment. If these measures fail and the pregnant woman continues to vomit almost everything she eats as well as everything she drinks she will rapidly become ill.

Hyperemesis gravidarum used to be considered a psychological condition in which a woman induced vomiting to obtain attention and a termination of her pregnancy. To stop this she would be told that on no account would her pregnancy be terminated. Today this is considered a somewhat dated approach and the whole management and treatment have changed. The woman is admitted to hospital and given special drugs which stop the vomiting within a few hours. Fluids containing sugar and other nutrients are fed into a vein until she is able to drink by mouth and take a light diet without vomiting. The condition is usually corrected within a few days. Hyperemesis gravidarum is today a rare condition and when it does occur it is usually connected with a multiple pregnancy or a hydatidiform mole or as a result of some hidden infection especially in the urinary tract.

Polyhydramnios

The normal amount of amniotic fluid at term is approximately 1 litre. If the amount is thought to exceed 2 litres then a condition of polyhydramnios is present. This is a potentially dangerous condition and occurs in about 3 per cent of all pregnancies.

Acute polyhydramnios

Acute polyhydramnios is rare and invariably starts at the 24th week of pregnancy. There is a sudden, rapid enlargement of the uterus so that the abdominal girth may increase by as much as 15 or even 30 cm in a few days. This is associated with a twin pregnancy and nearly always with a uniovular (identical) twin pregnancy. Rapid enlargement of the uterus may result in considerable abdominal discomfort or even pain. Should this happen the doctor must be notified.

The rapid uterine enlargement resulting from such a twin pregnancy usually continues for 7 to 10 days and then ceases. The pain and discomfort may be so severe that the woman has to be admitted to hospital for rest and special treatment. Premature labour may begin but the pregnancy usually continues satisfactorily and the twins, whose presence has been confirmed by ultrasonic scan, are delivered quite normally at the appropriate time.

Chronic polyhydramnios

Chronic polyhydramnios is usually first noted at about the 30th week of pregnancy, when the uterus enlarges to a degree greater than is expected. This is caused by the grossly increased amount of fluid within the uterus. The normal girth of a pregnant woman at term is approximately 100 cm but when polyhydramnios occurs the girth at 34 weeks may reach 100 cm, and at term may reach as much as 115 or 120 cm.

Chronic polyhydramnios results in a slow enlargement of the uterus and is not associated with pain or discomfort until the uterus becomes so large that its size creates discomfort.

The causes of chronic polyhydramnios are:

1 Unknown.
2 Twin pregnancy.
3 Diabetes.
4 Pre-eclampsia.
5 Congenital abnormality of the fetus.

Unknown. Approximately 50 per cent of women suffering from polyhydramnios have no specific cause for the excessive amount of fluid present. The large quantity of fluid over-distends the uterus and predisposes the woman to premature labour which is best avoided by rest and following the doctor's advice meticulously. If the baby is in a large amount of amniotic fluid it may not assume its correct position so that delivery should be in hospital where any abnormality of the baby's position can be corrected. Women with polyhydramnios are treated with special care during labour. The contractions of the over-distended uterus are relatively inefficient so that labour may be prolonged and an assisted forceps delivery may be necessary during the second stage of labour. Weak uterine contractions during the third stage of labour may predispose the woman to bleeding after delivery, and she is usually given injections of ergometrine or Syntocinon at the time of delivery rather than afterwards in order to prevent postpartum haemorrhage.

Polyhydramnios during pregnancy does not have a harmful effect on the development of the baby or on the woman after delivery, and there is no evidence to suggest that it will recur in a subsequent pregnancy.

Twin pregnancy. Acute polyhydramnios starts at 24 weeks in a twin pregnancy and chronic polyhydramnios usually develops at about the 28th or 30th week in a gradual manner. The problems of twin pregnancy are discussed in Chapter 30. In actual fact twin pregnancies do not really suffer from polyhydramnios since there are two normal fetuses each with a normal amount of liquor, but the total amount of amniotic fluid is greater than normal and symptoms are exactly the same as for an excessive amount of fluid in a single pregnancy.

Diabetes. Diabetic women who are carefully and rigidly controlled throughout their pregnancy have only a slightly increased incidence of polyhydramnios. If diabetes is uncontrolled or poorly controlled in pregnancy there is a much higher incidence of polyhydramnios and the excessive amount of amniotic fluid is a direct result of the unstable diabetes.

Pre-eclampsia. Some women with polyhydramnios develop pre-eclampsia. The reason for this is not known, but it may be that there is an association between the over-distended uterus and the blood supply to the kidney.

Congenital abnormality. Polyhydramnios is one of the most important signs of some varieties of serious congenital abnormality. Approximately

40 per cent of all single pregnancies which develop polyhydramnios do in fact harbour a baby suffering from a major degree of congenital abnormality. Polyhydramnios caused by congenital abnormality usually begins at about the 30th week and is indistinguishable from polyhydramnios resulting from other causes. Abnormalities of the central nervous system and of the spine of the baby may make its swallowing mechanism ineffective so that excess liquor accumulates within the amniotic sac. Abnormalities of the gullet, oesophagus or stomach may also result in defects of the swallowing mechanism and result in the formation of polyhydramnios.

Diagnosis of polyhydramnios

Polyhydramnios may be diagnosed if the uterus is found to be over-distended by amniotic fluid when the estimated duration of pregnancy is known to be correct. It is one of the indications for routine ultrasonic scan to see whether the cause is twin pregnancy or a congenital abnormality of the fetus. Modern ultrasound will demonstrate abnormalities of many fetal organs such as brain, bowel, bladder or kidney as well as the spine and other bones.

Treatment of polyhydramnios

Polyhydramnios may cause gross abdominal distension, discomfort, clumsiness, and the uterus sometimes grows so large that there is swelling of the legs and shortness of breath. Sleeping may become a problem owing to the difficulty of getting into a comfortable position. Treatment is rest, and mild sedation may be required.

If the scan reveals that a baby has a congenital abnormality the pregnancy may be terminated by inducing premature labour. This, however, is a decision to be taken by the doctor who knows all the facts in each individual instance.

Amniocentesis is the removal of a small amount of amniotic fluid for examination. The investigation is completely painless. An area of skin on the anterior abdominal wall is treated with local anaesthetic and a needle is gently introduced into the cavity of the uterus whence a small quantity of amniotic fluid is withdrawn. This may be done early in pregnancy at the 16th week in order to diagnose congenital abnormality (especially mongolism). It may be used later in pregnancy in the diagnosis of Rhesus incompatibility, for the diagnosis of other types of congenital abnormality, to estimate the baby's maturity accurately and to indicate the condition of the baby's lungs before inducing premature labour. In some instances of polyhydramnios, amniocentesis is performed to remove some fluid in order to relieve pressure within the uterus. It is not usually undertaken simply to establish the sex of the unborn baby by examining its cells.

Fibroids in pregnancy

Fibroids are rarely connected with pregnancy because the majority of women who become pregnant are under 30 whereas the majority of women who suffer from fibroids are over the age of 40. However, a few younger women do have fibroids, some of which occasionally interfere with the normal progress of a pregnancy.

The majority of fibroids are of no significance and have no effect upon a woman's fertility, her pregnancy or delivery. Some, however, impinge upon or distort the actual cavity of the uterus and may cause complications in pregnancy, as may a very large fibroid which by virtue of its size distorts the uterus and the other pelvic organs.

Fibroids that distort the cavity of the uterus and very large fibroids may occasionally cause infertility and, if this is considered to be so, they can be removed by an operation known as myomectomy in which the fibroids alone are removed and the conserved uterus is then carefully reconstructed. Similarly if it is considered that fibroids predispose a woman to recurrent or habitual abortion they are removed by myomectomy. Large fibroids may be responsible for the onset of premature labour. This is unusual, however, because they must be at least 10 cm in diameter to have this effect. They may occasionally predispose to an extra amount of bleeding after the baby has been delivered. The presence of such fibroids, however, is always known beforehand and precautions can be taken which will usually prevent any postpartum haemorrhage.

Abnormal presentation of the fetus

This is unusual but is a possibility where a very large fibroid is present in the lower part of the body of the uterus. Since there is no room for both the fibroid and the baby's head in the lower uterine segment, the baby's head is pushed to one side and does not present normally. This usually resolves itself spontaneously before the onset of labour because, with the stretching of the lower part of the uterus and formation of the lower uterine segment, the fibroid is drawn further up into the abdomen and the baby's head can descend into the pelvis. If the presentation does not correct itself spontaneously, the baby is delivered by Caesarean section. The fibroid may be removed at a later operation, if this is necessary, but it is not usually removed at the time of the Caesarean operation because of the danger of haemorrhage from the extremely vascular pregnant uterus.

Red degeneration

Red degeneration is a strange and peculiar condition in which a fibroid becomes very acutely inflamed. This usually happens about the middle of pregnancy and the fibroid suddenly becomes extremely tender and painful.

The amount of pain can be very considerable and it can be very difficult to arrive at an exact diagnosis. The treatment is admission to hospital, rest in bed, sedation and pain-killing drugs. The pain usually passes off spontaneously in about 48 hours (but may last for several days) after which the fibroid gets rapidly smaller and often causes no more trouble. It may be very difficult to differentiate between red degeneration and acute appendicitis. Because the danger of ignoring acute appendicitis is so great it may be necessary to operate in order to be certain of the diagnosis. If it proves to be red degeneration, the fibroid will be left in place and the abdominal incision closed without anything further being done. The disastrous consequence of failing to remove an acute appendix more than justifies the occasional 'unnecessary' operation.

Ovarian cysts in pregnancy

Ovarian cysts may occasionally be present during pregnancy. One of the main reasons for performing an internal examination at the beginning of a pregnancy is to ensure that the ovaries are normal as well as the uterus, vagina and the structure of the bony pelvis.

The ovaries always develop small cysts (up to 2 cm in diameter) during pregnancy and these are of no consequence. The corpus luteum also enlarges the ovary and may sometimes become cystic. Occasionally, however, a large ovarian cyst measuring several centimetres in diameter is found in early pregnancy. When a cyst of this size is discovered it is generally removed at the first reasonable opportunity. Because the cyst may be situated in the same ovary as the corpus luteum, and damage to the corpus luteum may cause miscarriage, the removal of the cyst by operation is usually deferred until after the end of the 14th week of pregnancy. By this time the placenta has taken over the hormone-producing functions of the corpus luteum. After the ovarian cysts are surgically removed the ovary is reconstructed so that it will again function normally.

Operation is advisable because ovarian cysts may undergo twisting or torsion, and if this happens later in pregnancy not only is the operation extremely difficult, but the woman might rapidly become very seriously ill before it could be performed. There is always a possibility that an operation for the removal of an ovarian cyst during pregnancy will precipitate a miscarriage. This does not often happen but it is a chance that has to be taken and is a much smaller risk to the woman and her baby than the danger of the cyst twisting at a later stage of the pregnancy.

Pre-eclampsia

Pre-eclampsia is a condition which is specific to pregnancy in which two of the three classical symptoms are present. They are:

1 A raised blood pressure.
2 Swelling of the feet, ankles or hands.
3 Protein in the urine.

More recently a fourth symptom, excessive weight gain, has been added to the above triad. This is not in fact a sign of pre-eclampsia, although it is nearly always a predisposing factor and a warning sign to which the incidence of pre-eclampsia can be directly related.

The cause of pre-eclampsia is still unknown despite a great deal of research. One aspect of the care of the pregnant woman in the antenatal clinic is always directed towards the prevention of pre-eclampsia.

Pre-eclampsia very seldom occurs before the 20th week of pregnancy, and is nearly always associated with extra weight gain. The essential change is a rise in blood pressure, but this is frequently accompanied by oedema, or swelling, of the ankles and feet as well as the hands and often the face. Oedema of the feet is easily recognizable because not only do shoes become tight, but the swollen part of the foot can be indented quite easily by pressing with the finger. Swelling of the hands is usually noticed when rings become too tight for comfort and have to be removed, and women usually complain of stiffness in the fingers or pins and needles in the hands, especially early in the morning.

Swelling of the face is nearly always part of the generalized weight gain, but oedema can be recognized by the general puffiness, especially around the eyes and neck.

The normal blood pressure in a healthy woman of 25 is 120/70 mm of mercury and does not alter greatly in normal pregnancy. The upper figure is the systolic blood pressure and the lower figure the diastolic blood pressure. The diastolic figure is the most important reading, because changes in this indicate a fundamental alteration in the body. The systolic blood pressure varies with emotion and exercise.

In pre-eclampsia the blood pressure rises until the diastolic pressure, which should normally be in the region of 60 or 70, has risen to 90.

As a result of a raised blood pressure protein is shed from the kidneys and can be detected in the urine. Routine urine tests are performed at every antenatal visit during pregnancy to detect the presence of sugar, ketones and protein. Pre-eclampsia is one of many reasons why protein is found in the urine during pregnancy.

Pre-eclampsia develops slowly and insidiously; the signs appear long before the symptoms, and can be detected by vigilant antenatal care long before the woman notices any abnormality. The importance of regular antenatal visits cannot be over-emphasized, since it is at these visits that the doctor is able to detect the very earliest changes which might, if unchecked, lead to pre-eclampsia, and he is then able to give advice and institute treatment to prevent its onset. The condition can almost always be avoided if the pregnant woman understands the importance of antenatal care, keeps her antenatal appointments religiously and carries out her doctor's instructions, especially those regarding her diet.

The reason for its development is not properly understood. A certain amount of swelling of the feet and ankles is normal in nearly every pregnancy, especially in the last 6 or 8 weeks. This usually appears during the day and generally disappears during the night, so that the feet and ankles have returned to normal by morning. This amount of swelling should not give rise to concern but ought to be mentioned to the doctor at the next antenatal visit. Some women have quite severe swelling of the ankles and also of the hands, abdomen and face without developing pre-eclampsia. Other women may develop a raised blood pressure without having any swelling of the feet or hands. It is normal for the blood pressure to fall in the early stages of pregnancy and to rise again at about the 20th week. There may be a further small rise in blood pressure towards the expected date of delivery and these minor changes in blood pressure are no cause for concern. The normal diastolic blood pressure of the non-pregnant woman, which is in the region of 70, may fall to 60, or even 50, in the first 12 weeks of pregnancy, rising again to about 70 by the 20th week of pregnancy. Further small rises may occur so that by the 36th week of pregnancy the blood pressure may have reached 80 or even 85. All these changes will be carefully recorded by the doctor, but do not cause any anxiety.

If the development of pre-eclampsia is allowed to continue unchecked the blood pressure will rise further and the oedema will increase. Headaches, especially over the eyes and across the forehead, begin, rapidly become more severe and do not respond to aspirin or the normal analgesics. Later the eyes are affected by blurring of vision and still later by the presence of flashing lights. Persistent headache and blurring of vision are very serious signs and must be reported immediately. This does not mean that every headache should be reported to the doctor but only those as described above which fail to respond to the usual remedies or those associated with persistent disturbances of vision.

If pre-eclampsia has developed then the treatment is admission to hospital, followed by bed-rest, sedation, daily urine tests, blood pressure taken four-hourly, observation of oedema and an accurate fluid balance chart. These simple measures usually control the condition but if they fail then treatment with drugs may be necessary. In very exceptional instances the condition continues to get worse despite rest and treatment and it may then be necessary either to induce labour before term or to perform Caesarean section.

Pre-eclampsia in itself does not do any lasting narm to the pregnant woman, so long as she is properly and efficiently treated. After delivery the swelling of the legs and hands goes, blood pressure gradually returns to normal although it may take several months, the kidneys return to their normal function and the protein will disappear from the urine Untreated pre-eclampsia, however, may develop into eclampsia, which is extremely dangerous but, as a result of modern antenatal care, is now a rare condition.

The real danger of pre-eclampsia is to the unborn baby. It has been estimated that in Britain approximately 7 per cent of women having their first babies and 3 per cent of women having subsequent babies suffer from pre-eclampsia. All in all a total of almost 5 per cent of all pregnant women develop the condition, sometimes with disastrous results to their babies. The danger to the baby varies directly with the height of the mother's blood pressure. Premature labour, either spontaneous or induced, results in a high proportion of small babies so that on an average 10 per cent of these babies fail to survive; that is 1 child in every 10 dying from a disease that is nearly always preventable. What a sin and what sorrow!

Eclampsia

Eclampsia is a most severe degree of a disease which in its mild form is called pre-eclampsia. Any woman who is suffering from pre-eclampsia runs a risk of developing eclampsia which is characterized by the occurrence of convulsions or fits. The fits last approximately one minute and are followed by a period of unconsciousness. Eclampsia occurs in late pregnancy or it may begin during labour or even after delivery. When a convulsion happens all the signs and symptoms of pre-eclampsia are present:

1 Raised blood pressure.
2 Generalized swelling or oedema.
3 Protein in the urine.
(4 Abnormally high weight gain.)

The woman also suffers one or more of the following symptoms:

Severe headache occurring characteristically over the front part of the head above the eyes and associated with an abnormal rise in blood pressure. It is persistent and is not relieved by aspirin or other normal 'headache tablets'.

Visual disturbances. These may be flashes of light before the eyes, coloured moving spots or blurring of vision and occasionally complete although temporary blindness.

Irritability. The woman is irritable, apprehensive and unable to tolerate noise or other mild disturbances.

Abdominal pain. Pain in the upper abdomen which may be mistaken for indigestion is usually severe, persistent and may be accompanied by actual vomiting which fails to relieve it.

The best treatment for eclampsia is its prevention Eclampsia is one of the most dangerous complications of pregnancy and even in the very best hands it may cause a patient's death. Even today approximately 1 in 20 women who develop eclampsia do not survive. The risk to the baby is even greater and approximately 1 in 5 babies fail to live. These figures show the reality of the danger of eclampsia which in the majority of instances should never happen. An isolated case is however bound to occur even with the most stringent antenatal care because the mother's blood pressure rises suddenly and without warning.

Prevention is the keynote and one of the many advantages of careful supervision during pregnancy has been the early recognition and adequate treatment of pre-eclampsia which in turn has virtually eliminated eclampsia itself in Great Britain.

Treatment

At the onset of eclamptic fits the patient is heavily sedated to prevent their recurrence. Expert nursing care in hospital is absolutely essential. If fits occur at home the doctor must be notified immediately and he will administer an appropriate sedative and arrange for the woman to be transferred to hospital. If labour starts spontaneously it may progress rapidly and easily while the fits are controlled by sedatives. If it does not, then, depending on the woman's condition, it may be necessary to induce labour or perform Caesarean section.

Placental insufficiency

A satisfactory and normal placenta is of course vital if a normal healthy baby is to be produced. The placenta reaches its full maturity at about the 32nd or 34th week of pregnancy. From this time to the end of pregnancy it slowly becomes more inefficient. This is a very gradual process and even at 40 or 42 weeks the placenta is capable of supplying a mature baby with all its requirements.

Complete failure of the placenta to develop will result in abortion at an early stage. Occasionally, however, the placenta grows but fails to mature properly and will produce less hormone than normal. This will have an influence upon not only the fetus but also the entire pregnancy. The size of the uterus will be consistently smaller than it should be for the duration of pregnancy. The mother's weight gain will be less than is normally expected. The baby itself will develop normally but will be small and there will only be a small amount of amniotic fluid present.

Such a dysmature placenta can only provide a restricted supply of materials and nutrition to the fetus with the result that the fetus develops normally but *slowly*, and is called a 'small-for-dates', or dysmature, baby. The problem with this situation is that eventually the placenta can no longer supply even the basic requirements and the baby becomes short of oxygen and may die *in utero*. This may be seen in babies who are abnormal or have suffered some infection *in utero*, or where the mother is malnourished, smokes heavily or suffers from some chronic illness such as renal or cardiac disease.

A second type of placental insufficiency may occur after the placenta has properly developed. This is because its rate of deterioration is most rapid after the 32nd or 34th week of pregnancy. This may be the result of unknown factors but may also occur in the presence of a raised blood pressure, pre-eclampsia, diabetes or after antepartum haemorrhage. When this secondary type of placental insufficiency occurs it results in a slowing down, and later a cessation, of the actual growth of the baby. First, the baby's liver and spleen stop growing, then less fat is laid down in its abdominal wall skin, and finally the head stops growing. This is always a sinister sign because it is associated with an increased risk of the baby dying *in utero*, as well as increased perinatal mortality and morbidity. The malnourished baby does not have sufficient glucose stores in its starved liver to withstand the stress of labour, and may become distressed. Some-times this may occur even before the woman goes into labour and a Caesarean section may be required as an emergency to save the baby's life. The immediate period after birth may be difficult for these babies and there is increasing evidence that as they grow older they are smaller in height and weight than they should be for their age, and that they may have learning difficulties.

The recognition of primary and secondary placental insufficiency is one of the main duties of the doctor and midwife at the antenatal clinic and modern scientific advances have made this easier. The definitive diagnosis is made with ultrasonic scanning evidence that the fetal growth is slowing down and the amount of amniotic fluid is abnormally small. The mother is admitted to hospital for rest, and regular monitoring of the fetus with hormone and other tests (see Chapter 22). The rest encourages blood flow to the uterus to increase and a sudden spurt of fetal growth may be seen on the next ultrasonic scan. On the other hand, if growth continues to fall, and other tests of fetal well-being are poor, it may be necessary to induce labour early rather than risk the baby dying suddenly *in utero*.

Death of the fetus in the uterus

On very rare occasions the baby dies in the uterus. If this occurs before the 28th week of pregnancy it will inevitably lead to miscarriage. If it occurs after the 28th week it will inevitably result in delivery occurring fairly soon. Most women at some stage of their pregnancy feel certain that their baby has died, especially if they do not feel it moving for some time. It must be remembered that even babies have periods of sleeping *in utero*, and so long as a woman feels her baby move on average ten times in a day at least, there is no cause for concern.

The causes of intrauterine death during late pregnancy are not properly understood. The majority of such deaths are caused by placental insufficiency where the placenta has either grown inadequately or become diseased so that it is unable to maintain an adequate oxygen and food supply to the baby. Other causes are premature separation of the placenta (abruptio placentae), congenital abnormalities of the fetus, Rhesus disease and accidents to the umbilical cord.

As soon as the baby dies the formation of progesterone and oestrogen is dramatically reduced with resulting diminution of the physical signs normally present during pregnancy. The sensation of being pregnant disappears quite quickly. The breasts decrease in size and the marks made by the veins under the skin of the breasts go quite rapidly. Any swelling of the fingers or ankles disappears and the uterus (together with the abdomen) gradually decreases in size. This shrinking of the uterus is due to the absorption of the amniotic fluid from around the fetus. Amongst the most dramatic of these signs is loss of weight previously gained.

The death of the baby in the uterus does not have any adverse effects on the mother's health, except in very rare instances when it may change her blood clotting mechanism. It is usual, therefore, when such a woman goes into labour, or has labour induced, for her blood clotting mechanism to be checked at the onset or immediately before the onset of labour. Any abnormality is corrected. The effect of an intrauterine death upon the mental state of a woman, however, is usually considerable.

Intrauterine death results in loss of weight, diminution of breast changes, reduction of venous engorgement on the breasts and the reduction of swelling of the ankles. Along with the signs mentioned above are two diagnostic ones. Although the fetal heart will not be heard by the doctor with a stethoscope, this can happen normally when the baby is lying in a certain position. However, when the baby is dead, no heart rate tracing can be obtained on an electronic monitor, and an ultrasonic scan will not detect a fetal heart beat. Changes do occur after death which can be detected on an X-ray, but only after 3 or 4 days.

When the diagnosis of intrauterine death has been made, the doctor or midwife must decide how to tell the woman, if she is unaware of it, and how to treat her. The majority of doctors and midwives are reluctant to inform her in an ordinary antenatal clinic that her baby is dead or is even suspected of being dead and she is generally asked to return with her husband or a responsible relative before discussing the problem.

When the woman and her husband have been told, their natural reaction is to ask for the dead baby to be removed as soon as possible. Until recently it was always considered best that labour should commence spontaneously and without interference. Today it can safely be induced in the same way as if the baby were alive. Often, the labour appears to be more painful and uncomfortable, and this is probably created by the tragic psychological effect on the woman of knowing that her baby is dead. In many instances, labour begins spontaneously shortly after the death of the fetus.

Mourning

The grief of losing a baby in this way may take many months to work through. The experience may seem unreal, especially if the woman does not see the baby after it is born, and if the hospital makes the arrangements for the baby's funeral. The love of her husband or partner and his support are absolutely vital at this time. Depending on the circumstances of the death, many hospitals will encourage the parents to see and hold their baby if they so want, and photographs may be taken.

The help of the general practitioner or health visitor in allowing a woman to talk of her grief may be very important after the woman goes home. Advice to have another baby soon is unhelpful, as it cannot replace the one that was lost. Many women have found great comfort by talking to other members of the Stillbirth Association. (The Stillbirth and Perinatal Death Association, Argyle House, 29–31 Euston Road, London NW1 2SD.

19 Ectopic Pregnancy

It normally takes the newly fertilized ovum 7 days to reach the cavity of the uterus after which it embeds itself in the endometrium. If for some reason the ovum has not reached the cavity of the uterus by the 7th day after fertilization it will embed within the Fallopian tube and become a tubal or ectopic pregnancy. Such pregnancies are rare, occurring approximately once in every 350 pregnancies. An ectopic pregnancy, however, cannot survive because it does not have the required blood supply nor is it protected by the thick muscular walls of the uterus. As the pregnancy grows and distends the Fallopian tube it may cause some lower abdominal discomfort or pain. The first indication that something is going wrong may be the onset of pain low down in one side of the abdomen. This is due to the Fallopian tube contracting in response to the stretching caused by the growing pregnancy within its lumen. Eventually, between the 6th and 12th weeks of the pregnancy, some bleeding occurs either from the outer end of the Fallopian tube, or from the Fallopian tube itself because the pregnancy has ruptured its wall. This results in quite acute and severe lower abdominal discomfort which may shortly afterwards be followed by some vaginal bleeding. This condition requires urgent admission to hospital and operation. It may be necessary to remove the affected tube together with the pregnancy that it contains, or occasionally it may be possible to remove the pregnancy and repair the Fallopian tube.

In its early stages an ectopic pregnancy cannot be differentiated from a pregnancy which is situated normally within the cavity of the uterus. It produces the same hormones as does a pregnancy within the cavity of the uterus and therefore a woman has exactly the same symptoms as she would have if the pregnancy were normally situated. However, when you attend the antenatal clinic for the first time an internal examination is performed by which the doctor will know if the pregnancy is normally situated in the uterus.

Women who have had one ectopic pregnancy and have had one Fallopian tube removed are naturally worried in case they develop an ectopic pregnancy in the other Fallopian tube. This is very rare but does happen in approximately 10 per cent of those women who have already had one ectopic pregnancy. If you have already had one ectopic pregnancy, as soon as you know you are pregnant you should visit the antenatal clinic so that you can be examined to check that the pregnancy is in the right place.

Secondary abdominal pregnancy

On very rare occasions an ectopic pregnancy survives for an indefinite length of time. This is peculiarly common amongst South African Negroes. The fertilized ovum embeds itself in the Fallopian tube and begins to grow without rupturing the tube until about the 7th or 8th week when the chorionic tissue surrounding the pregnancy gradually erodes its way through the wall of the Fallopian tube. This usually results in the death of the pregnancy and fairly extensive internal bleeding, causing pain. Very occasionally the erosion of the wall of the Fallopian tube is so gradual that there is only slight bleeding. The chorionic tissue then protrudes through the wall of the Fallopian tube and re-embeds itself in a surrounding structure from which it obtains a new blood supply. As more and more of the chorion erodes through the wall of the tube the new area of implantation is increased to such a size that it is capable of maintaining the pregnancy. The placenta can develop on almost any organ in the pelvis, including the posterior wall of the uterus, the walls of the pelvis itself, or even the intestine. The pregnancy continues to grow and to develop and all the symptoms are those of a normal pregnancy.

A secondary abdominal pregnancy is particularly dangerous because the baby is surrounded only by the amnion and chorion which do not form a very strong protection against external injury. Rupture of the amnion and chorion results in the amniotic fluid spreading throughout the abdominal cavity and consequently peritonitis. The diagnosis of an extrauterine pregnancy is extremely difficult and may only become obvious because the baby will not present normally when the pregnancy gets close to term. Suspicion may be aroused if the pregnancy fails to develop properly and is smaller than would be expected. It is occasionally possible for an extrauterine pregnancy to develop to term, and for the woman to go into a type of spurious, or false, labour which cannot, of course, result in delivery. An operation is performed to deliver the baby by opening the abdomen as soon as the diagnosis is assured. Extrauterine pregnancies are usually diagnosed by ultrasonic scan between the 12th and 30th week of pregnancy so that survival of the baby is extremely rare and in any event these babies usually suffer from congenital abnormalities, probably caused by the inadequate blood supply to the pregnancy which cannot be as efficient as that supplied to a pregnancy developing normally within the uterus. When an operation is performed for an extrauterine pregnancy, the baby is removed together with the amniotic fluid and as much of the amnion, chorion and the umbilical cord as possible. The placenta is usually left in place because its removal would result in considerable bleeding. The abdominal cavity will gradually reabsorb it over the ensuing months

20 The Rhesus Factor

The discovery of the Rhesus factor just over 40 years ago led to an understanding of why some babies used to become rapidly jaundiced soon after their birth and then sometimes died, while others suffered from a condition known as erythroblastosis fetalis which caused them to be still-born or die very soon after delivery. They suffered from gross swelling of all parts of the body and severe anaemia.

The remarkable story of how the Rhesus factor was first discovered, its importance understood, treatment devised for the women suffering from Rhesus incompatibility, advanced techniques developed for the treatment of the new-born babies (including the complete changing of their blood) and then, a few years ago, the discovery of the means to prevent this condition, reads rather like a detective story in a novel. It is a remarkable feat of modern medicine. The complete elimination of a disease has taken place within a space of 30 years which is within the working life of most people. Babies died from a strange condition, whose cause and origin were completely unknown. Slowly the pieces of a medical jigsaw have been put together until the complete picture is now available and, as a result, the condition is preventable in the majority of instances. It is a triumph of preventive medicine.

Approximately 85 per cent of European women are Rhesus positive and 15 per cent are Rhesus negative. About 94 per cent of Jews are Rhesus positive In order to understand what is meant by Rhesus positivity it is necessary to appreciate that the blood cells of every person possess six Rhesus factors—three inherited from the mother and three inherited from the father. These factors are labelled C, D, and E, and each factor may be either positive or negative. They are represented by small letters c, d, and e when they are negative, and large letters C, D and E when they are positive. Each person, therefore, has either a small 'c' or a large 'C', a small 'd' or a large 'D' and a small 'e' or a large 'E' from the mother, together with a small or large C, D and E from the father. The whole is written as c, d, e/C, D, E, if a person inherited a small c, d and e from the mother and a large C, D, and E from the father. Any combination of these small or large letters can exist.

A person is stated to be Rhesus positive when he possesses the factor known as capital or big D. Big D may be present on either side or on both sides. So far as the ordinary testing of the blood is concerned the only real interest is in D and the presence of one D makes a person Rhesus positive. To help understand Rhesus incompatibility and the Rhesus factor, we can forget both types of C and E and just concentrate on the factor D. If a woman possesses D/D or d/D, or D/d she is Rhesus positive. But if she possesses d/d she is Rhesus negative. The same applies to a man. If a man possesses D/D he is stated to be homozygous because every sperm which he forms must contain D. He will therefore pass D on to all his children, so that they will all be Rhesus positive as they will all contain D. If a man is d/D or D/d then he is stated to be heterozygous, and he can pass on either D or d to his children, so that, if the mother is Rhesus negative, 50 per cent will be Rhesus positive and 50 per cent Rhesus negative (see page 284). Only on very rare occasions do problems arise in relation to c/C or to e/E.

Rhesus sensitization

The Rhesus factor can only give rise to trouble when a Rhesus negative woman is carrying a Rhesus positive child. Throughout pregnancy, and especially at the time of delivery, blood cells from the child escape into the maternal circulation. The mother's body reacts to these positive cells by attempting to destroy them by forming an antibody, known as Rhesus antibody, but before she can form an antibody the organs which are destined to form that antibody have to be primed, sensitized, or given, as it were, an initial warning that a foreign substance is circulating in the blood stream. They are unable to make antibody immediately, but having received the initial warning, or sensitization, will immediately form Rhesus antibody should any further Rhesus positive cells enter the circulation. A Rhesus negative woman who is carrying a Rhesus positive child will, therefore, not make antibodies during her first pregnancy, but the cells which escape into her circulation during the first pregnancy will provide the sensitizing dose. Similarly, transfusions of Rhesus positive cells into a Rhesus negative person, or the injection of Rhesus positive blood into the muscle of a Rhesus negative person, will cause a similar sensitization following which any further injection will provoke the production of antibodies.

It is not known at precisely what stage in pregnancy a fetus is capable of sensitizing its mother. It is unlikely that pregnancies terminated before the 6th week can cause sensitization. It may, however, be possible for pregnancies after the 8th week to sensitize a woman and it is almost certain that pregnancies after the 10th week can.

Many attempts have been made to desensitize women who are already sensitized or who have circulating Rhesus antibodies. A new and exciting technique (plasmaphoresis) to remove Rhesus antibody from the maternal circulation is being developed and offers great hope in the future to affected women.

```
cde/cde  = Rhesus negative; does not contain D
CdE/CdE  = Rhesus negative; does not contain D
cDe/cde  = Rhesus positive; Heterozygous—contains one D
cde/cDe  = Rhesus positive; Heterozygous—contains one D
cDe/cDe  = Rhesus positive; Homozygous—contains two D
CDE/cDe  = Rhesus positive; Homozygous—contains two D
```

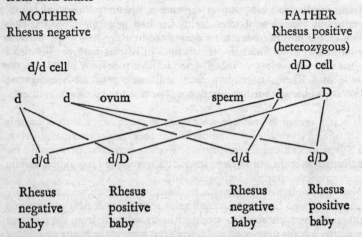

MOTHER
Rhesus negative

FATHER
Rhesus positive
(homozygous)

d/d cell

D/D cell

d   d   ovum   sperm   D   D

d/D   d/D   d/D   d/D

Rhesus positive baby   Rhesus positive baby   Rhesus positive baby   Rhesus positive baby

All the babies are Rhesus positive because they have all inherited D from their father

MOTHER
Rhesus negative

FATHER
Rhesus positive
(heterozygous)

d/d cell

d/D cell

d   d   ovum   sperm   d   D

d/d   d/D   d/d   d/D

Rhesus negative baby   Rhesus positive baby   Rhesus negative baby   Rhesus positive baby

50 per cent of babies are Rhesus negative and 50 per cent are Rhesus positive

Rhesus antibodies

Red cells escape from the circulation of the fetus into the mother's circulation in small quantities throughout pregnancy and in a woman who has been previously sensitized the escape of Rhesus positive cells from her baby into her circulation will provoke the production of Rhesus antibody to destroy the foreign circulating cells. Unfortunately, the Rhesus antibody so formed by the mother is capable of, and in fact does, cross the placenta into the baby's circulation where it commences to destroy the baby's own circulating Rhesus positive red cells.

If the mother makes a lot of Rhesus antibody it will form a high concentration in her blood and a high concentration will pass into the fetus, where it will cause massive destruction of the baby's Rhesus positive blood cells, with the result that the baby may die in the uterus from anaemia and heart failure (erythroblastosis fetalis). If the concentration is not so high the baby may be born alive but with severe anaemia and because the antibody already in his circulation continues the destruction of his red cells after birth, the baby will rapidly become jaundiced and may soon die. Such a baby would have his blood tested immediately at birth and will need to have his blood changed by an exchange transfusion. In this way most of the Rhesus positive cells are replaced by Rhesus negative cells which cannot be destroyed by the residual antibody within his system. These transfused Rhesus negative cells survive in the baby's circulation for approximately 40 days, during which time the baby will gradually eliminate all the Rhesus antibody from his system, and as he forms more of his own Rhesus positive cells they can no longer be destroyed. Although the baby's blood has been changed at birth from Rhesus positive to Rhesus negative, he will grow up to be Rhesus positive because his own blood forming organs can only make a Rhesus positive blood. Once the antibody has been washed out of his system he will come to no further harm and will develop into a perfectly normal child. Some babies may be only mildly affected at birth with only slight anaemia and a mild degree of jaundice. They require frequent tests, and careful observation but do not need exchange transfusions.

Blood groups

The statistical odds of a Rhesus negative woman marrying a Rhesus positive man and having a child with Rhesus disease are 0.2 per cent or 1 in 500. Only about 8 per cent of Rhesus negative women who are married to Rhesus positive men do in fact develop Rhesus antibodies and have problems with their children. For many years it was not known why only 8 per cent should be so unfortunate, nor could it be predicted who would be in the unhappy group. The answer to this problem depends upon the four major blood groups: O, A, B and AB, to one of which every person must belong. It is well known that people of one blood group cannot receive transfusions from people of certain other blood groups because for some unknown reason every person has an inbuilt mechanism to destroy any blood cells which do not belong to his own, or to a compatible, group. Let us now reconsider the Rhesus problem.

When a group B Rhesus negative woman is carrying a group A Rhesus positive baby the shower of the baby's red cells which enter the maternal circulation at delivery are incompatible with the mother's blood. They will, therefore, rapidly be destroyed by the mother's inbuilt mechanism to destroy any group A cells which enter her circulation, before they have had time to sensitize or even provoke the tissues of the mother into considering the production of Rhesus antibody. If on the other hand a group B Rhesus negative woman is carrying a Rhesus positive child who is also group B, the fetal cells which pass into the maternal circulation when the child is delivered are compatible with the mother's major blood group (they are both group B) and will not be destroyed but will continue to circulate until they have sensitized the mother who may later develop Rhesus antibodies.

A Rhesus negative woman can therefore be sensitized by receiving a quantity of Rhesus positive blood of a compatible or similar blood group either by transfer from her baby at the time of delivery or by the inadvertent injection of Rhesus positive blood. If these cells can be destroyed within one or two days (as happens when the blood group is not compatible) the woman is not sensitized. The Rhesus negative group B woman mentioned above who has been delivered of a group B Rhesus positive baby now has in her circulation group B Rhesus positive cells from her baby which, unless they are destroyed, will sensitize her to the production of Rhesus antibody.

If the woman who has compatible Rhesus positive red cells circulating in her system can be given Rhesus antibody shortly after her delivery it will destroy the Rhesus positive cells before they have had an opportunity to sensitize the maternal host and she need never develop any Rhesus antibodies. It is possible to isolate Rhesus antibody from a woman who has previously developed it to a high concentration in her blood. The Rhesus antibody can be extracted and purified and, as it is specific for the Rhesus D factor against which it was originally formed, it is known as anti-D immunoglobulin (see below). Rhesus disease is therefore controllable providing an adequate amount of anti-D immunoglobulin is given to the mother within 72 hours of delivery.

Prevention of Rhesus disease

Blood tests

Blood is taken at the beginning of pregnancy to test whether the woman is Rhesus positive or negative. If she is found to be Rhesus negative then a further test will be done to discover if any antibodies are present in her blood. Tests for Rhesus antibody will be repeated at intervals throughout pregnancy in any Rhesus negative person. It is not usual in Great Britain to perform tests on the husband's blood unless his wife develops antibodies. It is then important to know if the husband is homozygous or heterozygous so that the likelihood of his offspring being Rhesus positive or Rhesus negative can be assessed.

If antibodies are present they are expressed as a titre, that is the dilution of blood in which antibody can be recognized, and the titre is expressed as 1:4 or 1:8. As the amount of antibody increases in the blood so the dilutions in which it can be detected increase and if a large amount of antibody is present it may be detected in a dilution of 1:500 or even 1:1,000. Usually the antibody titre rises as the pregnancy progresses, but the outcome of the pregnancy is not directly related to the concentration of Rhesus antibody in the bloodstream. It is for this reason that other tests have been devised to judge more accurately how severely the baby may be affected.

Amniocentesis

The amniotic fluid which surrounds a baby suffering from Rhesus incompatibility contains a substance known as bilirubin which comes from the breakdown of the baby's destroyed red cells. The amount of bilirubin in the amniotic fluid increases as a greater number of the baby's red cells are destroyed and is therefore an accurate indication of the condition of the baby. A small amount of fluid is examined in the laboratory for bilirubin, with the result that accurate assessment can be made of the severity of the actual disease within the baby. Amniocentesis may be repeated at two or three weekly intervals. The results obtained are carefully plotted on a chart which, together with the patient's condition and antibody level, will determine the exact course of treatment to be adopted.

Treatment of affected babies

It is seldom that even mildly affected babies are allowed to proceed beyond the expected date of confinement. Moderately affected babies will almost certainly be delivered before the expected date, whereas severely affected babies may require special treatment before birth

Mildly affected babies will have a blood test performed on a sample of blood taken from the umbilical cord at the time of delivery so that their haemoglobin level can be estimated and the degree of anaemia and jaundice assessed. The tests are repeated at frequent intervals, but it is unusual for the baby to require any specific treatment.

Moderately affected babies also have a blood test performed immediately at birth. The degree of anaemia in these babies is such that they nearly always require an exchange transfusion. The umbilical cord is carefully preserved at the time of delivery and a very fine plastic catheter is threaded along its vein. The end of this catheter passes into the main vessel which returns the blood to the baby's heart. A small quantity of Rhesus positive blood is withdrawn from the baby and the same amount of especially prepared, fresh Rhesus negative blood is injected into the baby. This process of withdrawal and replacement is repeated taking 20 ml at a time until approximately 25 or even 30 lots of 20 ml have been withdrawn and each carefully replaced by Rhesus negative blood. By this method approximately 90 per cent of the baby's own blood is removed and replaced by Rhesus negative blood. It also has the advantage of removing from the baby's circulation most of the antibody which he inherited from his mother as well as a number of the harmful products causing the jaundice. Frequent blood samples are taken during the next four or five days to check that the newly injected blood cells are performing satisfactorily and that the level of jaundice is not increasing. Occasionally a second exchange transfusion, and in rare instances a third exchange transfusion, has to be given.

It takes approximately three days for an infant to excrete all the Rhesus antibody that he has acquired from his mother, so that generally speaking after the third day there is no further need for exchange transfusion, unless the level of bilirubin which causes the jaundice builds up within the baby's circulation to such a high level that his liver is incapable of excreting it. If this happens yet a further exchange transfusion may be necessary to remove it. Careful and repeated tests are performed on the bilirubin level in the baby's blood for the first six or even ten days after delivery because particularly high levels of bilirubin can cause damage to the baby's brain. This is the only method by which Rhesus babies can be permanently affected and doctors therefore continuously monitor the bilirubin level and take prompt action before it can become dangerous.

The majority of children who fall into the category of Rhesus incompatibility do survive and are perfectly normal, healthy infants and adults.

Severely affected babies present a most difficult problem. It is nearly always possible to foretell the severity of their affection from the result of amniocentesis. If a severely affected baby is left alone it will die in the uterus. It must therefore either be delivered before it dies or be treated while still in the uterus. It is always possible to deliver a baby prematurely but if it is too premature it will fail to survive. If, on the other hand, it is not delivered prematurely it may die inside the uterus from anaemia. The technique has therefore been devised by which a transfusion can be given to the baby while it is still in the uterus. This is a highly complicated and complex procedure achieved by passing a needle through the abdominal wall of the mother, through the wall of the uterus and into the abdomen of the baby. A small catheter is threaded through the needle and a carefully calculated quantity of specially prepared Rhesus negative blood is injected into the baby's abdomen over a carefully prescribed length of time. The catheter is then withdrawn. The Rhesus negative blood cells are absorbed from the baby's abdomen into his circulation. Since they are not destroyed by the Rhesus antibody present in his circulation they help the baby to survive. Such transabdominal transfusions may be repeated as frequently as two-weekly intervals until the pregnancy reaches the 34th week, when delivery may be induced with a reasonable chance that, by exchange transfusion after delivery, the child will survive and be normal.

The premature delivery of babies affected by Rhesus incompatibility is now very commonplace. There are, of course, hazards in the premature delivery of any baby, but the doctors weigh these very carefully against the hazards of leaving the baby in the uterus with the continuous passage of Rhesus antibody into his circulation. The modern methods that are available calculate scientifically the exact date at which delivery can be most safely undertaken. This is not pure guesswork.

Anti-D immunoglobulin

Anti-D immunoglobulin is purified Rhesus antibody obtained from people who have a high circulating antibody level. When injected into a person it will rapidly destroy Rhesus positive cells. Anti-D immunoglobulin is given to Rhesus negative women by injection after the delivery of a Rhesus positive child to prevent them being sensitized.

Blood is taken from the baby immediately on delivery and from the mother about 30 minutes after delivery. Both blood groups, Rhesus factor and haemoglobin levels are checked. If the two blood groups are not compatible then the mother will immediately destroy the baby's red cells that have escaped into her circulation. During pregnancy small numbers of red cells from the baby's circulation escape into the mother's circulation but at the time of delivery there is usually a large shower of fetal red cells escaping into the maternal circulation. When the blood groups of the mother and baby are not compatible these red cells are rapidly destroyed before the Rhesus factor which they contain can sensitize the mother. If the baby's blood cells are compatible with the mother's they will remain in her circulation where they can be detected by the Kleihauer test. This indicates that the Rhesus negative mother will become sensitized by the circulating Rhesus positive cells and an injection of anti-D immunoglobulin is given within 72 hours of delivery to prevent sensitization There are no known toxic or side effects from the injection.

The administration of anti-D immunoglobulin is carefully controlled because its use prevents women becoming sensitized and, therefore, prevents them from producing Rhesus antibodies thus automatically reducing the source of supply. In order to make absolutely certain that sensitization does not occur it is now the usual practice to give anti-D immunoglobulin to all Rhesus negative women shortly after delivery or abortion

Zygosity

The difference between a heterozygous and a homozygous man is explained on page 283. If a man is heterozygous half his offspring will be Rhesus positive and half Rhesus negative. Those children who are Rhesus negative will be unaffected even if they are produced by a woman who has been previously sensitized or who has actually developed antibodies. The very presence, however, of a Rhesus negative baby may provoke a higher concentration of Rhesus antibody in the mother. The reason for this is now known. Tests performed upon the amniotic fluid of the baby will show conclusively if the baby is positive or negative. If the child is Rhesus negative then it can be allowed to go to term and be delivered in the normal way despite the presence of antibodies in the mother's circulation

A-B-O incompatibility

In very rare circumstances incompatibility occurs between the major blood groups of the mother and the baby. These are usually concerned with the mother being group A and the baby being a different group. A-B-O maternal fetal incompatibilities are rare and mild, so that the babies are not severely affected and little or no treatment is necessary before delivery. The baby may become jaundiced and slightly anaemic and may require repeated tests during the first seven or ten days of life.

Kell incompatibility

As well as the major A-B-O blood groups and the Rhesus factor there are many minor blood groups and factors, one of which is called Kell. People are either Kell positive or Kell negative. A Kell negative woman may be sensitized by a Kell positive child, in a manner similar to that in which a Rhesus negative woman is sensitized, so that she develops Kell antibodies. Kell antibodies, however, are relatively weak and while they may cause some jaundice and a mild degree of anaemia in the baby after birth, they seldom affect the infant severely. The formation of Kell antibodies is extremely rare.

Now that the proportion of Rhesus-D affected babies is decreasing, more are found affected by antibodies to C and E antigens. The mothers in this situation carry the D antigen and are therefore Rhesus positive, but become sensitized to the fetus which carries the C and E antigens. In virtually all cases the women have been sensitized previously by a blood transfusion. It is now recommended that all young women be given blood which is not only matched for the D antigen, but also C, E and Kell antigens.

21 Medical and Surgical Conditions during Pregnancy

Pregnancy is very often the first opportunity available to the doctor for complete examination of an apparently healthy, normal young woman. Occasionally disease or abnormalities are detected for the first time and it is therefore important that a woman should have a complete physical examination as early in pregnancy as possible. Should the doctor find anything unusual he will consider, firstly, the effect of the pregnancy on the disease, and secondly the effect of the disease on the pregnancy. It is not the intention of this book to be involved in detailed study of these diseases; it gives a broad outline of the way in which they may be associated with pregnancy.

Heart disease

Heart disease is either congenital or acquired. About 65 per cent of the instances of heart disease in women are of the acquired type. Most of these result from rheumatic fever from which they have previously suffered, usually in childhood. The remainder are from congenital abnormalities of the heart. Modern medical care ensures that women with heart disease come to no harm either during or as a result of their pregnancy, except those who suffer from a most severe form of heart disease and in whom pregnancy is not advised. Pregnancy is seldom terminated today because a woman is suffering from heart disease.

There are four grades of cardiac disease in the international classification:

Grade I. There is no limitation to normal activity, no shortness of breath on performing ordinary household duties, climbing stairs or shopping.

Grade II. Some limitation; shortness of breath is present on simple exertion such as climbing stairs or shopping, or excessive household work like scrubbing and polishing.

Grade III. Serious limitation; there is shortness of breath during ordinary mild activity.

Grade IV. Very serious limitation; there is shortness of breath while a person is at rest in bed, and special care and attention are obviously necessary.

The main problem with respect to pregnancy associated with cardiac disease is that the amount of extra work the heart has to undertake is increased by between 25 to 40 per cent at about the 30th week of pregnancy. Cardiac disease presents the ideal (if there be an ideal) condition for the demonstration of good antenatal care. The first essentials are meticulous and frequent supervision, and extra rest to prevent any extra strain on the heart. Extra rest means that the pregnant woman should stay in bed for 12 hours each night and have at least two 2-hour periods of rest during the day. Special care must be taken to avoid anaemia and excessive weight gain and to guard against infections, especially flu and the ordinary common cold. Swelling of the hands or feet, or the onset of cough or shortness of breath, should be reported immediately to the doctor. At the first sign of any infection or a rise in temperature she should go to bed and notify the doctor at the earliest reasonable opportunity. This is particularly applicable to coughs and colds. The time of greatest increase of work load on the heart during pregnancy is at about the 30th week and most obstetricians encourage their cardiac patients to take more bed-rest for the remaining few weeks. Such bed-rest is usually in hospital, but if home facilities are adequate there is no reason why a woman should not rest quietly at home. Most women feel much stronger after 2 weeks in bed. Infected gums and bad teeth present a particular danger to the pregnant cardiac patient and she must visit her dentist regularly. If any dental extractions are necessary during pregnancy a short course of antibiotic is given.

A number of years ago the standard treatment of the pregnant cardiac patient was induction of labour at 36 or 38 weeks. This is now considered unnecessary interference unless there is some other indication for inducing labour. For some unknown reason labour itself in women with heart disease is nearly always rapid and easy. An antibiotic is usually given during labour and for the first day or two after delivery. Women with Grade II or III cardiac diseases are admitted to hospital at about 38 weeks in order to have further rest before the onset of labour.

It has been repeatedly emphasized throughout this book that the normal outcome of a pregnancy depends just as much on the pregnant woman as it does on her medical or nursing advisers. A woman with heart disease should be aware of the possible problems that her disease may present, understand the reasons for the extra care and attention that her pregnancy requires, and if she obeys the rules she will come to no harm.

Heart operations on women suffering from cardiac disease are avoided if possible during pregnancy although they cause little or no increase in danger to the mother or her baby.

The question of breast-feeding by cardiac patients is one that can only be answered after individual discussion. Generally speaking there is no reason why a woman with mild cardiac disease should not breast-feed her baby if she wishes. Many doctors, however, discourage women with severe cardiac disease from breast-feeding unless they are really determined to do so.

Diabetes mellitus

It is most unusual for an untreated diabetic woman to become pregnant and if she does the death rate for both mother and infant without treatment is extremely high. Diabetes mellitus is a disease that has been transformed as a result of the discovery of insulin, and, more recently, by drugs which may be taken by mouth, and its improved control in young people has made women with the disease a relatively common finding in the antenatal clinic.

Diabetes may become unmasked for the first time during pregnancy and a pregnant woman's urine is therefore tested for the presence of sugar at every antenatal visit. Generally speaking women with diabetes are interested in their disease and they understand it extremely well. The main problem concerning the diabetic who becomes pregnant is the meticulous and exact control of her diabetes. The diabetic woman and her baby are exposed to many difficulties during pregnancy which do not affect the non-diabetic woman. Most of these problems can be avoided if the diabetes is kept under very strict control by meticulous care and attention throughout the whole of the pregnancy. The drug requirements of the diabetic patient vary during pregnancy so that a woman who is taking insulin will have her dosage changed several times throughout the pregnancy. Careful stabilization of both drugs and diet is of the utmost importance as the uncontrolled diabetic has an increased danger of miscarriage, of developing pre-eclampsia, or polyhydramnios, of going into premature labour, of having a congenitally abnormal infant or of being delivered of a dead baby. The need for exact control of the diabetes cannot be over-emphasized, because nearly all the above complications are a direct result of instability of the diabetic state.

Up to fairly recently the majority of diabetic women were delivered at the 36th or 37th week of pregnancy because their babies tended either to die in the uterus as a result of the adverse affect of the diabetes on the placenta, or to grow to a very large size.

Estimations of oestriol and other hormone levels will indicate those babies which are at risk of dying in the uterus and also the time at which they should be delivered. Excessively large babies may be delivered by Caesarean section at 38 or 39 weeks. Labour in a diabetic woman is usually uncomplicated and its management not difficult. Whether delivery be by Caesarean section or by normal labour, a special intravenous drip of glucose solution controls the diabetic condition accurately during labour and delivery. Even with all this care and attention the newly delivered baby of a diabetic mother may still have a difficult time during the first

24 or 48 hours, and requires careful supervision by specially trained staff during the first two days of life.

Sugar is frequently found in the urine of a normal pregnant woman because the kidneys allow the passage of sugar at abnormally low levels during pregnancy. This is known as low renal threshold. It is a perfectly normal phenomenon and does not indicate that a woman is suffering from diabetes. Further special blood tests have to be undertaken in order to establish a diagnosis of diabetes.

Anaemia

The prevention of anaemia is one of the most important aspects of antenatal care. The degree of anaemia is assessed by measuring the haemoglobin level in the blood. The haemoglobin is the protein within the circulating red cells which is responsible for transferring oxygen from the lungs to the tissues in the body and in a pregnant woman, to the placenta and therefore to the fetus. When the haemoglobin level falls so does the ability of the body to transfer oxygen. What is probably more important is the fact that when the haemoglobin level in the blood is measured, only one constituent of the blood is being estimated and a fall in haemoglobin level also implies a fall in all the other factors which constitute normal blood.

The normal haemoglobin level in the adult male is approximately 100 per cent (14.7 g) whereas in the average adult female the average haemoglobin level is accepted as being 90 per cent (13 g). The level is lower in the female than in the male because of the constant and repeated loss of blood at menstruation. The repeated menstrual loss may also gradually diminish the iron and protein reserves in the female body so that even in the non-pregnant state a woman may become anaemic purely because of iron shortage. It is obvious that pregnancy may produce anaemia simply because the pregnant woman has already lost most of her reserves at menstruation and has no resources to meet the demands of the growing fetus.

During pregnancy there is an increase in the volume of blood circulating through the body which is an automatic response of the body to the increasing demands of the uterus for a greater blood supply. The blood volume increases by as much as 30 per cent and this is brought about by a rise in the plasma or fluid content of the blood which necessarily causes dilution of the red cells. Thus there are two factors causing anaemia in pregnancy. Firstly, a lack of reserves and resources from which to manufacture new cells or haemoglobin, and secondly, a dilution of the blood already present.

The symptoms of anaemia are slow in onset and are recognized only very gradually. Tiredness, lethargy, lack of energy, inability to perform ordinary household chores leading to untidiness, bad temper and irritability are the classic symptoms of anaemia. Pallor or whiteness of the skin together with a tired look makes the diagnosis obvious.

One of the main aims of antenatal care is to prevent anaemia by two basic principles. Firstly, the control of weight gain; the more weight that is gained in pregnancy, the more blood will be required in the body and therefore the greater will be the dilution of the blood already present. There is excessive dilution of blood together with an extra work load on the heart when the weight gain exceeds 9 kg. A pregnant woman who develops pre-eclampsia also retains an extra quantity of fluid so that her blood is further diluted with resulting anaemia. Secondly, the provision of all the factors that the body requires for the manufacture of new blood cells and haemoglobin; these are mainly iron, a reasonable diet, vitamins and folic acid. A reasonable diet contains all the materials that are required for the normal production of blood cells and haemoglobin and the dietary supplements cope with the extra demand during pregnancy.

Causes of anaemia

Pre-existing anaemia. It is surprising how many women commence their pregnancy with a haemoglobin level of less than 90 per cent. This is probably because they have never taken supplementary iron or vitamins to offset the loss of blood at menstruation, so that their body stores are depleted. It is obvious that such a woman is going to become anaemic during her pregnancy when extra demands are placed on her circulation.

Iron deficiency. Some women who are fit and healthy before the onset of pregnancy may have sufficient iron reserves and stores in their body to meet all the demands of pregnancy without requiring any additional iron therapy. Since it is impossible to measure the actual reserves of iron in the body it has become standard practice to give iron tablets to all women during pregnancy. A normal person cannot have an excess of iron. These tablets must be taken regularly as prescribed. Anaemia due to iron deficiency may develop because:

1 The iron tablets are not being taken. A pregnant woman must take her iron tablets or iron can be given by injection. It is well known that some iron tablets do upset the digestion and the bowels but if this happens alternative iron preparations which will not cause any disturbance can be given.
2 The iron tablets have been taken but the iron is not being absorbed from the intestine. This condition sometimes occurs but is not properly understood. When it does happen the iron can be given by injection.
3 The iron has been taken and absorbed, but the body is unable to use it because it lacks some of the other essentials for making haemoglobin and red cells, such as magnesium, copper or thyroid. These so-called

trace elements are usually contained within the iron or the vitamin pills.

Other diseases of the blood. There are a group of diseases either of the blood or of the blood-forming tissues which predispose a patient to a persistent and lifelong anaemia. Thalassaemia and sickle-cell disease are generally found in people from the West Indies, Asia, Africa and Mediterranean countries. Such conditions require special care and treatment during pregnancy.

Folic acid deficiency causes megaloblastic anaemia which is characteristic of pregnancy and is present in 5 to 10 per cent of all pregnant women, especially in those who have had repeated pregnancies or a twin pregnancy. Folic acid is now administered regularly to all women during pregnancy.

Infection is one of the factors that will cause anaemia in an otherwise normal pregnancy because some infections, especially those in the urinary tract, do result in a depression of the bone marrow which stops functioning satisfactorily. Furthermore such infections may have gone on for some time and may be without symptoms. In addition, people who have recently been, or come from abroad may have infection with parasites in the bowel which leads to a chronic loss of blood and consequent anaemia.

Anaemia used to be considered normal during pregnancy. This is no longer accepted. Anaemia can do nothing but harm and must be rigorously treated as soon as the first signs appear. Anaemia should be prevented so that pregnant women do not go into labour whilst anaemic. The prevention and treatment of anaemia, however, do demand the full cooperation of the pregnant woman without which it is impossible to undertake the repeated blood tests necessary for the diagnosis, or to undertake preventive or curative treatment.

Hypertension

Blood pressure is always expressed as two figures, such as 120/60, measured in millimetres of mercury. The higher is the systolic blood pressure which is the pressure reached within the blood vessels at the height of a heart beat and varies considerably with exercise, fatigue, excitement and emotion. The lower figure is the diastolic blood pressure which is the minimum level to which blood pressure falls between heart beats and this is of the greatest significance because it only varies as a result of some fundamental change in the circulation. The blood pressure normally rises with age but it is unusual for an otherwise normal woman to have a raised blood pressure during the childbearing period of her life. If her blood pressure is raised (hypertension) this is generally the result of some pre-existing condition

A woman suffering from hypertension, that is a diastolic blood pressure of 90 or more when she is resting, should consult her doctor about the advisability of becoming pregnant. Pregnancy itself causes a further rise in blood pressure and hypertension tends to reduce the blood supply to the uterus and therefore to the placenta and the baby, with the result that the baby is small, dysmature and may even fail to survive.

Providing all the appropriate tests and investigations have been performed and a woman with hypertension is properly looked after there is no absolute ban on her becoming pregnant, but she must realize that the restrictions placed upon her will be greater than those placed upon a woman who does not have a raised blood pressure before the onset of pregnancy. Hypertension does present an increased hazard to her baby and to herself and the number of her pregnancies should therefore be limited. Each individual woman must be judged on her merits after the widest consultation and consideration.

Kidney disease

The main kidney disease that may be present before the onset of pregnancy is chronic nephritis. This is a condition where the blood pressure is usually raised and a woman's fertility is reduced. Any woman who is known to suffer from chronic nephritis should consult her doctor before contemplating pregnancy. Urinary tract infections may also exist and are discussed below.

Urinary tract infection

Urinary tract infection (commonly known as cystitis) is the term which is now used to describe all infections that occur in the bladder and the kidney, replacing the previously used diagnoses of cystitis, pyelitis and pyelonephritis. It is one of the commonest types of infection to occur during pregnancy.

About 20 per cent of women have bacteria normally present in their urine and although the reason for this is uncertain, it is known that this particular group of women are very liable to develop urinary tract infections during their pregnancies. Special specimens of urine are taken at the onset of pregnancy to detect those women who are liable to develop infections. The final factor that leads to the onset of a urinary tract infection is not known. The action of the hormone progesterone causes some stagnation of urine within the urinary tract and this always predisposes to infection.

Urinary tract infections do not have any effect upon the pregnancy itself or on the baby, but occasionally an acute attack of pyelonephritis causes a high temperature which may precipitate premature labour.

Cystitis

An inflammation or infection of the bladder is known as cystitis. The symptoms may be sudden or gradual in onset and are frequency of passing urine, together with pain or stinging, or a certain amount of urgency, lower abdominal discomfort and occasionally blood in the urine.

Pyelonephritis

An infection involving the kidneys is termed pyelonephritis. There is usually severe pain in the loin associated with either the right or the left kidney accompanied by a sharp rise in temperature, shivering attacks and a definite feeling of illness. The symptoms of cystitis are often present.

Cystitis should be reported to your doctor or to the antenatal clinic as soon as convenient but acute cystitis or pyelonephritis should be reported as a matter of urgency. A mid-stream specimen of urine is collected and sent to the laboratory so that the infecting organism can be cultured and its sensitivity against various antibiotics assessed. A course of antibiotics or sulphonamides is given and the symptoms usually subside within 24 to 48 hours, but treatment must be continued for four or five days.

Recurrent urinary tract infection

Occasionally urinary tract infections recur during pregnancy and it is then usual to give the pregnant woman a prolonged course of treatment extending over several weeks or even months and sometimes to continue treatment until the end of pregnancy. Recurrent urinary tract infections usually merit extensive investigations but since these nearly always involve X-rays they are not undertaken until after delivery.

Vaginal discharge

A small quantity of mucoid vaginal discharge is usually present in early pregnancy and is frequently one of its earliest symptoms. The vagina normally contains a certain amount of moisture which arises from the glands in the cervix, as a secretion through the vaginal wall, and also from the glands at the entrance to the vagina. This moisture should never be very obvious or create a discharge which stains underwear or causes discomfort. A discharge is only normal during pregnancy, immediately before and immediately after a period, at the time of ovulation, as a result of sexual excitement, occasionally during puberty and the menopause, and in some women who are given hormone treatment such as some types of contraceptive pill. A small amount of mucoid discharge may also occur as a result of tiredness, stress, strain, during illness and also when the temperature is raised. Otherwise vaginal discharge is never really normal. However, a large number of women do, in fact, have a certain amount of vaginal discharge for which no adequate cause can be found and which is, therefore, accepted as being normal. It is extremely doubtful if it should be considered normal.

A certain amount of colourless mucoid discharge is a symptom of early pregnancy. The rise in hormone levels results in congestion within the reproductive organs in the pelvis which in turn results in an increase in the secretion through the vaginal walls. As pregnancy advances the discharge tends to increase but it should never become offensive nor should it cause any irritation. This type of mucoid vaginal discharge is often known as leucorrhoea, a word usually reserved for vaginal discharge of normal origin which does not cause any symptoms.

Cervical erosion

The normal rise in hormone levels during pregnancy provokes active growth of the glands within the cervical canal as well as an increase in secretions which is responsible for an increasing discharge as pregnancy advances. Occasionally excessive discharge from the cervical canal causes an 'erosion' or ulcer to form on the vaginal part of the cervix. The erosion itself continues to secrete mucus, the quantity of which is proportional to its size. Cervical erosions occur in about 75 per cent of all pregnancies and usually heal spontaneously after delivery, although occasionally they may persist and then require treatment. An erosion sometimes becomes infected by ordinary organisms which are normally present within the vagina or in the vulva and then the discharge becomes yellow and offensive. Any infected discharge may also result in soreness or actual irritation at the entrance to the vagina. Any soreness or irritation should be reported to the doctor or midwife at the next antenatal visit. Erosions are not usually treated during pregnancy because the treatment may predispose to an abortion or early labour. Vaginal infections have no effect on the baby because the contents of the uterus are protected by the plug of mucus in the cervix.

A small amount of yellow vaginal discharge does not usually warrant treatment but if it becomes profuse, offensive or causes discomfort, it should be treated. A swab of the discharge is taken for culture and subsequently treatment with a pessary or cream is prescribed which reduces the amount of infection present within the erosion. The quantity and offensive nature of the discharge will rapidly diminish. Vaginal douches should not be used during pregnancy because some of the fluid may pass through the cervix into the uterus causing infection, abortion or premature labour.

Blood-stained discharge

If any blood is present in the vaginal discharge you must go to bed and notify the doctor or midwife immediately.

Trichomonas infection

Infections of the vagina by the trichomonas vaginalis organism cause a profuse, yellow or greenish discharge associated with intense irritation and soreness, and sometimes frequency and pain on passing urine. The organism can be seen by examining a smear from the vaginal discharge under the microscope. The infection usually affects the husband as well as the pregnant woman. A seven day course of tablets, such as Metronidazole, is given to both partners and symptoms should be relieved within three days.

Monilial vaginitis

Infection of the vagina by candida albicans otherwise known as monilia (or thrush) is fairly common during pregnancy. The reason for this is not properly understood although the fungus itself thrives because of the relatively high glycogen content of the cells lining the vagina during pregnancy. It may be a new infection contracted during pregnancy or it may simply be a flare-up of a dormant infection which has not previously caused any symptoms. Pregnancy, diabetes, a course of antibiotics and some types of the contraceptive pill are all factors that predispose to fungus infections of the vagina.

Monilia causes a thick, white vaginal discharge associated with intense irritation of the vulva and the entrance to the vagina as well as a soreness and burning in the vagina itself. The irritation may cause great distress and it can be so severe that it wakes the woman at night or prevents sleep.

The modern treatment of this condition is a course of pessaries that contain an antibiotic which acts specifically on the fungus and on the yeast-like organisms which are also frequently present. The rather old-fashioned remedy of painting the vagina with half per cent aqueous solution of gentian violet is still very efficient. The insertion of a colourless and odourless pessary or cream has replaced this rather messy procedure. The symptoms should be relieved in one or two days after starting treatment. The fungus has the unhappy habit of suddenly reappearing later in pregnancy; any woman who has had an attack during her pregnancy is well advised to ask if she can keep a spare supply of treatment.

New-born babies sometimes develop thrush (fungus) infections in the mouth. These are recognized as white patches surrounded by a mild reddened area on the tongue and gums and are nearly always caused by the fungus getting into the baby's mouth from the mother's vagina at the time of delivery. The hospital and nursing staff are very often blamed, quite incorrectly, when a baby gets thrush in his mouth. A course of medicine will cure the baby very quickly without any permanent damage.

Venereal disease

Syphilis

When the pregnant woman first visits the antenatal clinic, a blood test is taken to determine her blood group, Rhesus factor, haemoglobin and also to perform a Wassermann test. This test is used to diagnose syphilis and is performed as a routine on all women at their first antenatal visit. Various refinements of the Wassermann test (known as the WR) are now also performed for the accurate diagnosis of syphilis because some diseases, such as glandular fever, may give a false positive result. The importance of diagnosing syphilis in early pregnancy is that the causative organism (treponema pallidum) does not cross the placental barrier until the 20th week of pregnancy, and it can be completely cured before then by the administration of antibiotics. If not treated until after the 20th week the organism crosses the placenta and infects the baby. It is a tragedy if this disease remains undetected in the mother when it is so easily curable during her pregnancy. Untreated syphilis may result in death of the baby in the uterus or in premature labour and will certainly result in the delivery of a child suffering from congenital syphilis.

Gonorrhoea

Gonorrhoea is comparatively rare during pregnancy because the infection usually causes an acute inflammation of the Fallopian tubes, resulting in considerable damage to the tissues, blockage of the tubes and eventual infertility or sterility. If the disease is treated in its very early stages, before the tubes have been damaged, it can be completely cured and will not affect a subsequent pregnancy. On rare occasions, however, women do become pregnant when they are suffering from gonorrhoea, or they contract the disease during pregnancy. The organism is harboured in the vagina and cervix and infects the eyes of the new-born infant during delivery. Unless this is rapidly recognized and treated it may result in blindness.

If a diagnosis of gonorrhoea is made the woman is usually referred to a special treatment centre and her husband or partner should also attend.

Tuberculosis

Tuberculosis of the lung may occasionally be associated with pregnancy. Modern medicine has done a great deal to reduce the incidence of lung tuberculosis, so much so that many clinics and hospitals today no longer expose their pregnant women to the once routine chest X-ray for its diagnosis, except where the incidence of tuberculosis remains an important local problem. The importance of BCG inoculation of all children cannot be over-emphasized because this is the main method of conferring immunity to tuberculosis and thus preventing people acquiring or spreading the disease.

If a woman who is pregnant has developed tuberculosis of the lung the pregnancy will not interfere with her treatment either by drugs or, if necessary, by surgery. The tuberculosis itself will not have an adverse effect on the pregnancy or the delivery. The few women who suffer from active tuberculosis are usually advised against breast-feeding and may have their babies isolated and given BCG inoculations as soon as they are delivered. Once a baby has developed immunity to the tubercle bacillus he may be returned to his mother, but not for breast-feeding.

Surgical emergencies in pregnancy

Surgical emergencies during pregnancy are comparatively rare, but when they do occur they are treated on the same principles and in the same manner as in the non-pregnant patient.

Acute appendicitis is extremely rare in pregnancy. It is difficult to diagnose and may be confused with round ligament pain occurring in the lower right side of the abdomen or an infection of the right kidney. If acute appendicitis is diagnosed in pregnancy then the appendix must be removed immediately.

Acute intestinal obstruction, which is the name given to the condition where a stoppage occurs in the intestine, is also rare during pregnancy, but must be operated upon.

Strangulation of a hernia or rupture is unlikely after the 20th week of pregnancy because the enlarging uterus prevents intestine from entering the hernia. Strangulation causes severe local tenderness.

Ovarian cysts. When an ovarian cyst is found during early pregnancy it should be left until after the 14th week, when it is surgically removed by enucleating the cyst from the ovary. It is important that such operations should not take place before the 14th week because the affected ovary may contain the corpus luteum upon which the pregnancy is dependent. After this, however, the hormones required for the maintenance of pregnancy are no longer produced by the corpus luteum but by the placenta, and if the corpus luteum is then removed the pregnancy will continue in the usual way. On rare occasions ovarian cysts undergo a twisting, or torsion, during pregnancy causing very acute pain and immediate operation is essential.

Haemorrhoids seldom present an acute condition during pregnancy and their treatment is left until after delivery. On rare occasions, however, a haemorrhoid prolapses outside the anus and becomes swollen and filled with a blood clot. This thrombosed prolapsed haemorrhoid is extremely painful and can be temporarily relieved by injecting the haemorrhoid with local anaesthetic, making a small incision over it and removing the clot. This is a simple procedure and results in complete relief of the severe pain.

Other operations may be necessary for a variety of acute emergencies which are as likely to occur during pregnancy as at any other time. Under modern surgical conditions and with modern anaesthesia these operations are performed without danger to the pregnant woman or to her baby. It is, nevertheless, true that on rare occasions the general response of the body to an acute emergency which results in operation also causes uterine contractions and occasionally abortion or miscarriage. Modern anaesthetics are administered with high concentrations of oxygen which protects both the mother and the fetus from any harmful effects.

Dental emergencies

All pregnant women should visit their dentist as soon as possible in pregnancy and should notify him of their pregnancy. Dental hygiene is of the utmost importance. If removal of teeth or fillings is required it may be performed under local anaesthesia without any danger to the woman or her baby. If general anaesthesia is necessary this may also be given, but in these instances most dental surgeons prefer to admit the woman to hospital. It is a common belief that local anaesthesia should not be used for dental extraction or fillings during pregnancy but there is no argument against its proper use.

22 Monitoring the Fetus

The high-risk pregnancy

Childbirth has always been associated with some risk to both mother and child, and midwives and obstetricians have always recognized that there are some women in whom the risks may be increased. It is only in the last 30 years or so, with improved collection of records and statistical analysis, that a pattern emerges of what factors might place the fetus at higher risk of being unwell, premature, unduly small or even still-born or dying soon after birth. Some of these factors such as social class or biological differences in women cannot be easily altered, whereas pathological conditions may be treated if detected. The major aim of antenatal care is to identify risk factors as they may apply to individual women. This is why such a detailed social history is taken at the first visit, and why doctors insist on the pregnant woman having an examination at least monthly during pregnancy. Sadly, it is often the women with the greatest number of risk factors who have the poorest antenatal care.

It has been known for many years that the age of the mother, her social class and her parity (the number of children she has borne) all bear decisively on the risk to her baby. The perinatal mortality is four times higher in social class V women as compared with social class I women. Perinatal mortality is higher in the woman under 20 years or over 30 years, and in the woman who is by herself and unsupported. Finally, the child who is the second-born in a family has the best fetal outcome compared with his other brothers and sisters. If there has been a previous premature delivery or still-birth, then there is a much higher risk of the same thing happening again.

In some hospitals in Great Britain, a 'risk card' is given to the mother, and contains information about those factors which may have an adverse effect on the outcome of the pregnancy. A list of some of these factors is presented below. It must be emphasized however that it is the accumulation of a number of factors which puts a pregnancy in a high-risk category. It does not necessarily mean that the baby will be born sick or still-born, but is simply a means of alerting the midwife and doctor to the fact that extra means of assessing the health of the fetus *in utero* may be required.

Which factors are important?

Most of these factors are chronic and can be identified early in pregnancy. However, some are acute (e.g. problems which arise in labour, or in response to sudden pathology in the mother such as infection).

Factor	Potential adverse effect
Maternal age less than 18 years	woman may be unsupported and pregnancy unplanned premature labour pre-eclampsia
more than 35 years	higher incidence of Down's syndrome (especially after 40 years) pre-eclampsia placental insufficiency
Social class V	pre-eclampsia placental insufficiency premature labour
Parity more than 5	placental insufficiency malpresentation of the fetus ante- and post-partum haemorrhage
Weight less than 45 kg	placental insufficiency
greater than 85 kg	hypertension gestational diabetes operative delivery thrombo-embolism
Height less than 152 cm (5 ft)	cephalopelvic disproportion
Events in early pregnancy vaginal bleeding	spontaneous abortion

Factor	Potential adverse effect
Events in early pregnancy	
conception after taking fertility drugs	multiple pregnancy spontaneous abortion
conception with intrauterine device *in situ*	spontaneous abortion premature labour
more than 2 previous terminations of pregnancy	cervical incompetence
emergency surgery	spontaneous abortion
Events in later pregnancy	
previous premature labour	premature labour (depends on cause)
previous still-birth or neonatal death	still-birth or neonatal death (depends on cause)
antibodies in previous pregnancy	recurrence in next pregnancy
small-for-dates baby	placental insufficiency
large-for-dates baby	gestational diabetes operative/traumatic delivery
smoking	placental insufficiency
alcohol excess	premature delivery addicted baby
heroin addiction	placental insufficiency addicted baby
infection	premature labour infection
chronic maternal illness (anaemia, renal disease, hypertension, cardiac disease)	premature labour placental insufficiency
pre-eclampsia	placental insufficiency

Factor	Potential adverse effect
Events in later pregnancy	
diabetes	congenital abnormality
	premature labour
	sudden death *in utero*
multiple pregnancy	placental insufficiency
	premature labour
malpresentation	operative delivery
post-maturity	placental insufficiency
Events in previous labour	
uterine scar (Caesarean section or other operation)	uterine rupture
labour less than 4 hours	neonatal asphyxia
post-partum haemorrhage or retained placenta	recurrence in next pregnancy

Monitoring fetal growth in the antenatal clinic

The general examination made at each visit is a simple yet important way of assessing the good health of the mother and her baby. Questions are usually asked about how actively the baby moves and how often. The doctor or midwife palpates the abdomen and observes the size of the uterus, whether it is growing uniformly, the size of the fetus, and how much amniotic fluid it moves in. A more accurate yet simple way of assessing growth is to measure the length of the uterus, from the top of the fundus to the pubic bone. After 30 weeks, the length in centimetres roughly corresponds to the gestation in weeks, and a good proportion of small-for-dates babies may be diagnosed in this way. Also after 34 weeks the girth measured in inches round the umbilicus roughly corresponds to the gestation in weeks.

Ultrasound and its use in pregnancy

High-frequency sound waves are directed through the mother's abdomen into the uterus. As they are reflected off the fetal bone and other tissues of different density, a pictorial representation of the baby is obtained. This is shown on a screen which looks like a radar screen. In fact, ultrasound was used during the Second World War to detect submarines and flaws in metal.

Ultrasound has transformed obstetrics because it can give important information quickly and very accurately. Sometimes this information could only otherwise come from blood tests which might take a number of days, or from special X-rays with their associated dangers. Very extensive research has been undertaken and, so far as is known, ultrasound does not harm the fetus. It is usually performed at least once in early pregnancy in most women having their babies in the larger teaching or district hospitals. The woman is asked to keep her bladder very full, oil is rubbed on her abdomen, and then the radiographer passes the arm of the ultrasound machine gently across her stomach, backwards and forwards. The mother can then see a picture of her baby on the screen. In the more modern machines ('real-time scanners') the fetal movements, breathing patterns and heart beat can all be clearly visualized. A very experienced radiographer can determine the weight of the baby, the volume of amniotic fluid, and even the sex of the older fetus.

In modern obstetric practice ultrasound is used to:

1 Confirm a pregnancy before clinical tests can be used, since the gestation sac can be visualized from 6 weeks and the embryo from 7 weeks.
2 Establish if a pregnancy is still viable when bleeding occurs in early pregnancy, since the fetal heart can be seen between 7 and 8 weeks.
3 Establish the length of gestation, by measuring the length of the fetus up to 12 weeks, and then the diameter of the head after that time. Up to 30 per cent of women do not know when their last period occurred, or have irregular cycles, and ultrasound before 10 weeks is accurate to within 5 days and before 24 weeks is accurate to within 10 days.
4 Detect multiple pregnancies since each gestation sac can be seen at an early stage. This is important in women who have been treated with fertility drugs.
5 Identify certain fetal abnormalities of the spine (spina bifida), head (hydrocephaly with a grossly enlarged head, or anencephaly where no brain or skull forms), kidney and bowel. In Rhesus-affected babies, ultrasound can even detect if they are in heart failure.
6 Assess fetal growth. The clinical impression of a baby that is small-for-dates can be confirmed with ultrasound which shows loss of growth in the liver and abdominal wall and finally the fetal head. It also shows a decrease in the amniotic fluid. Conversely, ultrasound can also show if a baby is growing larger than it should, as in poorly controlled diabetes. It is far more accurate than palpation by the doctor or midwife.
7 Localize the placenta. Women with an ante-partum haemorrhage must

have the placenta localized before a vaginal examination is performed, in case the bleeding is being caused by placenta praevia where the placenta covers the cervical os. Before ultrasound, very special X-rays had to be performed to localize the placenta. Ultrasound also has the added advantage of showing if there is any haemorrhage behind the placenta.

8 Confirm the fetal position. This is very important in early pregnancy when amniocentesis is being performed, to ensure that neither the placenta nor fetus is in the path of the needle. Later in pregnancy the same situation prevails. Babies affected by Rhesus disease, who would die if prematurely delivered, can now be transfused *in utero*. Prior to ultrasound, high amounts of radiation were given as X-rays were taken to localize the baby's abdomen in which the blood containing catheter is inserted.

9 Identify any remnants of placental tissue which may remain in the uterus after a spontaneous abortion or delivery.

10 Detect and measure the size of ovarian cysts, fibroids or any other pelvic swelling in early pregnancy.

Ultrasound has transformed modern obstetrics. It can be used to make a diagnosis about the state of the pregnancy much earlier than was previously possible, and also about the state of the fetus. This means that a baby with a gross abnormality incompatible with life can be detected early, and the pregnancy terminated if the parents so wish. Later in pregnancy, accurate knowledge of an abnormality before birth allows the medical team to plan the delivery better, and prepares other people such as paediatricians or surgeons for any intervention which may be required on their part. In fact, it has been possible recently to 'operate' on babies *in utero* who have obstruction in their urinary tracts. The distended bladder, detected by ultrasound, can be drained by a tiny plastic catheter whose other end remains in the amniotic fluid. In this way an attempt is made to prevent chronic damage to the kidneys by the build-up of urine under pressure.

Alphafetoprotein screening

Alphafetoprotein (AFP) is a protein, about the size of albumin, which is produced by the fetal liver in early pregnancy, and finds its way into the mother's circulation in increasing amounts. A breach in the baby's skin which exposes its blood vessels allows very high levels to pass into the amniotic fluid and also the mother's blood. This can occur in spina bifida where the spinal column does not close properly over the spinal cord, and anencephaly (see above). Some abnormalities of the baby's abdominal wall and kidney abnormalities can also give raised AFP levels, as can twins or a threatened abortion.

The blood test to detect levels of AFP is most accurate between 16 and 18 weeks. If the level is high another blood sample is taken and if that too is high, an amniocentesis is recommended. AFP screening in this way will detect 85 per cent of all babies with spina bifida.

Amniocentesis

The amniotic fluid in which the baby lives (see Chapter 4) contains cells from the fetal skin as well as chemicals which the fetus passes out in its urine and in the fluid bathing its lungs. These living cells increase in number from about 12 weeks to reach a maximum at 22 weeks. Amniocentesis involves tapping off some of this fluid, and is therefore only done after about 16 weeks.

A small amount of local anaesthetic is injected into the woman's abdominal wall, after the placenta has been localized with ultrasound. A hollow needle is then passed through the numb area into the amniotic sac and up to 20 ml of fluid is drawn off. A small adhesive plaster is placed over the needle hole, and another ultrasound scan ensures that the baby is moving normally. Part of the fluid may be tested for various chemical substances. The rest is used to grow the fetal cells. Special techniques are used to 'harvest' these cells subsequently, and they are then used for their assigned purpose. The process of growing cells takes 3 to 4 weeks and may sometimes fail.

Tests on the fluid include:

1 Chromosome analysis of the cells. There are an abnormal number of chromosomes in some conditions associated with congenital abnormality and mental retardation. The commonest of these is mongolism (Down's syndrome) and its incidence increases with the mother's age. Women over 37 years are offered amniocentesis for this reason. It may sometimes be important to know the sex of the baby when the mother is a carrier of a serious X-linked recessive disorder, such as haemophilia or muscular dystrophy. In this situation only the male child is affected, and has a 50 per cent risk of inheriting the disease.
2 AFP level when two blood samples have been elevated. If this too is abnormally high, there is a very great chance that the baby has spina bifida. Ultrasound scanning may detect the abnormal area.
3 Enzyme levels in a number of hereditary diseases called inborn errors of metabolism. These diseases affect the normal production of fats, proteins or carbohydrates in the body such that severe mental and physical handicap can result. Most of these diseases are rare but in certain groups they may be more frequent, for example Tay-Sachs disease in Ashkenazi Jews. The biochemical abnormality can be detected in the fetal cells obtained from amniotic fluid.

4 Bilirubin levels in Rhesus-affected babies (see Chapter 20). As fetal red blood cells are destroyed by the mother's antibodies against them, bile pigment increases proportionally. By examining the level in amniotic fluid every two to three weeks, and using specially prepared graphs, the obstetrician can decide when the baby can most safely be delivered.

5 Chemicals associated with maturity of the fetal lungs. Once the lung has matured, chemicals which act rather like detergents, increase rapidly and prevent the lungs from collapsing once the baby has been born. It may be important to know this if a doctor is contemplating early delivery, for example in a woman with a small-for-dates baby, where the risk of prematurity and breathing problems must be balanced with the risk of the baby dying *in utero*.

Amniocentesis therefore has a number of important uses extending throughout pregnancy. Its main risk, apart from damage to the fetus or placenta, is the onset of premature labour or a spontaneous abortion. This risk is about one per cent, but even less if ultrasound facilities are always used.

Fetoscopy

Under local anaesthetic it is possible to insert a very fine telescope through the mother's abdominal wall into the uterus. The baby can be directly visualized. This has been used where there is a risk that babies may suffer from hereditary skin disorders, cleft palate or abnormalities of the fingers and toes. Blood samples may also be taken and this is important where there is a risk of sickle-cell disease or thalassaemia which are blood disorders seen in Negroid people and those from around the Mediterranean. Fetoscopy is only done in a very few centres in Britain, and carries a 10 per cent risk of precipitating an abortion.

Hormone assays

There are two important hormones which are produced from the placenta in increasing amounts throughout pregnancy. Human placental lactogen (HPL) is a protein hormone which is detected in the mother's blood in increasing amounts as pregnancy advances, the levels depending very much on the size of the placenta. Low levels after about 32 weeks' gestation are associated with a higher incidence of fetal distress, small-for-dates babies and even still-birth. HPL is useful for monitoring women with high blood pressure or placental insufficiency.

Oestriol is a form of oestrogen which increases one-thousand-fold in the pregnant woman. It is produced by a number of steps that occur in the fetal adrenal gland, the fetal liver and then finally the placenta. Hence it is a good indicator of both fetal and placental health It can be measured in maternal urine (collected over 24 hours) or in maternal blood.

In many hospitals where women are in-patients with blood pressure or other complications of pregnancy, these two hormones are assessed twice weekly. As with HPL, low levels of oestriol are associated with a higher incidence of still-birth, fetal distress and a low-birth-weight baby. A fall in levels, which persists, is generally considered sinister and may warrant delivery of the baby.

Fetal movement recording

Fetal movements usually decrease and stop some hours before fetal death. Hence a mother's observation of how active her baby is, is a good means of assessing fetal well-being. The mother is asked at nine o'clock each day to count up to ten fetal movements, and mark on a chart the length of time it takes to reach this number. In most women fetal movements decrease from about 32 weeks to term, but at least ten in 12 hours should be noticed.

Antenatal cardiotocography

The baby's heart beats at a rapid rate between 120 and 160 beats per minute. As in the adult, an electrocardiograph of the baby's heart rate can be taken. A healthy baby shows an increase in the heart rate following fetal movement or uterine contraction. A distressed baby will often show a fall in the heart rate after movement or uterine contraction, or even in the absence of any stimulation. Other abnormalities may also be seen.

The ECG recording is simple to perform. The mother lies partly on her side and the device which records the fetal heart rate is strapped to her abdomen over the side where the heart beat is heard loudest with the ordinary stethoscope. The tracing of the heart rate appears on a special chart and the woman marks on it the times when she feels the baby moving.

In women in hospital with complications of pregnancy, a fetal heart rate tracing may be performed over 20 minutes or even an hour each day. In conjunction with other test results such as HPL or oestriol, and evidence of fetal growth on ultrasound scanning, doctors can try and reach decisions on whether it is safer to deliver a baby early than risk its sudden demise *in utero*.

Although the use of 'high technology' has its critics, most mothers feel immensely reassured when they see a tracing of their baby's heart rate and hear it beating, or see their baby moving or even 'breathing' on an ultrasound scanner. The improvement in perinatal mortality in recent years has been caused not simply by a general improvement in maternal nutrition and social welfare, but by increasing ways of recognizing when the fetus may be at risk *in utero*.

X-rays

There are fewer and fewer indications for X-rays now that ultrasound facilities are available. However, pelvimetry, an X-ray which is taken in such a way as to allow measurement of the woman's pelvis, may still sometimes be ordered in late pregnancy. Where the pelvis is abnormally small or malformed (for example, following a fracture in an accident), it may be necessary to perform a Caesarean section. In hospitals where breech vaginal deliveries are performed (see Chapter 27), the measurement of the pelvis must always be known. Some doctors will also order X-rays late in pregnancy for their diabetic patients, or women carrying twins.

23 The Fetal Position

The position of the baby lying at rest in the uterus is known as the fetal position (see fig. 24). The head is bent forwards with the chin resting on the chest, the arms are crossed so that the right hand rests on the left shoulder and the left hand rests on the right shoulder. The legs are bent at both the hip and the knee, so that the feet are crossed over the genitalia. The feet themselves are turned inwards so that they do not protrude outside the line of the body. The baby does, of course, move within the uterus and, especially in mid-pregnancy, it has great freedom to stretch and extend both its arms and legs. Frequent movement of all its muscles is essential in order to promote and maintain their development.

The lie

The 'lie' of the baby refers to the manner in which it is lying in the uterus.

Longitudinal lie

If one end of the baby is lying over the pelvic brim or is engaged within the pelvis itself so that its spine is almost parallel to the mother's spine, then the lie is stated to be longitudinal. In early pregnancy the baby can lie in any position and is free to twist and turn around inside the uterus as it wishes. At about the 28th week it begins to assume the longitudinal lie with one end lying immediately over the pelvic brim. In approximately 98 per cent of all pregnancies the lie is longitudinal.

Oblique lie

In approximately 1.5 per cent of instances the lie is oblique where the lower part of the baby lies just above the groin with its spine lying obliquely in relation to the mother's spine. This usually occurs only in women who have had several children and in whom the muscles of the abdominal wall have been slackened by repeated pregnancies, or where there is an excessive amount of fluid and therefore the baby is allowed to move around inside the uterus with comparative freedom. In nearly every instance an oblique lie will be converted spontaneously to a longitudinal lie at or before the onset of labour.

Transverse lie

In approximately 0.5 per cent of pregnancies the spinal column of the baby lies at right angles to that of the mother. This may happen when a woman has had many pregnancies which have resulted in slackness of both the abdominal wall and the uterus, or in the presence of an excessive quantity of amniotic fluid. In very rare instances transverse lie may be caused by fibroids, or any other space-occupying tumour or cyst which prevents the baby from assuming a longitudinal lie, and it is corrected to a longitudinal lie by the doctor performing external version either before or immediately after the onset of labour. Very occasionally this may be impossible and Caesarean section is performed. Transverse lie, however, is a rare complication.

Presentation of the baby

The presentation of the baby refers to that part of the baby which overlies the brim of the pelvis or the entrance to the birth canal. Nearly all babies are eventually converted into a longitudinal lie so that either the head or the bottom of the baby presents at the pelvic brim and the presentation is either head first (cephalic) or bottom first (breech).

At about the 28th week of pregnancy most babies are breech presentations with the head lying in the fundus, or upper part, of the uterus near the ribs. At about the 32nd week in a woman having her first baby, or at about the 34th week in a woman having subsequent children, the baby turns round spontaneously so that its head presents and it becomes a cephalic presentation. Neither the reason for this somersault nor the mechanism used to effect it is known. Ninety-six per cent of babies eventually assume a cephalic presentation, while the other 4 per cent remain as breech presentations.

The position of the baby's back is also important because a well flexed baby will always lie with its back to the front of the abdomen in what is known as an 'anterior' position. The back may be just to the right or to the left of the mid-line. A posterior position is when the baby's back is towards the mother's spine and it may, similarly, be right or left. A posterior position, which sometimes occurs in a first pregnancy, is not very favourable because the baby cannot assume an attitude of complete flexion, so that the head does not fit satisfactorily into the pelvic brim and may not engage, resulting in premature breaking of the waters and sometimes a long labour.

Cephalic presentation

In cephalic presentation the head presents. It is normally well flexed, which means that the chin is pressing down towards the chest. In 99 per cent of cephalic presentations the posterior part of the head, or vertex, is the part which actually descends first and will be delivered first. Such presentations are frequently known as vertex presentations. In the remaining 1 per cent the head is extended, so that instead of the baby having its chin tucked on its chest its head is bent as far back as possible, so that it looks directly into the pelvis and the birth canal. This is known as a face presentation. From a purely mechanical point of view a face presentation is only slightly more difficult than a vertex presentation. Whatever part of the baby's head presents a certain amount of swelling, known as the caput, forms over the area which lies immediately above the dilating cervix. This swelling can be fairly extensive and may distort the head, or the lips, nose and cheeks of a face presentation, so that the baby looks quite ugly immediately after delivery. The swelling soon disappears and the baby's features rapidly return to normal with no ill effect.

Breech presentation

As stated above, the majority of babies are breech presentations until approximately the 32nd week of pregnancy, after which they spontaneously rotate through 180° to cephalic presentations. Approximately 4 per cent of babies, however, fail to undergo this rotation and remain breech presentations.

External cephalic version

It is very much easier and safer for both the mother and her baby if the child is delivered head first. An important part of antenatal care is to ensure that the baby assumes the correct position at the right time and antenatal attendances are therefore usually arranged at two-weekly intervals from the 30th week. If by the 32nd week in a primigravida, or by the 34th week in a woman having a subsequent pregnancy, the baby has not yet assumed its cephalic presentation, the obstetrician may decide to turn the baby from a breech to a cephalic presentation, and this is known as external cephalic version (ECV). This sounds very dramatic but is in fact extremely simple and entirely free from pain or discomfort.

The woman lies on an examination couch with her feet slightly raised. She is asked to relax completely. Her abdomen is gently powdered and the doctor, using both hands, will slowly rotate the baby by exerting gentle pressure on it so that the baby's body is pushed up on one side of the uterus and the baby's head is gently pulled down the other side. This is frequently practised in antenatal clinics and has helped reduce the incidence of breech presentation from its normal 4 per cent to less than 1 per cent. External cephalic version may be performed on several occasions if necessary. There is no danger of the baby becoming entwined within his umbilical cord or of knots forming during this procedure. Remember

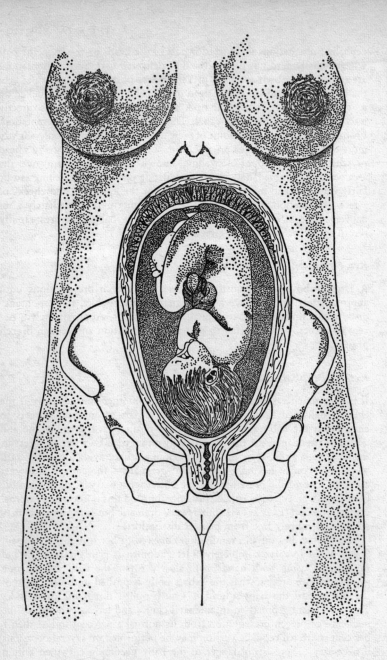

Fig. 24 Cephalic presentation

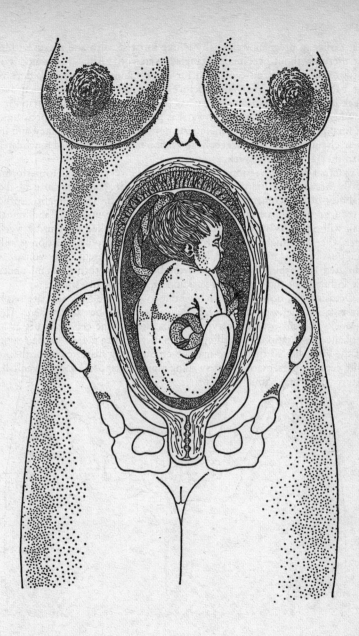

Fig. 25　Breech presentation

that earlier in pregnancy the baby is free to twist, turn and rotate within the uterus without becoming entangled in its cord. After this manoeuvre the woman remains on the couch for a few minutes and the position of the baby is confirmed by the doctor. It is usual to see the woman one week later to ensure that the baby has remained in its new presentation.

When an excessive amount of water is present the baby may not assume its final presentation within the uterus until very late in pregnancy and in these circumstances external cephalic version may be performed much later than the 32nd or 34th week.

External cephalic version can occasionally be very difficult to perform, partly because the uterus will not relax and also partly because of the inability of the woman to relax her abdominal wall. There might also be a reduced amount of amniotic fluid present. If the uterus or abdominal wall will not relax sufficiently the woman will be asked to return a week later when she might be more relaxed. If external cephalic version is still not possible the use of anaesthesia may be considered. The woman is admitted to hospital overnight and the baby gently turned round under the influence of the complete relaxation of a general anaesthetic.

Occasionally, however, it is impossible to rotate the baby so that breech presentation persists and breech delivery has to be undertaken. The buttocks present over the cervix and dilatation of the cervix occurs as in cephalic presentation. A swelling, or caput, will form mostly in the region of the genitalia, so that these may be considerably distorted at birth. As with cephalic presentation, this swelling rapidly disappears and the genitalia return to normal within 48 hours.

24 Labour

The cause of labour

The reason why labour starts is not known although there is today an increasing amount of evidence to show that the fetus, or the placenta (which is under the control of the fetus), produces the hormone which leads to the onset of labour, and thereafter controls the course of labour. The average duration of pregnancy is 40 weeks, but as has been explained in Chapter 7 this may vary, not only from woman to woman, but from one pregnancy to another, and, as it depends also on the father of the baby, it may vary if a woman marries for a second time. Quite apart from this, each pregnancy is a law to itself and each pregnancy arrives at maturity at an individual time. Forty weeks, or 280 days, is merely an average, and normal maturity may be at any stage from the 36th week to the 44th week, although if labour starts before the 38th week it is generally referred to as premature, and after the 42nd week as postmature. Nevertheless premature and postmature labours are perfectly normal.

It is a well accepted fact that all muscle must contract and relax fairly frequently, otherwise it will waste away. This applies to every muscle in the body and one only has to consider the muscles in an injured arm or leg after they have been encased in plaster to realize how rapidly muscles will waste if they are not used. The uterus is no exception and muscle in the uterus contracts regularly throughout life and although a woman is not normally aware of these contractions she may occasionally notice them as pains associated with the menstrual period. Uterine contractions occur throughout pregnancy at slightly irregular intervals every 15, 20 or 30 minutes and last for about 25 seconds. The uterus can be felt to harden either by an examining hand or by the woman herself. While the pregnant woman may be aware of these contractions they are not painful. They were described many years ago by Braxton Hicks and are known as Braxton Hicks' contractions. As the pregnant woman nears term they become more obvious and may occasionally become uncomfortable, but never painful. When labour commences the Braxton Hicks' contractions become regular, stronger and more forceful.

The medical definition of the onset of labour is 'the onset of regular, painful, uterine contractions'. This is really an appalling definition and guaranteed to frighten any pregnant woman. Furthermore it is not true. The modern teaching and theory are to refer to uterine contractions as 'contractions' and not to call them 'pains', although they have been so called for centuries. The onset of labour is in fact marked by the onset of uterine contractions occurring every 15 to 20 minutes, which can be timed by the clock to be regular, and which are uncomfortable, but are not necessarily painful. They are accompanied by a definite hardening of the uterus, which can easily be felt by a hand placed on the abdomen. Whereas Braxton Hicks' contractions last for 20 to 30 seconds, the contractions at the onset of labour last for 40 seconds or more.

Labour can be induced either by breaking the waters and therefore altering the pressures within the uterus itself, or by administering drugs and hormones, which have a direct contracting effect on the uterus. The induction of labour is discussed in Chapter 25. But even when labour is artificially induced the exact reason or cause of the onset of labour is not known.

Time of day

The majority of people believe that most babies arrive at night. This is not strictly true. With very small variations, approximately 4 per cent of babies arrive each hour of the day and night.

There are various reasons for this belief. Perhaps, because during winter the hours of darkness are longer than the hours of daylight, the darkness is interpreted as night. Even during summer any baby which arrives between 8.0 p.m. and 8.0 a.m. is thought in many people's minds to have arrived during the night. The average length of labour is from 6 to 12 hours and, therefore, it is highly probable that part of the labour will occur during the night, either the disturbance of the onset, or the excitement of the delivery, but it is the wakening at four o'clock in the morning which sticks in people's minds and not the arrival of the baby at midday

Time of year

There is certainly a slight variation in the birth rate throughout the year with a peak of arrivals during March, April and September. A possible reason for this is that conception is related to summer holidays in the previous June or July and to Christmas.

False labour

The uterus contracts about every 15 to 20 minutes during pregnancy. The contractions last about 20 to 30 seconds and may be felt occasionally as a tightening of the uterus or abdomen. They play an important part in allowing the uterus to grow during pregnancy and are very useful in assisting the circulation of maternal blood to the placenta Braxton Hicks' contractions inevitably become stronger and more regular towards the end of pregnancy. Occasionally, if a woman is apprehensive, or lives a long way from the hospital or has no adequate means of conveyance, she may become extremely anxious that she reaches the hospital in time for her baby to be delivered, and this may lead to an exaggerated appreciation of the uterine contractions, so that they become confused with the onset of true labour. This is termed a false labour. After a woman in false labour has been admitted to hospital, uterine contractions will get less strong and less frequent and will gradually resume the normal pattern of Braxton Hicks' contractions. It is usual under these circumstances to keep the woman in hospital overnight and to let her return home the following day.

If you are in doubt as to whether you are in labour you should telephone your doctor or midwife and be prepared to answer the following questions: How long have the contractions been present? At what intervals are they occurring? How long are they lasting? Have you had a 'show'? If the labour is true the contractions will have been present for some time and occasionally for several hours. The interval between contractions will be 20 minutes or less. The duration of the contractions will be 40 seconds or more. While the passage of some blood-stained mucus, or 'show', is not essential to diagnose the onset of labour, its presence nearly always indicates that labour is commencing.

The majority of women who are admitted to hospital in false labour are very dejected, disappointed and upset when they are allowed to return home the next day. They feel ashamed that they should not have realized that they were only in false labour, and despite the reassurances of the medical and nursing staff it is extremely difficult to remove this natural feeling of guilt. This feeling is groundless, because it is very often difficult for doctors and midwives to differentiate between true and false labour, and indeed many women who are qualified doctors and midwives are frequently admitted to hospital in false labour themselves.

The onset of false labour has no ill effect on either the mother or her baby.

The mechanism of labour

The mechanism of labour and the expulsion of the fetus by the uterus is considered in three stages and it is necessary to treat each stage separately.

Stage I, or the first stage of labour, is from the onset of labour to full dilatation of the cervix (when the neck of the uterus is stretched sufficiently to allow the baby's head to pass through).

Stage II is from full dilatation of the cervix to completion of delivery of the baby.

Stage III is from completion of delivery of the baby to completion of the delivery of the placenta or afterbirth.

In order that the human race should not die out, every woman must be capable of having at least two children. The essential part of the subtle mechanism of labour is the process whereby the baby can be expelled from the uterus which then returns to normal so that a subsequent pregnancy can occur, not only on one occasion but on ten, or even twenty, occasions if so desired.

The uterus is composed of an upper uterine segment, a lower uterine segment and a cervix. The lower uterine segment develops during the last few weeks of pregnancy and is formed by Braxton Hicks' contractions of the upper uterine segment actually pulling against and stretching the lower part of the uterus, with its resulting thinning and formation of what becomes known as the lower uterine segment. The cervix itself is closed, in so far as the canal is approximately 2 or 3 mm in diameter and 2.5 cm in length. Forceful contractions of the uterus might result in tearing, or splitting, of the cervix which would not then be able to return to normal for subsequent pregnancies. This sometimes results in incompetent cervix.

The first stage

Uterine contractions are designed to eliminate the canal of the cervix without damaging its muscle; this is done by the muscular contractions of the upper uterine segment pulling on the lower uterine segment, which in turn pulls on the upper part of the cervix (fig. 26) so that it is incorporated into the lower uterine segment and the cervical canal is obliterated. Point O, which was the internal os of the cervix, is gradually taken up to become part of the lower uterine segment, and X, which was at the lower part of the cervix (external os), is gradually shortened and then dilates. When uterine muscle contracts in a Braxton Hicks' contraction, it reacts in the same manner as other muscles pulling against adjacent structures. During labour, however, the upper uterine segment, consisting almost entirely of muscle, produces a unique property, known as retraction, by means of which it is able to slightly shorten itself after every contraction and thus increase the force exerted upon the lower uterine segment; it is then capable of maintaining this shortened length and yet relaxing completely between contractions. This ability during labour of the muscle fibres of the upper part of the uterus to maintain a shortened length and yet to relax completely is not found in any other muscle of the body. The strength of the contractions in the upper uterine segment is quite considerable. The lower uterine segment does not contain so much muscle, having been previously stretched, but it transmits the pull of the upper uterine segment to the upper part of the cervix. This process of elimination of the length of the cervical canal is known as effacement, or 'taking up of the cervix'. The

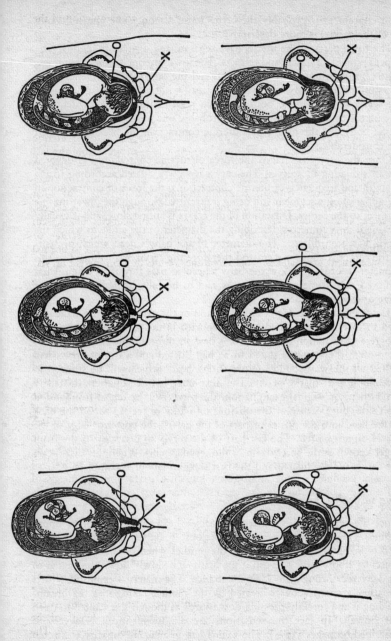

Fig. 26 Effacement of the cervix: O internal cervical os; X external cervical os

term effacement is probably the better term, although the phrase 'taking up of the cervix' is more descriptive.

The three parts of the uterus have separate and distinct functions. The upper segment contracts and retracts. The lower uterine segment contracts a little but does not stretch or retract, and the cervix itself stretches only. Thus full dilatation of the cervix is achieved without any damage to either the cervix or the uterus, both of which return to normal after delivery. The uterus contains the biggest and probably one of the strongest muscles in the body. At the height of a uterine contraction the pressures created are considerable.

Once the cervix is effaced the force of uterine contractions is devoted towards dilating the cervix. The cervix is slowly dilated according to the strength and frequency of uterine contractions, the force of contraction in the upper uterine segment still being transmitted through the lower uterine segment to the cervix. Dilatation of the cervix is at first slow, and is usually measured in centimetres describing the diameter of the circle to which the cervix has been dilated. The diameter of the baby's head which presents to the cervix is about 9.5 cm and therefore the cervix has to dilate to this diameter in order to allow the baby's head to pass through. When it has achieved this diameter the cervix is said to be fully dilated and the first stage of labour is ended.

Description of the degrees of dilatation of the cervix must be standardized so that they can be accurately reported in the patient's records. The progress of dilatation of the cervix is described in centimetres up to 4 cm. At 5–6 cm the cervix is stated to be half dilated and a rim of cervix will be felt all the way round the presenting head, which will be situated in the middle part of the pelvis. The next stage is three-quarters dilated (7 cm), when, on vaginal examination, the cervix will be felt in front and at each side, but because of the obvious difficulty of feeling round the back of the head into the posterior part of the pelvis, the posterior edge of the cervix cannot be felt. The last part of the cervix to disappear is the front edge, known as the anterior lip of the cervix (8 cm). When this disappears the cervix is fully dilated and the first stage of labour is complete.

The second stage

Once the cervix is fully dilated the baby's head can pass into the upper vagina. The force of uterine contractions, together with the expulsive efforts involuntarily produced by the mother when the head reaches the muscular floor, serve to push it gradually and slowly down the vagina to be delivered through the vaginal entrance. The maternal expulsive efforts are usually spontaneously created by the mother taking in a big breath, holding it and forcibly pressing downwards as though she wanted to open her bowels. In fact the sensations are almost identical. (Delivery is described on pages 337–8). The vagina has an amazing capacity to stretch and enlarge during the latter part of pregnancy so that the passage of the baby's head (which is 9.5 cm in diameter) causes no injury or damage. As soon as the baby has been delivered the second stage is complete.

The third stage

The third stage of labour is defined as that time between the delivery of the baby and the completion of delivery of the afterbirth or placenta. The uterine contractions recommence shortly after the delivery of the baby. The placenta separates from its attachment on the inner surface of the uterus and is expelled into the upper part of the vagina. The descent of the placenta into the vagina is accompanied by an apparent lengthening of the umbilical cord, a show of blood and the contracted uterus rises in the abdomen. The placenta can now be delivered either by gentle traction on the umbilical cord or by expulsive effort of the mother.

Length of labour

It is difficult to describe the length of normal labour for the simple reason that it is different in every woman and for each pregnancy in the same woman. Furthermore, it is actually difficult sometimes to diagnose the onset of labour. The definition of onset of labour as the start of 'regular, painful uterine contractions' is not entirely satisfactory as it does not take into account the efficiency of those contractions in dilating the cervix. A young woman, especially if anxious and nervous, may respond with pain to Braxton Hicks' contractions and feel she is in labour. On the other hand, women who have attended relaxation and psychoprophylaxis classes may sometimes be 5 cm or more dilated before they appreciate their contractions as painful. Many obstetricians would say that, if a cervix is less than 2 cm dilated, it is unlikely that a woman is in active labour.

On average, the cervix during labour dilates at the rate of 1 cm every hour. Initially the dilatation is fairly slow and this is called the latent phase of labour; once the cervix has dilated to 3 cm the active phase of labour begins and the contractions tend to be stronger, thus causing the cervix to dilate at a more rapid rate.

One way in which doctors and midwives attempt to detail objectively the progress of labour is to use a partograph. This is a simple graph depicting the normal rate at which the cervix dilates in most women. During labour women are examined by a doctor or midwife every four hours, and the dilatation of the cervix is plotted on the graph. In this way any delay in the normal progress of labour can be detected early

Primigravidae

Primigravidae are women having their first child and the length of labour is expected to be longer than in subsequent pregnancies. The average length of labour for the majority of women having their first baby is about 12 hours. The range, however, varies from 2 or 3 hours to 18 or 24 hours. It has been shown by many studies that short labours are associated with the best possible outcome for the baby, and the least risk of either a forceps delivery or Caesarean section. On the other hand, the longer a labour, the higher the risk of fetal distress or some sort of operative delivery by the obstetrician.

The great advantage of detecting delay in labour early is that attempts to improve contractions can be started before either the mother or the fetus has become stressed. This is usually done by the use of an intravenous infusion of Syntocinon, a synthetic form of the body's natural hormone (called oxytocin) which causes the uterus to contract. Improved contractions decrease the likelihood of the baby having an extended head and so not rotating in the pelvis in the normal way (see later).

Most women, when they are admitted in labour, will also have their membranes artifically ruptured. This has been shown to decrease significantly the length of labour and also the need for drugs like Syntocinon. A recent study in Liverpool showed no evidence of harm to the fetus by this procedure.

It is impossible to anticipate the duration of labour before its onset or to make any prediction until it is actually established, and even then most obstetricians obey the golden rule: 'Never predict the date of delivery or the time of delivery because if you are right you get no credit since everyone expects you to be right, and if you are wrong everyone thinks you are no good.' It is in fact a 'heads you win, tails I lose' bargain.

Multigravidae

Multigravidae are women having their second or subsequent baby. The onset of labour in a multigravid woman is usually more easily recognizable than in a primigravid woman and therefore the duration of labour can be accurately recorded. Labour is at most always shorter and easier, with an average duration of 6 hours. Delay in the progress of labour is far more likely to be due to disproportion between the size of the baby and the mother's pelvis than in the primigravid patient and should always be taken very seriously indeed. This is because a uterus which has functioned normally in a previous labour is unlikely to suddenly function inefficiently in the next labour. The cause of the delay is not poor contractions but obstruction which prevents the fetus descending through the pelvis (see Chapter 26).

Fear

The fear, pain, tension syndrome which has been recognized for many years, but was reiterated and again made popular in this country by Dr Grantly Dick-Read in his book *Natural Childbirth* (fifth revised edition, *Natural Childbirth*, edited by L. Snaith and A. Coxon. Heinemann Medical Books, 1968), undoubtedly exerts a very great influence upon the duration of labour. Fear, which engenders the tension and pain syndrome, is nearly always due to ignorance, and nothing but good can come from education during pregnancy, especially when that education includes careful instruction concerning the mechanism of labour together with the various reasons for its management.

Most women have a certain amount of fear or apprehension of labour which is usually:

1 For the health and welfare of their baby.
2 For their own health and welfare.
3 For the discomfort or pain of labour.

Most of the complications of labour can be successfully treated and therefore result in no permanent harm to either the woman or her baby, but it must be emphasized that the management of labour begins with good antenatal care, including instruction about labour and the postnatal period as well as the management of the baby.

Labour and maternal age

Maternal age undoubtedly plays a part in the duration and ease of labour. The 'elderly primigravida' is generally considered to be a woman over the age of 35 who is having her first baby. It is really inexcusable to call her elderly, but she is just entering the last third of her reproductive life and it is for this reason and for this reason alone that she is termed an elderly primigravida. Pregnancy and labour present certain risks to the elderly primigravida, but with proper antenatal care and good supervision during labour these are negligible. Indeed maternal age should never be used as a deterrent to establishing a pregnancy, and strangely enough a lot of women who are having their first baby over the age of 40 have, for some unknown reason, an extremely easy labour. Generally speaking, however, the length of labour increases about 1 or 2 hours for every 10 years, so that, on average a woman of 33 has a labour between 1 or 2 hours longer than one of 23. Of course, the whole process of natural selection must also be taken into account in this context and some women deliver more easily and rapidly, whereas there are those who were destined from their very beginning to have a longer labour.

Number of contractions per delivery

It is not known exactly how many contractions are required to deliver a baby. The main problem of estimating this in labours which begin spontaneously is that a number of contractions have obviously occurred before the woman is aware that she is in labour, and indeed the greater her confidence, faith and understanding, the more contractions will she have before she appreciates this. The number can be estimated with relative ease if labour is induced in hospital although this is a rather artificial standard. Nevertheless, at a rough working estimate, it probably requires about 150 contractions to deliver a first child, about 75 for a second or third child, about 50 for a fourth or fifth child and between 30 and 40 contractions to deliver subsequent children.

There are many women who have had more contractions than those listed above and many others who have delivered their baby with only one or two contractions. One famous doctor recounts the story of how a patient of his who was expecting her fifth child sent for him one evening but he found her to be in false labour. Knowing that she delivered her babies very quickly he decided to stay with her. He sat up most of the night. At 5.00 a.m. when he was feeling rather tired and as no further uterine contractions had occurred, he went downstairs to the kitchen to have a cup of coffee and to smoke his pipe. When he arrived in the kitchen the midwife called to him to return immediately to the patient's room, and on returning he found his patient was already delivered, having had two strong contractions within the space of three minutes. Both mother and child were quite satisfactory and he delivered the placenta without incident.

Signs of labour

Many women who are expecting their first baby are worried that they will fail to recognize the symptoms indicating the onset of labour but the vast majority of women do recognize the early symptoms easily and know that labour has started. Labour usually begins in one of three distinctive ways:

1 The onset of powerful, regular uterine contractions.
2 Rupture of the membranes.
3 The passage of a small quantity of blood: the 'show'.

Uterine contractions

The first stage of labour begins with the onset of regular uterine contractions which can be felt. Braxton Hicks' contractions are the normal contractions which occur in the uterus throughout pregnancy every 15 to

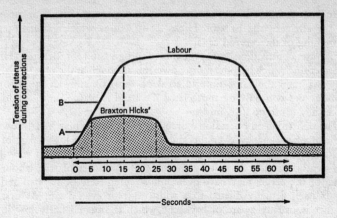

Fig. 27 The relative strengths and durations of Braxton Hicks' contractions and contractions during labour
A   level at which contractions can be felt with a hand
B   level at which discomfort occurs

20 minutes, and while they may be appreciated by the mother during the later stages of pregnancy they rarely cause any discomfort.

Uterine contractions in labour have a definite pattern which is easy to recognize. As will be seen from fig. 27 the uterine muscle normally exerts a mild amount of pressure or tone. When a uterine contraction commences the pressure within the uterus rises relatively slowly. A hand placed on the uterus is able to detect the contraction before the mother becomes aware of its presence. It continues to increase in power until it reaches a maximum where there is a plateau, or levelling out, lasting for anything between 30 and 50 seconds. The uterine contraction then disappears relatively rapidly. Each woman's pain threshold varies and while most women are aware that the contraction is present soon after its onset, actual discomfort may not be felt until the contraction has been present for up to 10 seconds.

Braxton Hicks' contractions follow a slightly different pattern. From fig. 27 it will be noticed that the uterine pressure during a Braxton Hicks' contraction increases gradually and maintains a plateau for about 20 seconds after which it disappears at about the same speed as that at which it arises. The first stage of labour ends when the cervix, or neck of the womb, is fully dilated. The process of dilatation, or opening, of the cervix, is the longest part of labour. Throughout most of pregnancy the length of the cervical canal is approximately 2.5 cm. It is filled with a plug of mucus which prevents infection from the vagina entering the uterus. The actual diameter of the canal varies from 2 to 3 or 4 mm. The hormone changes in the body during early pregnancy cause a softening of the cervix, and from about the 36th week onwards it is further softened, or ripened, by the effect of the Braxton Hicks' contractions which gradually cause shortening of the cervical canal.

Uterine contractions are probably a progression of Braxton Hicks' contractions which become more powerful, although at the onset of labour they maintain the same time interval of approximately every 20 or 30 minutes and will only be appreciated if a hand is placed on the abdomen since they cause no discomfort.

The tightening and occasional dragging pains which may be felt towards the end of pregnancy over the abdomen, or over the lower part of the abdomen, are in fact achieving quite a considerable result in a very quiet and gentle manner, so that by the time of the onset of true labour the canal of the cervix may have been almost completely obliterated and the cervix itself actually dilated to a width of 1 or even 2 cm. At first the mother is usually aware of backache which is situated fairly low in the back, is central, rather nagging in character and intermittent. The backache occurs at the same time as the uterine contractions and lasts only while the contraction is present. If she places her hand on her abdomen she will probably feel the uterus contracting at the same time as she experiences the backache, at regular, rhythmic intervals every 20 or 30 minutes and lasting for 30 or 40 seconds. This type of backache may continue for several hours and eventually progress into true labour. Alternatively, it may disappear after a few hours only to reappear after a few days or even a week. It may recur or continue several times before it is converted into true labour. When true labour does commence the backache tends to become more annoying. The uterine contractions occur every 15 to 20 minutes. It is at this stage that the woman may pass the mucous plug from the cervix, or she will notice the 'show' which will appear as a pinkish, slightly blood-stained mucous discharge. Either of these signs often heralds the onset of true labour and invariably ensures that true labour has started or is going to begin within a relatively short time.

As the uterine contractions become stronger, the discomfort usually radiates round into the lower part of the abdomen. This movement of discomfort from the back into the lower abdomen is usually a sure sign that labour is established. Gradually the pain and discomfort are transferred from the back into the lower abdomen where they are only felt during a uterine contraction. This type of discomfort may continue for anything up to 2 or 3 hours with the uterus contracting about every 15 minutes. It is at this stage that the cervix is being gradually effaced if this has not been previously achieved by Braxton Hicks' contractions.

After the cervix has been effaced it begins to stretch or dilate. As the contractions become stronger, they will be felt over the lower half of the abdomen and their frequency will gradually increase to about once every 10 minutes. For an hour or two they will probably increase in strength so that they are felt over the whole of the uterus and occur about every 5 minutes. The cervix is now about 3 cm dilated and the longest and latent part of labour is over. The contractions will continue to be felt over the whole of the abdomen or uterus, and will gradually increase in frequency until they occur about every 3 minutes, and at this stage the cervix is about 6 cm dilated. As the cervix approaches full dilatation, uterine contractions may occur every 2 to 2½ minutes and are still felt over the entire uterus or abdomen. The degree of dilatation of the cervix can usually be assessed from the timing and frequency of the contractions. For instance, the low backache is usually associated with gradual effacement of the cervix. When the uterine contractions cause discomfort to spread over the whole uterus they are usually occurring at 10 minute intervals and the cervix is about 2 cm dilated. When the stronger contractions are spaced 5 minutes apart, the cervix is approximately 3 cm dilated.

The head may not become engaged in the pelvis before the onset of labour. If not, then it will usually do so during the first stage of labour. As the head engages in the pelvis discomfort may be felt in the lower abdomen, or in the pelvis, and as the head is gradually pushed lower a sensation of pressure is felt in the lower part of the pelvis.

At some stage during the labour the membranes will rupture. You will be conscious that something has popped or burst inside followed by the drainage of water from the vagina. It is at this stage that you need quite a lot of reassurance that everything is satisfactory, especially since you have no knowledge whether the initial gush of fluid is water or blood. When this sensation happens it is always water which is coming out; such a dramatic rush of blood never occurs during labour.

As the end of the first stage is reached and the second stage begins you will feel an entirely different sensation. The uterine contractions are no longer as uncomfortable as they were a very short time previously. A pressure is felt in the pelvis and there is an almost uncontrollable desire to push or bear down. This is usually greeted with some relief because, having spent several hours relaxing and breathing during uterine contractions, you are now able to do something positive and definite. The contractions become a little more frequent, every 1 or 2 minutes, and this together with the automatic desire to push means that the worst of the labour is over.

Quite a high proportion of women are nauseated towards the end of the first stage of labour and vomiting is not at all unusual at the start of the second stage. It is accepted by experienced doctors and midwives as one of the signs of full dilatation of the cervix.

The mucous plug

The mucous plug, or operculum, which lies within the cervical canal protecting the cavity of the uterus throughout pregnancy, is usually dislodged as soon as the cervix is fully effaced or 'taken up' The mucous plug may appear before the onset of actual labour, especially if quite a lot of backache has been experienced. Usually, however, it comes away early in the first stage of labour and can be easily recognized as a lump of thick, fairly solid, clear, rather sticky mucus which measures 1 or 2 cm in diameter and may occasionally be tinged with a small amount of blood giving it a pinkish colour.

The 'show'

The passage of a small quantity of blood known as a 'show' is one of the commonest signs of the onset of labour. The show which heralds the onset of labour is nearly always a small amount of pinkish blood mixed with mucus. It is seldom pure blood and it is seldom bright red. The show may appear without any previous sign or warning, although it can be associated with rather forceful uterine contractions or low backache. It is important to remember that a show either at the onset or in the early part of labour is a perfectly normal phenomenon and is nearly always associated with the passage of the operculum. Any bleeding is coming from the uterus and is not the baby's blood, nor does it in any way adversely affect the baby. The passage of the blood from the vagina at any stage in pregnancy should be immediately reported to whoever is responsible for your care, and the presence of the show is no exception.

The bag of waters

The baby lying within the uterus is surrounded completely by amniotic fluid which is contained within the uterus by the membranes which completely line its inner surface. As the cervix gradually dilates the chorion and amnion are exposed as a shiny membrane which fills the centre of the dilating cervix. The baby's head is situated just above the dilating cervix and the membranes, but in between the head and the membranes is a quantity of liquor which is still held within the uterus by the intact membranes. The liquor which lies in front of the baby's head is known as 'the bag of waters' or the forewaters. This was once considered essential to normal labour and a prerequisite for satisfactory dilatation of the cervix, and this is the reason why, when the membranes ruptured early and the forewaters were no longer present, women were supposed to have a long and difficult labour. This is not true. Indeed today many doctors believe that the head itself will dilate the cervix more efficiently than the forewaters and if a bag of waters is still present after the cervix has reached 3 cm in dilatation they will purposely rupture it with a special pair of forceps so that labour can proceed more rapidly.

It is unusual for a baby to be delivered with unruptured membranes completely covering its head and face, and it is then said to be born in a caul (David Copperfield was born in a caul which was preserved and which he later sold). This used to be considered lucky and to denote that the baby would never suffer death by drowning at sea. If the membranes are intact they are ruptured as soon as the head is delivered to prevent the baby breathing in amniotic fluid when it takes its first breath.

Rupture of the membranes before the onset of labour

If the head is not engaged in the pelvis or is situated just in the pelvic brim, the membranes may rupture before the onset of labour. When this happens quite a large quantity of fluid escapes from the vagina. This is an indication for going to hospital immediately or notifying the doctor or midwife who is responsible for your care. The actual rupture causes no sensation as there are no nerves in the membranes. Many women consider it a wise precaution to put a sheet of thin polythene on the bed between the mattress and the bottom sheet in case the waters break while they are in bed.

Quite a few pregnant women have a genuine fear that the membranes will rupture while they are out doing the shopping, on a bus or walking in the street. If the fetal head is engaged then rupture of the membranes results in the loss of only a very small amount of liquor, so little, in fact, that it is unlikely to cause embarrassment. It is only if the membranes rupture when the head is not engaged that relatively large quantities of liquor can suddenly and dramatically be lost from the vagina. It is understandable that this accident causes acute embarrassment, but in the circumstances everyone is willing to help and to provide somewhere to rest until help can be obtained either from relatives or by sending for the midwife or the ambulance.

Rupture of the membranes is followed after an interval by the onset of labour. The interval varies according to the duration of pregnancy. Generally speaking the earlier in pregnancy that the membranes rupture spontaneously, the longer will be the latent period before the onset of labour. The membranes rupture spontaneously and without warning at about the 20th week of pregnancy when the woman has an incompetent cervix. Abortion follows after a few hours or days. Between the 28th and 36th week of pregnancy rupture of the membranes is said to be premature. At the 30th or the 32nd week of pregnancy this is followed by an interval of a few hours, a few days or a few weeks before the onset of labour. The treatment of a woman who ruptures her membranes at this stage of pregnancy is admission to hospital and bed-rest. Indeed the onset of labour may be discouraged by the administration of sedatives, special drugs or alcohol given by an intravenous drip. The survival rates for delivery at the 30th week of pregnancy are less than at the 36th week, and it is most important for a pregnancy to continue as close to the 36th week as possible. Each day that the onset of labour can be delayed when a woman is only

30 or 32 weeks pregnant may make all the difference between success and failure, and a delay of weeks or even a month will almost certainly make the difference between a live and possibly a dead child.

At the 38th week of pregnancy and onwards rupture of the membranes nearly always results in the onset of labour within 6 or 12 hours and it is therefore an indication for admission to hospital. The fluid which leaks away is watery, with a distinctive smell, and is not normally blood-stained. The leakage may be confused with the passage of small quantities of urine but simple tests are available in the hospital which can rapidly differentiate between amniotic fluid and urine. The cells lining the amniotic membrane secrete and absorb approximately 1 litre of fluid per hour in a continuous cycle, so it is not surprising that slow leakage of quite a considerable amount of fluid should continue from the vagina after the membranes have been ruptured.

Many women fear that should the membranes rupture before the onset of labour, or alternatively if they rupture in the early stages of labour, they will suffer from a 'dry labour', which is thought to be difficult, tedious, prolonged and painful. This is not true, although when the baby is in the occipito-posterior position the labour may be prolonged and the membranes do tend to rupture early. This position, however, only occurs in a relatively small percentage of women having their first baby. There are also one or two other rare conditions such as transverse lie and brow presentation when the membranes may rupture early and where labour is going to be prolonged anyway, but there is no evidence whatsoever to suggest that a 'dry labour' is anything other than normal. Since the cells lining the amniotic membrane continue to secrete amniotic fluid at the rate of up to a litre per hour, even when the membranes have ruptured, a 'dry labour' as such does not really exist and a comparatively large quantity of fluid drains from the vagina during labour. This rate of production of liquor continues throughout normal labour even when the membranes are intact, the liquor being absorbed from the amniotic sac in exactly the same manner as during the latter part of pregnancy.

The membranes do not usually rupture spontaneously until labour is well established, when the cervix is about 3 cm dilated or almost fully dilated. Following spontaneous rupture of the membranes during labour the woman is usually examined internally to assess the progress of labour, the state of the cervix and the position of the baby's head. Occasionally the membranes remain intact until the very end of the first stage, that is when the cervix is fully dilated, and they show at the vulva as a distending bag of water which ruptures spontaneously, or is ruptured by the doctor or midwife.

The second stage of labour

At the onset of the second stage of labour the uterine contractions undergo a very subtle and yet very definite change and are associated with a desire to push or bear down. This expulsive desire is at first present only at the height of a contraction, but gradually becomes more noticeable.

The change from the first to the second stage of labour is usually recognized by your midwife because, unfortunately, you may not only feel sick, but you may also actually vomit. This is fairly common although the reason is not known. Also you will begin to make expulsive efforts, which will be apparent from your holding your breath and probably grunting when you breathe out. If you have been instructed at antenatal or relaxation classes you will readily recognize this transition to the second stage of labour, but even the woman who has never had any instruction in labour will automatically begin to bear down and bend up her knees to make her expulsive efforts more efficient.

The uterine contractions continue every 1 or perhaps 2 minutes lasting approximately 1 minute. As the baby's head gradually descends in the vagina and reaches the pelvic floor, the desire to push becomes greater When the baby's head reaches the pelvic floor (the levator ani muscles) the back of the head rotates round to the front of the pelvis and starts to stretch the pelvic floor, causing a sensation of fullness or pressure in the rectum so that the desire to push becomes almost uncontrollable.

The baby's head continues to descend and stretches the pelvic floor further so that it comes into contact with the muscular outlet of the pelvis, known as the perineum. This causes an even greater desire to push. As the perineum is slowly distended by descent of the head the mother often feels some discomfort, frequently described as a tearing sensation as if everything were splitting wide open. This never happens and the sensation is purely the result of normal stretching and distension of the perineal muscles. The baby's head can be seen at the entrance to the vagina when it begins to distend the perineum. When the entrance to the vagina is about 3 or 4 cm dilated by the baby's head, the neck is situated just behind the front bone of the pelvis (the symphysis pubis) and from this time on the completion of delivery is by the baby extending his head over the perineum from the bent position against his chest. First the brow and then the nose, face and eventually the mouth and chin are delivered over the perineum by this movement, while the neck remains in approximately the same place.

The baby is delivered with the back of his head uppermost and his face sweeping over the perineum but as soon as the head is delivered the baby's shoulders rotate in the pelvis spontaneously, so that the baby looks at either the right or left thigh of the mother The eyes, nose and mouth are wiped with clean gauze and gentle aspiration of the mouth and nose removes any fluid in the upper air passages. After the baby's head has

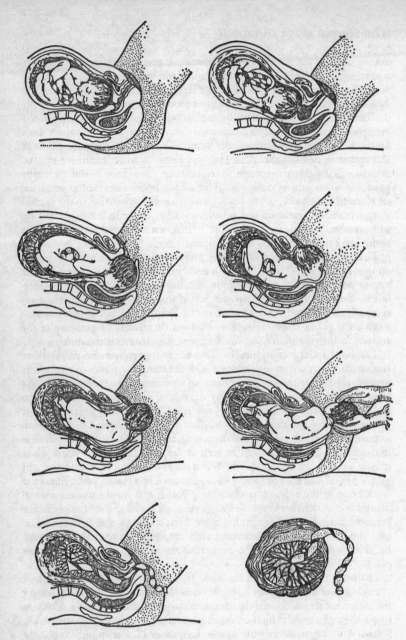

Fig. 28 Labour

been delivered uterine contractions stop for a short while and when they begin again the first requires only a slight expulsive effort to push down one shoulder, so that it can be seen at the vaginal entrance. Further bearing down results in delivery of the other shoulder which sweeps upwards and over the perineum in much the same way as the forehead and face were delivered. Now that both shoulders have been delivered the remainder of the baby slides out more or less spontaneously. First the hands appear and then the trunk, and the rest of the body is delivered by lifting the baby's head and shoulders up towards the mother's abdomen. This movement of lateral flexion of the baby's body will enable you to see him as soon as he is delivered. The duration of the second stage of labour is usually 30 to 60 minutes for a first baby and, on average, less than 20 minutes for subsequent babies.

You must not be surprised when you first see your baby because he will probably be quite a bright blue colour, his head, face and body will be partially covered with a white, greasy, cheesy looking material known as vernix; he will be wet and slippery and may have a few streaks of blood on his head, face and body. His hair will be plastered down on to his head by the vernix and his face will probably be screwed up in an angry grimace just prior to taking his first breath. His head will be a peculiar shape, caused by moulding and the formation of a caput.

As soon as your baby is delivered he will be placed on your abdomen where you can touch him and feel him, unless he requires resuscitation. His mouth, throat and nasal passages will be gently aspirated to suck out any liquid that they contain. When this has been done and the baby has started to breathe normally and then perhaps to cry, his colour will turn from a darkish blue to a nice bright pink. The umbilical cord is then divided with a pair of scissors between special metal clamps placed about 15 cm from the baby's umbilicus. Your baby is now free and from now onwards has to live an entirely independent existence. The metal clamps prevent any bleeding from the vessels in the umbilical cord. The cord is tied or a special plastic clip applied, after which the clamp attached to the baby's end of the umbilical cord is removed. The clamp on the placental end of the umbilical cord prevents any blood loss from the placenta itself. It is the baby's blood which circulates through the umbilical cord and the placenta. Your blood and your baby's blood do not mix. If, after delivery of the placenta, a specimen of the baby's blood is required it can easily be collected from the cord attached to the placenta by gently removing the clamp. By this method up to 50 or even 60 ml of blood are available without having to take any from the baby himself.

Usually within a few seconds of the delivery of the baby's head, or certainly within a few seconds of the completion of delivery, he takes his first breath. As soon as he does this his lips and then the surrounding area, followed by his chest and abdomen, turn from blue to pink. Gradually the rest of his face and then his arms and legs turn pink. The breathing is

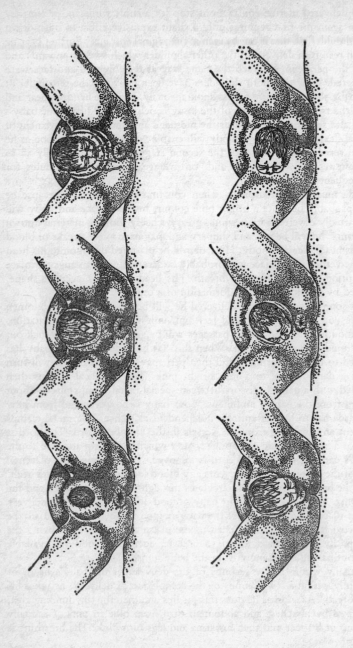

Fig 29 Delivery of the baby's head

at first somewhat irregular and he may cough and splutter, indicating that there is a further collection of liquid in his throat which is promptly aspirated by the midwife. Within a few seconds at least, or a few minutes at most, he begins to cry. This may start as a weakish whimper or with a full blown angry cry. This is the moment you have been waiting for and you will remember it for ever. As your baby's crying rapidly becomes established you will see that his body has turned completely pink, his arms are outstretched and each hand clenched into a fist; that his legs are partly bent and his face is screwed up in a grimace of anger as he literally screams as hard as he can. This angry cry is very much encouraged by both midwife and doctor because it means that the lungs are fully expanded and all the baby's vital functions will begin to work satisfactorily. It also means that the changes in the circulation of the baby's blood, which are so essential for survival after delivery, have been accomplished satisfactorily and safely. Hearing a good healthy cry is not only a moment of relief and happiness for you, but is also a moment of considerable relief and thankfulness on the part of your nurse and doctor that the transition from intrauterine to extrauterine life has been satisfactorily accomplished. You should have great pride in your accomplishment and they experience satisfaction and pleasure in having helped you achieve it.

The third stage of labour

The third stage of labour is that time from the delivery of the baby until the completion of the delivery of the placenta or afterbirth. In anticipation of the third stage of labour the midwife usually gives the mother an injection either as soon as the baby's head is born or as soon as the first shoulder is delivered. This intramuscular injection makes the uterus contract thus hastening the third stage of labour so that excess bleeding is prevented. The injection is either ergometrine 0.5 mg or syntometrine, which acts more rapidly and contains 0.5 mg of ergometrine and 5 units of Syntocinon, or Syntocinon alone. The uterus contracts quite powerfully about 4 minutes after it has been given. You will feel this but it is neither painful nor unpleasant. You will also be aware that the uterus is expelling the placenta into the vagina because you will feel the vagina being distended as the placenta is pushed from the uterine cavity into the upper part of the vaginal passage.

The midwife usually delivers the placenta by a procedure known as controlled cord traction. She gently pulls on the cord while pushing the uterus in your abdomen gently upwards and backwards. This helps to free the placenta from the uterus and once you feel the placenta in the vagina itself you have another, and what is destined to be your final, urge to push. By a very gentle expulsive effort the placenta is expelled from the vagina into the hands of the waiting midwife. As soon as the placenta, together with its membranes, is delivered the third stage of labour is complete.

In fact there are still plenty of things which you have to do before you can really consider that the delivery has been completed. If a perineal tear has occurred or if an episiotomy has been performed, a few stitches will have to be inserted. Your blood pressure and other recordings are made. You need a bath and a change of clothes; to put on some make-up and tidy your hair, and in fact there are hundreds of little things which still remain to be done.

For several years the third stage has been conducted by the routine use of drugs to make the uterus contract, given before the actual delivery of the placenta itself. The previous method of conducting the third stage depended upon the spontaneous return of uterine contractions and some people still favour this method. Usually after an interval of 10 or 15 minutes following delivery the uterine contractions again start spontaneously. These are at first rather sluggish and weak, but after a further 10 or 15 minutes they become quite strong and are sufficiently powerful to separate the placenta from the inner lining of the uterus and to push it down into the upper part of the vagina. The placenta will be delivered with one gentle expulsive effort, after which the midwife gives the mother an injection of either syntometrine or Syntocinon to contract the uterus and prevent haemorrhage.

Relief of pain in labour

History

The history books of any country abound with horrifying tales and stories of women who either suffered agonies during labour or actually died during childbirth. They contain little information about those many women who had easy, safe, spontaneous and natural deliveries and who suffered little or no discomfort in the process. This is probably because nobody believed them and their stories were disregarded as being untrue or not sufficiently dramatic to recount.

Different civilizations have used various methods in their attempts to control or alleviate the pains and discomforts of labour. The majority of these ideas have, as their basis, the use of a simple faith in some type of supernatural thought, hence we find the use of charms, witchcraft and the creation of special gods or deities to take care of women who are either pregnant or in labour.

In the past women were generally looked after by older women who had themselves borne children and who therefore understood the problems involved in childbirth and who could provide the suffering labourer with a degree of sympathy and understanding that she would be unlikely to obtain elsewhere. In 1847 James Young Simpson administered ether for the first time to a patient for delivery in Edinburgh and although anaesthetics had been previously administered, credit for the first obstetric anaesthetic must go to Simpson. Later in 1847 he used chloroform, also for the first time, and so he introduced an era of obstetric anaesthesia which, very sadly, 140 years later has not yet achieved its full recognition nor its true potential.

Today there are various methods which may be used to diminish, control, alleviate or completely eliminate pain and discomfort during labour. These methods fall broadly into the following categories:

1 Suggestion, which includes relaxation, psychoprophylaxis and hypnosis.
2 Drugs to alleviate either anxiety or pain.
3 Local or regional anaesthesia.
4 General anaesthesia.

Suggestion

Suggestion is a very powerful factor in the control of discomfort or pain in labour. Consider the tremendous and disastrous psychological damage that may be done to a 6-year-old girl who has to listen to her mother undergoing the 'agonies of labour'. When this unfortunate experience is further supported and fortified by dramatized and harrowing descriptions of the horrors of labour in print and on film and television screens, it is small wonder that the young girl views her own future labour with some apprehension. It must, therefore, be obvious that the psychological or mental preparation for labour should begin at a very early age and many years before sexual maturity. Even if nothing positive is done, every care should be taken to ensure that the young girl is not indoctrinated with the false horrors of childbirth which can create such a deep impression on the young and highly sensitive personality that subsequent attempts at its correction, even after the onset of pregnancy, are almost doomed to failure.

Sex education of girls at home as well as at school should include complete and honest descriptions and explanations of pregnancy and labour specifically designed to create confidence and to remove any deep-seated apprehension which may already have been implanted in the young and impressionable mind.

The various and different methods of suggestion that are available for women during the antenatal preparation for childbirth are based on a correct attitude to labour. They frequently involve a series of classes which include exercises specifically designed to encourage relaxation during uterine contractions and also to strengthen muscles which may be required at the time of delivery. It is beyond the scope of this book to deal in detail with these various methods but their main aims are briefly outlined.

The main principles behind the majority of these methods are that childbirth can be a pleasurable and happy experience, and that education and the creation of self-confidence will partially if not completely eliminate apprehension and fear. In order to achieve a correct attitude to labour it is necessary to educate the woman herself and also those nearest and dearest to her. The converse is likewise true; the interfering female imbecile who insists on recounting, and who seems to take a great delight in retelling, numerous and invariably false or horrifying stories of her own and her friends' experiences in childbirth can do immense damage in a few seconds.

The respective merits of the various methods of suggestion and preparation are so difficult to assess that opinions on their relative values vary from the completely converted to the rude and derisory. Above all, the inherited and acquired tribal, racial and social influences will dictate the response of each individual to a particular regime although the influence of an enthusiastic and dedicated instructor will be of immense importance in overriding and eliminating previous prejudices. The fundamental fact that it is you who are pregnant and it is you who are going to have the baby cannot be repeated too often. If you have confidence in those who are looking after you, as well as confidence in your own ability, then you require very little else, although most people would agree that you will only gain this confidence from further education in and an understanding of the whole process of pregnancy, labour and delivery. For your confidence and peace of mind you must be in harmony with those who are in charge of your welfare during your pregnancy and labour, and if you wish to undertake some special or particular psychological preparation for labour it is important that your doctor and midwife should not only agree with this, but should themselves be familiar with its basic principles and practice. An analysis of the various regimes shows that their mechanism of action is uncertain. Faith in one's own ability, an understanding of what is happening, a certain amount of distraction which is achieved by the performance of various exercises, all combine to alter favourably a labouring woman's response to the painful stimulus of a uterine contraction. No one should believe that labour is truly painless. Although there are many women who have had babies and who will testify that labour can be painless, it would nevertheless be foolhardy to promise anybody in advance that she will have a painless labour. Suggestion and education (or psychoprophylaxis) undoubtedly result in an appreciable reduction in the amount of pain experienced in labour and this form of antenatal instruction should be considered essential to every pregnancy.

A certain amount of antagonism is said to exist between those people who believe in natural childbirth and psychoprophylaxis and those who believe in the administration of drugs during labour. There is no earthly reason why you should not benefit from both approaches, combining them in your best interests and to your own advantage. You should have no hesitation in accepting analgesic drugs or an epidural block if you find the process of labour becoming more uncomfortable than you had anticipated. You must also remember that occasionally conditions do arise in labour which may make labour unnecessarily prolonged or unduly painful if adequate analgesia is not administered at the correct time.

Antenatal classes

Antenatal classes usually include a course of six or more lessons given to women while they are attending the antenatal clinic and they include instruction in the elementary physiology of pregnancy, labour and lactation, as well as instruction and mothercraft classes. Some classes are devoted to exercises designed principally to teach you to relax during labour and especially during uterine contractions, and may also instruct you in the special breathing techniques that should be performed during uterine contractions in both the first and the second stages of labour. (For further information write to the National Childbirth Trust, 9 Queensborough Terrace, London W2.)

There are two main schools of thought regarding the type of antenatal instruction that should be given, and while the supporters of each method undoubtedly believe that their own is vastly superior to the other, they do appear to have a great deal in common and it is for this reason that the majority of hospital and private instruction classes combine a mixture of both methods in varying degrees. The two different methods are classed as (1) natural childbirth, and (2) psychoprophylaxis.

The principles of both natural childbirth and psychoprophylaxis have been known and obeyed in varying degrees for many centuries throughout different civilizations. To Dr Grantly Dick-Read, however, must go the credit for bringing natural childbirth very much to public notice. Psychoprophylaxis has become popular as a result of the recent work of Lamaze and Vellay.

Natural childbirth is based upon the principle that fear, tension and pain are linked together. Fear itself is caused by ignorance and a lack of knowledge concerning pregnancy, childbirth and delivery, and may even be enhanced by incorrect beliefs in the terrors of pregnancy and delivery. Fear produces tension. The tension may be both mental and physical. Physical tension causes pain in muscles. This is especially marked in the muscle of the uterus and in particular in the cervix when the muscle refuses to relax with the resulting prolongation of labour and increase of pain. The mental tension and its associated anxiety result in an increased appreciation of pain and therefore fear of further pain.

A vicious cycle of fear, tension and pain is thus established and according to the Grantly Dick-Read teaching this can only be broken by removing the fear that initiates this syndrome. Grantly Dick-Read taught that by simple instruction, education and explanation during pregnancy, the whole process of birth could be changed from a frightening and fearful process to a pleasurable and joyful occasion. He also believed that women who had not acquired a fear of labour would not experience or suffer much of the pain or apprehension that is normally associated with childbirth in a civilized society. Unfortunately Grantly Dick-Read's method of natural childbirth was claimed by some as 'painless childbirth'. Far too much was sometimes claimed for the method and of course when painless childbirth was not achieved the method was castigated by those who did not believe in its principles and it gradually fell into disrepute. Only the occasional woman will in fact have a pain-free labour. If a woman is falsely indoctrinated into believing that she will have a painless labour, she may react in an adverse manner when she inevitably experiences pain during labour.

Natural childbirth is not synonymous with painless childbirth.

Natural childbirth has today resumed an important role in the antenatal instruction of patients and this philosophy is usually accompanied by a course of instruction in muscular relaxation and in relaxation exercises which are practised at antenatal classes so that they can be put into effect during labour.

Psychoprophylaxis. The whole principle of psychoprophylaxis is based upon work that is believed to have been undertaken in Russia and has probably been practised for a long time. It accepts the underlying principle of the conditioned reflex; that most women believe that labour is painful and therefore they experience pain. The primary task is therefore to decondition them to such an extent that this belief is no longer held and then recondition them to the principle that uterine contractions in labour need not be painful. This is accomplished in two ways. Firstly by careful instruction, and secondly by active patient participation. The patients receive fairly extensive instruction in both the normal and abnormal physiology of pregnancy, labour and delivery, and this is accompanied by a series of active exercises, many of which are breathing exercises of different types to be used during uterine contractions throughout the different stages of labour. One of the more important aspects of psychoprophylaxis is that it teaches that abnormalities may occur and also that labour may be painful, and amongst women who practise psychoprophylaxis there is ready acceptance of analgesia if labour becomes more painful than they had anticipated.

It must be emphasized very strongly that the majority of instructors conducting antenatal and relaxation classes do not conform strictly to either the pure natural childbirth or the pure psychoprophylaxis method of instruction but do in fact utilize a combination and adaptation of the two methods which they consider to be best suited to their own particular unit. Whatever instruction you receive you should never have any sense of failure if some untoward abnormality occurs during labour.

Hypnosis

Hypnosis or hypnotic aid for the relief of pain during childbirth has been employed experimentally for many centuries and has advantages as well as disadvantages. The pregnant woman is particularly susceptible to hypnotic influences and may be very receptive to hypnosis.

Hypnosis carries with it a certain amount of mystique and although the exact mechanism whereby hypnosis is produced is not known there is nothing mysterious about the technique that is used. Any interested person can easily learn it. The patient lies down and makes herself comfortable. The room should be quiet and the patient should be mentally relaxed. The hypnotist will then suggest a state of further relaxation and sleep and, as a condition of increased suggestibility is produced, the suggestions are gradually changed to commands and the woman is instructed regarding labour and is told that it will be relatively pain-free or much less painful than she had previously believed. There is a close comparison between the principles followed in the technique of hypnosis and the underlying principles of most relaxation classes.

Only willing volunteers are suitable subjects for hypnosis during labour, and about 50 per cent of these can be trained and hypnotized to a level at which they will not experience pain.

There are two main problems involved in the utilization of hypnosis during labour. The first is the difficulty in organizing satisfactory classes of instruction for such a relatively small number of patients. It is very time-consuming and quite impossible for any one person to devote so much time to a comparatively small group. The second major disadvantage is that very occasionally a state of relatively deep self-hypnosis may be induced which can produce undesirable effects in a woman who is psychiatrically or emotionally disturbed.

Drugs

There is an almost endless list of drugs which have been, or which still are, used during labour. Drugs are used for one or more of three main purposes.

1 A sedative or tranquillizer. A sedative drug is one which relieves anxiety and induces a feeling of calmness or drowsiness, whereas a tranquillizer only relieves anxiety and does not cause drowsiness or sedation.
2 A hypnotic is a drug which induces sleep.
3 An analgesic is a drug which relieves pain without necessarily inducing sleep although large doses of an analgesic will usually cause loss of consciousness.

The majority of drugs administered during labour will cross the placenta and therefore enter the baby's circulation where they will exert an effect similar to that which is exerted upon the mother herself. It necessarily follows therefore that the amount of a drug administered to a woman during labour must be very carefully controlled.

There is a correct dose of every particular drug for the individual patient at each different stage of labour and the proper dose can only be judged when the labour itself is viewed as a whole and the condition of both the patient and her baby is taken into consideration along with the progress of the labour. There is, therefore, no 'correct dose' for any drug during labour. The optimum dose lies somewhere between one which is too small to be of any significance or therapeutic value and one which is effective but associated with too many unpleasant or even dangerous side-effects. Thus 25 mg of pethidine, for example, is a completely safe but very ineffective dose whereas 250 mg of pethidine will produce excellent pain relief which may be accompanied by loss of consciousness, depression of respiration and a lowering of the blood pressure resulting in depression of the baby's breathing if it is delivered within 2 or 3 hours of the dose being administered.

The ideal drug for the relief of pain in labour would be one which acts on the mother alone and does not cross the placenta to the baby, but unfortunately no such drug exists nor is there any likelihood that one will be found in the near future.

There is no single technique for managing pain in labour which is better than any other. The aim, however, is the same for each woman—to make the pain and discomfort of her contractions *acceptable to her*. All women are excited and anxious when in labour, especially if it is the first time. Antenatal classes and education, a happy atmosphere in hospital and the presence of husband, partner or friend can all contribute in making a woman more relaxed during labour. If, however, she is frightened and distressed with pain, and this is not alleviated, the labouring woman will lose confidence in her attendants, will not happily participate in her labour and the delivery of her child and may even have adverse feelings towards that child or her husband or partner. Her distress may prolong her labour and add to her unhappiness even more. It will not be the unique experience of love, mystery and wonderment that it can be.

Not all women will need drugs during labour, especially if they have had a previous child. The choice of drug and the time of its administration will depend on a number of factors, the most important of which are:

1 The individual needs of the woman. The relaxed woman may not require any pain relief until she is in the last part of the first stage of labour, just prior to complete dilatation of the cervix. On the other hand, the woman who is frightened and anxious may need a mild sedative even before she is in established labour. Patient preference also has something to do with the choice of pain relief. Some women dislike intensely the state of 'disassociation' from themselves that can occur with pethidine;

other women will want to have only pethidine. Some women will refuse to contemplate the thought of an epidural anaesthetic, because of something they have heard or read about it. Other women will want an epidural even before their contractions are truly painful!

2 The progress of labour. A sedative would clearly be most inappropriate if a woman were nearing the second stage of labour, whereas it would be very helpful in early labour. Similarly, all drugs given to the woman late in labour will be present in significant concentrations in the baby's blood, if given within one to three hours of the baby being born.

3 Any obstetrical or fetal complications. There are certain situations, for example, high blood pressure, in which an epidural anaesthetic is recommended (see later). There are also absolute contra-indications for its use. Likewise, all drugs must be used with considerable caution if the baby is premature or small-for-dates, because the baby's liver will be immature, and it is here that most drugs are broken down and eliminated from the body.

4 The facilities available. All midwives are entitled to administer inhalational analgesics or pethidine to women in labour. Not all hospitals, however, are fortunate enough to have around-the-clock anaesthetists, and therefore epidural anaesthetics cannot be offered in many smaller hospitals.

Sedatives and hypnotics. In the early part of the first stage of labour, sedatives and hypnotics may be administered, especially if the woman is unduly anxious or if the early part of labour coincides with the late evening or early night. In the latter circumstance it may be considered advisable for the woman to relax and perhaps sleep during the early part of her labour. The sedatives that are used are variations of chloral hydrate which may be given as a mixture or as tablets of Tricloryl or Welldorm. They are very safe in early labour. The hypnotics are predominantly medium-acting barbiturates such as pentobarbitone (Nembutal), amylobarbitone (Amytal), butobarbitone (Soneryl) and quinalbarbitone (Seconal). Like all barbiturates, they cause depression of the central nervous system and in larger doses, or if followed by other drugs such as pethidine, can lead to a fall in blood pressure and respiratory depression. Barbiturates are only slowly eliminated from the baby after it is born and can cause the baby to be drowsy and sluggish. They used to be given in large amounts to women with pre-eclampsia, in order to sedate them and prevent eclamptic fits, but because of their effects on the fetus are no longer used for this purpose.

It must be reiterated that sedatives and hypnotics should only be given in very early labour. They are not analgesics and, if given to a woman in pain, will only cause her to become restless and uncooperative.

Tranquillizers. The phenothiazine group of drugs act on the central nervous system to relieve anxiety and tension. They also have excellent anti-emetic properties and are therefore useful to treat vomiting. Promazine (Sparine) and promethazine (Phenergan) are commonly used in obstetrics in combination with pethidine.

Diazepam (Valium) is an excellent tranquillizer and anti-convulsant and has the advantage of causing amnesia. It is used in the treatment of eclamptic fits, and also in place of pethidine during the later part of the first stage of labour, or to provide relaxation for a forceps delivery. Unfortunately it is slowly eliminated from the fetus and can cause drowsiness, problems with temperature control and poor feeding.

Hyoscine (scopolamine) was used for many years as a sedative and to provide amnesia, it being argued that pain control is not important if the patient has no memory of it. When used with morphia, it produced 'twilight sleep', which sometimes worked well, and sometimes caused the woman to become physically violent and uncontrollable. It is no longer used.

Analgesic drugs, pethidine and pentazocine, are used after labour has become established and are given to relieve, alleviate or lessen the pain experienced during uterine contractions. Most of these drugs are given by intramuscular injection, although a slowly running intravenous infusion can be used. This has the advantage that it can be controlled once the correct level of analgesia has been achieved, and in actual fact the total dose of drug given is less than with repeated intramuscular injections. After the onset of established labour the stomach does not empty very rapidly with the result that the absorption of drugs taken by mouth is extremely slow and unreliable.

The usual dose of pethidine is from 100 to 200 mg given by intramuscular injection. The drug begins to act about 15 minutes after the injection and not only is it very efficient at relieving the pain of uterine contractions but it also induces a sensation of euphoria and well-being. The action of pethidine continues for approximately 4 hours. Although pethidine is a drug of addiction the possibility of producing addiction by its administration to a woman during labour is negligible. Pethidine does not prolong labour once it has become established. Indeed a timely and opportune injection of pethidine will frequently ease and quicken labour because of the beneficial relaxation which follows the relief of pain. Morphine may also be used to relieve pain during labour but its place has been taken almost entirely by pethidine.

Fortral (pentazocine) is a comparatively new synthetic analgesic drug with properties very similar to those of pethidine.

All narcotic analgesics cross the placenta and may cause respiratory depression in the baby if it is born within one to three hours of the drug being given. This is particularly important in a baby who is premature or has been distressed during labour. Drugs which are direct antagonists of the narcotic drugs can be given to the baby.

Inhalation analgesia

Inhalation analgesics are administered intermittently during uterine contractions at the end of the first stage of labour and during the second stage of labour. The two main inhalation analgesics used in this country at present are:

1 Nitrous oxide.
2 Trichloroethylene (Trilene).

Nitrous oxide, otherwise known as 'laughing gas', has been used as an inhalational analgesic during labour for many years but has now been replaced by a mixture of nitrous oxide and oxygen. The Entonox apparatus is the standard method of administering nitrous oxide and oxygen. Fifty per cent nitrous oxide and 50 per cent oxygen are previously mixed in a cylinder. The apparatus is a small machine expecially designed for the self-administration of the pre-mixed gases and has replaced all previous methods of self-administration of nitrous oxide.

Nitrous oxide itself does possess a comparatively strong analgesic, or pain-relieving, action. When it is combined with 50 per cent oxygen the level of analgesia is satisfactory for most women during normal labour and delivery, especially if a dose of pethidine has been previously administered. It provides a remarkable amount of relief from the discomfort of uterine contractions although complete relief should not be expected. Consciousness is not lost and the mixture of half nitrous oxide and half oxygen is completely free from side effects even if administered for as long as 12 hours.

Although nitrous oxide does cross the placenta to the baby, the increased level of oxygen present in the mixture is of benefit to both the mother and her baby and the advantageous effects of the oxygen far outweigh any possible theoretical disadvantages of nitrous oxide. The mixture itself is not explosive but because it contains 50 per cent oxygen it should obviously be kept away from naked flames or fires.

Most courses of antenatal instruction held by maternity units include the method of use of the Entonox apparatus. It thus follows that the majority of women will be familiar with the machine and will be confident about using it when they eventually require to do so in labour. There is a fairly long piece of flexible tubing attaching the apparatus to the face mask which is triangular in shape. The base of the triangle fits over the chin and the apex of the triangle fits over the bridge of the nose. Unless the mask is properly fitted on to the face then the gas will not flow out of the cylinder. Usually the method of application of the mask to the face will be demonstrated to you by a member of the staff of the maternity department and afterwards you will be invited to try it out for yourself. The smell of the rubber tube may be slightly objectionable but the gas mixture has no smell. If you press the face mask firmly on your face and inhale you will automatically draw the mixture of nitrous oxide and oxygen from the cylinder and as soon as the gas begins to flow a hissing noise can be heard so that you now have complete control over your own inhalational analgesia. Since you hold the mask yourself you can remove it whenever you wish and suffocation, which many women fear, is impossible. Furthermore, you also have complete control over the level of analgesia because the deeper and more rapidly you breathe, the more nitrous oxide and oxygen mixture you will inhale and therefore the greater will be the effect of the analgesia. Analgesia itself starts about 20 seconds after first inhaling the nitrous oxide, reaching its maximum after about 45 to 60 seconds. In order to obtain the most efficient use of the apparatus you should breathe fairly deeply and at a normal rate. Rapid and shallow breathing is not very efficient because the gas and oxygen mixture does not get down into the lungs whence it can be absorbed into the blood stream.

The proper use of inhalational analgesia is to begin the inhalation before the actual discomfort of the uterine contraction is felt. A uterine contraction does not normally become uncomfortable or painful until 15 to 20 seconds after its onset. If you start inhaling the analgesic mixture as soon as the uterine contraction begins, the analgesic itself will become effective at the same time as, or even before, the uterine contraction becomes uncomfortable or painful. This is the most efficient method of using inhalational analgesia. The technique during the first stage of labour is to begin breathing with deep but regular breaths as soon as a uterine contraction becomes apparent and continue deep and regular breathing until it has passed.

In the second stage of labour the technique must be altered because you have to hold your breath in order to make expulsive efforts. You will be told to take several deep breaths of the gas mixture immediately before the onset of a uterine contraction so that you will derive the maximum amount of analgesia throughout the uterine contraction itself. You will be instructed in advance not to push when the head is showing or actually being delivered but to breathe easily and gently without making any expulsive effort. Continuous breathing of the nitrous oxide and oxygen mixture through the Entonox apparatus at this time is most beneficial because it discourages the unwanted pushing efforts and increases the amount of analgesia.

The satisfactory use of the Entonox machine probably depends on satisfactory antenatal instruction in its use so that when you go into labour you will not be unfamiliar with what it looks like or with how to use it.

Trichlorethylene (Trilene) is an inhalational analgesic which in high concentrations can be used as an anaesthetic. It is administered during labour via either the Tecota or the Emotril automatic inhaler. Both these machines have been carefully designed and tested under all circumstances so that they allow only a safe concentration of 0.5 per cent or less of

Trilene vapour in air to be administered. There is no danger that the concentration of Trilene can be increased because automatic compensation adjusts for any temperature changes that may occur in the surrounding atmosphere and for different rates of breathing. The machines themselves are strong and will operate in any position since the contents are unspillable.

The indications and the technique for Trilene analgesia are essentially similar to those described for nitrous oxide and oxygen analgesia. If the machine is used in the department to which you are being admitted, then you will be shown the Trilene inhaler at one of your antenatal classes. A similar piece of flexible tubing connects the face mask to the machine. The face mask is exactly the same as that used on the Entonox machine and should be pressed over the face as previously described and is held by the woman herself so that there is no possibility of suffocation or receiving an overdose. Here again breathing should be normal and regular since rapid and shallow respiration does not result in satisfactory analgesia.

Trilene possesses one important property lacking in nitrous oxide. The elimination of Trilene from the blood and tissues is comparatively slow because Trilene is not exhaled immediately by the lungs and the concentration of Trilene gradually increases in the body following each successive inhalation. As a result of this there is a mild build-up of analgesia after you have inhaled Trilene for the first few contractions. Following this you will need less Trilene with the succeeding contractions but the same principle applies: you should commence the inhalation as early as possible after the onset of the contraction and before it becomes uncomfortable or painful. Trilene is a powerful analgesic agent with a well-maintained action in low concentrations. It can be used with air so its use is not limited by the availability of gas and oxygen cylinders.

The very fact that there are two different types of inhalation analgesia is sufficient to indicate that neither is superior to the other. Extensive studies have been undertaken but have not produced any decisive advantage in favour of any one of these. A theoretical disadvantage of the Entonox apparatus is that it does require a cylinder of pre-mixed nitrous oxide and oxygen. While such cylinders may not be readily available for domiciliary midwifery, they are usually available in most maternity units. The choice of method therefore rests usually with the obstetric unit concerned who may favour any one single type of inhalational analgesia or may utilize all three in order that the staff (especially the midwives during their training) may become accustomed to and proficient in the use of all three different types of apparatus.

It should be emphasized that inhalational analgesia plays an important part in the relief of pain in labour if used in appropriate circumstances. It is particularly useful for the painful contractions of a rapid labour especially in multigravidae, or for the transition from the first to the second stages of labour. If inhalational analgesia is used over a longer time the mother will soon become dehydrated and exhausted because of the excessive deep breathing necessary for adequate pain relief. If prolonged analgesia is necessary, pethidine or epidural anaesthesia should be considered.

Local analgesia

Local infiltration of the perineum for episiotomy. When an episiotomy is necessary the perineum is injected with local anaesthetic. This is a very simple and easy procedure. The injection itself is completely painless and since the local anaesthetic works almost at once, the episiotomy can be performed immediately without causing any pain or discomfort. Repair of the episiotomy after delivery may require a further injection of local anaesthetic but this causes no discomfort and the episiotomy can be sutured without any pain whatever. Should any discomfort be felt while the stitches are being inserted, then a further small injection of local anaesthetic can be placed in the particular spot that has not been completely anaesthetized by the previous injections.

Pudendal nerve block is a type of local or regional anaesthesia performed, in some instances, immediately before forceps delivery. The pudendal nerves supply sensation to most of the perineum, the vulva and the vagina as well as to the muscles of the pelvic floor. The block is performed by injecting the nerves in the side wall of the pelvis with local anaesthetic. The injection itself is completely painless and results in immediate anaesthesia and loss of sensation in the vagina, perineum and vulva. An easy and painless forceps delivery is thus possible without the administration of a general anaesthetic. A pudendal nerve block is also used when a general anaesthetic is better avoided, such as for those who suffer from advanced cardiac disease.

Paracervical block is a form of local analgesia that is most effective during the first stage of labour. A diagram of the nerve supply to the uterus is seen in fig. 30. Most of the nerves that supply both the uterus and the cervix are collected together in a ganglion, or plexus, adjacent to the cervix. If local anaesthetic is injected into the plexus all the uterus will become insensitive to pain and pain associated with the first stage of labour will be either completely relieved or certainly reduced without affecting uterine activity. The nerve supply to the vagina, perineum and vulva which travels via the pudendal nerve remains unaffected when a paracervical block is performed.

A paracervical block can only be performed during the first stage of labour when the cervix is less than 5 cm in diameter. It is easy to perform and gives total relief in approximately 90 per cent of instances for 3 or up to 4 hours. It is widely used throughout the United States and Scandinavia but has not received wide acceptance in the United Kingdom.

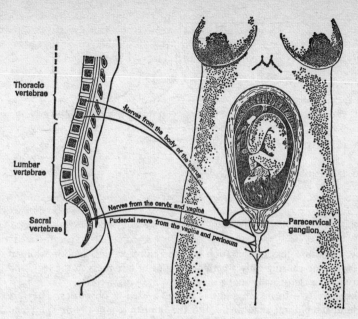

Fig. 30   The nerve supply to the uterus, cervix and vagina

Epidural analgesia

A representation of the sensory nerve supply of the uterus and birth canal is seen in fig. 30. The nerves that carry pain from the uterus to the brain arrive at the spine in the lower thoracic and upper lumbar regions. The nerves carrying pain from the cervix arrive in the spinal column in the sacral region together with those carrying the nerve supply from the vagina, the perineum and the vulva.

The extradural (syn. epidural) space is continuous from the base of the skull to the tip of the spinal column. It contains the spinal nerves as they enter and leave the spinal cord with fatty tissue and blood vessels. Local anaesthetics that are injected into the extradural space will cause anaesthesia in the spinal nerves, the extent of which will vary according to the amount of local anaesthetic injected and the position of the woman when the injection is made.

The nerves that carry sensory fibres (pain) are very much finer and more sensitive to the effects of local anaesthetic agents than are the nerves that carry motor function (movement). Epidural anaesthesia therefore is more effective against the nerves that carry sensation of pain than it is against the nerves that carry motor function or movement. It is thus possible, and it frequently happens, that injections of local anaesthetic into the epidural

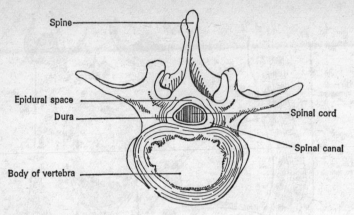

Fig. 31   A cross section through the spinal cord (lumbar vertebra)

space will cause loss of sensation and therefore painless labour while at the same time causing only a certain amount of heaviness in the legs, and most women can usually move their legs quite satisfactorily.

There are two forms of epidural analgesia used in obstetrics. They are the lumbar epidural anaesthetic into the lumbar region of the spine and the caudal anaesthetic (into the tip of the spine in the region of the coccyx), either of which may be used as a single injection or as a continuous injection technique. When the continuous injection technique is used, a fine polythene catheter is inserted into the extradural space so that further injections of local anaesthetic can be given when required. The technique of epidural anaesthesia is highly specialized but the injection itself and the insertion of the catheter for continuous epidural anaesthesia are painless although they may cause a certain amount of discomfort. An epidural anaesthetic is given either at the onset of labour or when contractions become sufficiently painful. The woman is usually placed on her left side with head bent and the knees up towards the chest. Some local anaesthesia is injected into the skin of the back and also into the deeper tissues. A needle is then introduced as illustrated in fig. 32 until the epidural space is reached. A single injection can then be given, or if a continuous epidural anaesthetic is required a fine catheter is threaded down the needle, while it is withdrawn, and the catheter is then strapped to the woman's back so that repeated injections of local anaesthetic can be given at intervals which vary from 2 to 4 hours when the pain recurs.

Towards the end of the first stage of labour or during the second stage of labour the woman may experience pain in the vagina or perineum and anaesthesia of this area can be achieved by sitting her up and injecting a further amount of anaesthetic. Gravity alone will allow the anaesthetic agent to spread slowly down the epidural space until it reaches the nerves

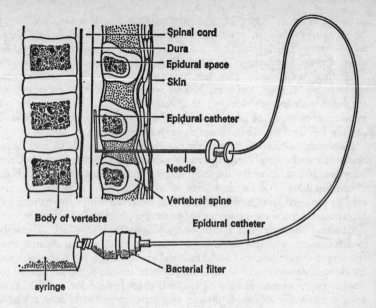

Fig. 32 Epidural catheter

as they enter the sacral part of the spinal column and thus effectively produce anaesthesia of the vagina, perineum and vulva.

It is important to emphasize that an epidural anaesthetic is not a spinal anaesthetic. In spinal anaesthesia the dura is pierced and the anaesthetic is injected into the space immediately surrounding the spinal column. Spinal anaesthesia has certain complications which do not apply to epidural anaesthesia.

Indications for epidural anaesthesia

Epidural anaesthesia is probably the most efficient method of obtaining relief of pain and discomfort in labour and it has the immense advantage that it has absolutely no ill-effects whatsoever upon the baby. Absolute or total relief of pain cannot be obtained in 100 per cent of instances; occasionally epidural anaesthesia may fail on account of some technical reason or even when it is accomplished the relief of pain may not be complete. However, in over 90 per cent of women the relief of pain is complete and the woman can then enjoy a labour absolutely free from pain.

Epidural anaesthesia may be required when the woman has failed to receive adequate relief of pain from other analgesic drugs or in some instances such as placental insufficiency where the use of more conventional analgesic drugs is restricted. Pre-eclampsia or hypertension, prolonged labour, uterine inertia, persistent posterior position of the baby's head, are all factors which might indicate that an epidural anaesthesia should be given. Lastly, but perhaps the most important, is the mother's choice.

Epidural anaesthesia does not prolong labour or decrease uterine contractions. It does, however, lead to an increase in the need to deliver the baby with forceps. Ideally, its effects should be allowed to wear off in the second stage of labour, so that the woman regains sensation and can use her own expulsive efforts to push the baby out.

Increasing numbers of women are having epidural anaesthesia for Caesarean section. Not only can the mother participate in the birth, but the baby needs less resuscitation than when a general anaesthetic has been given. Similarly, it is an ideal form of analgesia when a forceps delivery may be required, as in a twins or breech delivery, or where special rotation forceps are needed for a baby in the posterior position.

Epidural anaesthesia is a time-consuming procedure which is usually undertaken by a skilled anaesthetist who has spent a great deal of time training in the technique. Caudal epidural anaesthesia may be administered by either anaesthetists or obstetricians. There are not sufficient anaesthetists for every woman to have an epidural anaesthetic if she so wished, or even if medically indicated, though epidural anaesthesia is now available in most of the larger maternity units throughout the country. It is a method of anaesthesia, however, which is growing in popularity, and there seems little doubt that it will gradually continue to do so providing there are sufficient doctors and nurses available.

Complications of epidural anaesthesia

A fall in blood pressure (hypotension) is the commonest complication of epidural anaesthesia and occurs in approximately 5 per cent of instances. In order to detect this complication the blood pressure is taken at frequent intervals after an epidural anaesthetic has been given. A fall in blood pressure is quite easily corrected by turning the woman on to her side.

The dura itself, that is the membrane immediately surrounding the spinal cord, is perforated in approximately 1 per cent of women and when this is detected no epidural anaesthetic is given. In rare instances, approximately one per thousand, an injection of local anaesthetic may be given after the dura has been pierced in which case a spinal anaesthetic will result. So long as this is recognized it is not harmful but it will result in the temporary loss of motor power as well as sensation in the legs.

Other complications, such as infection, are virtually unknown.

Epidural anaesthesia is sometimes blamed if weakness or loss of sensation somewhere in the legs, or weakness or lack of control of the bladder, follows labour. Such complications are almost unknown after epidural anaesthesia. Weakness of the bladder or an inability to pass urine shortly after delivery, or an inability to control the bladder satisfactorily for the first few postpartum months, does sometimes follow normal labour and is more frequent after a difficult vaginal delivery, especially if forceps have been used. Loss of sensation in parts of the lower limbs or occasional weakness in the legs may also follow difficult or prolonged labour.

Spinal anaesthesia

Spinal anaesthesia is the single injection of a local anaesthetic solution into the tissue space which immediately surrounds the spinal cord. This type of injection can be given once only during labour. It is a very efficient anaesthetic which may be used for the relief of pain during labour, for Caesarean section or for forceps delivery. It lasts for approximately 2 hours. Spinal anaesthesia for childbirth is not very popular in Great Britain because some pregnant women so treated used to develop quite severe headaches which occasionally lasted for several days. Other forms of anaesthesia have proved equally if not more efficient.

Recent advances in spinal anaesthesia during labour, however, have reduced the complications and adverse reaction so that it is regaining popularity especially for Caesarean section.

General anaesthesia

General anaesthesia for any purpose associated with pregnancy or childbirth is administered by a specialized anaesthetist and not by a midwife or obstetrician. There is no reason why a pregnant woman should not be given a general anaesthetic at any stage during her pregnancy, for an operation not directly associated with her pregnancy, which cannot reasonably be left until after the end of the pregnancy. Anaesthetics do not harm the pregnant woman or her baby but all drugs including anaesthetics are better avoided in pregnancy if possible.

General anaesthesia may be required during pregnancy in order to perform external cephalic version (if this cannot be performed when the mother is conscious), for the induction of labour or to perform Caesarean section before the onset of labour. General anaesthesia may also be required at any stage during labour or at the time of delivery, especially if forceps delivery or Caesarean section is necessary.

A short note of warning about what to expect if you do have a Caesarean section. Immediately before most operations an injection of drugs known as premedication is usually given, which induces drowsiness, a sense of well-being and allays apprehension. Such an injection usually contains morphine or one of its derivatives, which are not given immediately prior to Caesarean section, together with a drug such as atropine which reduces the secretions from the chest, throat and nose during anaesthetic. Before a Caesarean operation is performed only the atropine-like substance will be given to you so that when you go to the operating theatre you will be completely awake and will not feel at all sleepy or drowsy. This is for the protection of your baby because if drugs are given to make you feel drowsy then your baby may also be drowsy immediately after delivery. Sometimes an antacid is given orally before general anaesthesia to reduce any feeling of sickness. It is also possible that before the anaesthetic is started you will be asked to breathe some oxygen from a mask for one or two minutes. This is not intended to put you to sleep but gives your baby an extra supply of oxygen immediately before the anaesthetic is administered. You may well be asked to hold the mask on your face as for the inhalation of gas and oxygen during labour; the mask should be pressed firmly on your face and you should breathe evenly and normally. The anaesthetist will tell you exactly what he is going to do and nothing sudden or unexpected will happen. After a few minutes you will be given a small injection into a vein in the arm and will drift off gently to sleep. When you wake up you will be back in bed and it will all be over.

Care of women in labour

When to call the midwife

If you are having your baby at home you should discuss with your midwife well in advance exactly when to call her. While there are rough guiding rules, each woman is treated as an individual and the midwife will have slightly different requirements for different mothers. As you are having your baby at home it is assumed that you have already had at least one baby and that the pregnancy and delivery were normal. You will, therefore, be aware of the three signs of the onset of labour:

1 The onset of uterine contractions at regular intervals occurring every 20 or 30 minutes and associated with discomfort in the abdomen or lower back.
2 Rupture of the membranes.
3 The passage of the 'show'.

Notify your midwife as soon as labour commences or the membranes rupture but remember that she is on duty 24 hours a day and you should be as cooperative as possible. For instance, if you wake at 3.0 a.m. with some tightening in the abdomen and some low backache and you find that this is repeated at 3.30 a.m. and again at 4.0 a.m. so that you are fairly sure you are in early labour, there is no need to notify the midwife immediately, but you can wait until the contractions have become more frequent and she has had a chance to complete her night's sleep. Similarly, if at 9.0 p.m. you believe that you are starting labour, it would be a kindness to notify your midwife as soon as possible, rather than delaying it until midnight or 1.0 a.m. Of course, no doctor or midwife likes being called out of bed unnecessarily in the middle of the night, but all agree that they would rather make a hundred unnecessary journeys than fail to be called for one necessary one.

When to go to hospital

You should go to hospital as soon as you are sure that labour is properly established, or when the membranes rupture, or if you have any sort of vaginal bleeding. Well over 99 per cent of women who are due to be delivered in hospital arrive there in plenty of time. If there is any doubt concerning the onset of labour, or if you are worried about your condition, do not hesitate to phone the hospital. There is always someone on duty, even in the small hours of the morning, who is well trained in the rapid assessment of the situation.

If you are fairly certain you are in labour tell the sister in charge exactly what has happened and she will undoubtedly instruct you to send for an ambulance and to go to hospital as soon as possible. You will have been given a card with the telephone number of the ambulance service and when you speak to the ambulance station you must make it perfectly clear that you are a maternity patient in labour and also state the hospital to which you are going. The ambulance service is extremely busy and has many calls, some more urgent than others. Women in labour do have some priority and the ambulance will call for you as soon as possible.

Preparing to go to hospital

No one can know what time you will be going to hospital so it is essential to have everything prepared beforehand.

1 Make adequate arrangements for the house, the children and your husband or partner to be looked after during your absence.
2 Make arrangements for your own transport to hospital.
3 Prepare and pack everything that you will need so that you just have to pick up the case when you are ready to go.

The house and family. You should make arrangements for someone to come and look after the children, or for the children to stay elsewhere. If they are going away it should be arranged for about a week before the expected date of confinement. If you go into labour at 3.0 a.m. it is not very easy to get the children up, dressed and off to their destination as well as getting yourself to hospital. In any event, you may wish to arrange for someone to do some cleaning and to look after the house. They will need to have a list of the names and addresses of the shops that you usually use, as well as the name and address of the doctor. A note about the amount of bread and milk usually delivered and the time of deliveries is helpful, as well as a list of where to find things, such as tea, coffee, soap and toilet paper.

Arrangements for your transport to hospital will depend on your circumstances and the distance that your home is situated from the hospital. Even if you have a car it might be too long a journey there and back for your husband or partner. The ambulance drivers and their assistants are very skilled in dealing with all emergencies and you will be in very safe, capable hands. When you attend the antenatal clinic the hospital will give you instructions on how to call the ambulance as well as a card to give the ambulance driver so that he will know exactly where to take you. If you are making arrangements for your husband, partner or a friend to drive you to hospital, they must be certain how to get there and which entrance to take you to on arrival. The car should always have sufficient petrol for the journey there and back.

Packing your case to go to hospital. Everything should be packed and ready to take with you at least two weeks before the baby is expected. Most hospitals provide a list of essentials that they expect you to take with you. If you do not wish to put things actually into the suitcase, they should be gathered together in a drawer so that you can pack them in just a few moments. If you do not do this in good time, you will have to do it in a hurry after labour has begun and will almost certainly forget something. The most important things to take are: nightdresses, which should be easily washable and you should have three or four for frequent changes; a light dressing gown and a pair of bedroom slippers, since you will probably get out of bed either on the day you have your baby or on the following day; a bedjacket and toilet requisites as well as your make-up. You should take two nursing brassieres, as well as two sanitary belts or a supply of disposable pants. The hospital provides special maternity sanitary towels.

You will be surprised how your time will be occupied while you are in hospital, but there may be some time for reading and writing letters and you should not forget to take books, some writing paper and a pen. If you receive flowers or letters of congratulation it is much easier to write thank you letters while you are in hospital; when you return home you will have even less time. Finally, remember a photograph of your husband or partner as well as any other small ones that you might especially want with you.

Admission to hospital

If you have been attending antenatal classes at the hospital you will have visited the wards, the admission room and the delivery rooms. You will also have been told about the routine or the organization for your admission When you enter the hospital you are received by the midwife and taken to the admission room. You should have telephoned to say that you are coming and she will be expecting you. When you are undressed and in bed the contents of your case are transferred to your bedside locker and your clothes carefully packed in the case for your husband or partner to take home. You are then examined either by the midwife on duty or by the house surgeon. Your notes are already available and a short history of the onset of labour will be taken together with any other symptoms that you may have experienced. Your blood pressure, pulse and temperature are recorded. A careful note is made of any vaginal bleeding or loss of water. It may or may not be necessary to perform a vaginal or rectal examination to ascertain the position of the presenting part in the pelvis and the dilatation of the cervix. A specimen of urine is obtained and tested for protein and sugar.

After these essential preliminaries, an enema is given in some instances, while in others it is not advisable. Broadly speaking, an enema is administered if labour is in its early stages, since emptying the lower bowel makes subsequent delivery easier and cleaner, and an enema also encourages the progress of labour. A bath or shower is usually advised for all those women in labour but may not be if the membranes have ruptured.

Examination on admission. The abdomen is carefully examined to assess accurately the condition of the mother and her uterus as well as the condition of her baby, and the stage to which labour has proceeded. The uterus is palpated with care to find any areas of tenderness or pain. The frequency, duration and strength of uterine contractions are carefully noted and recorded. The position of the baby is ascertained and the presenting part is palpated. Finally, the fetal heart is listened to. The progress of labour is estimated by the degree of dilatation of the cervix or the descent of the presenting part which will be the head or the breech. It is obvious, therefore, that both the dilatation of the cervix and the position of the presenting part should be known and recorded as soon as possible in order that further progress can be estimated.

Vaginal examination is performed early in labour and careful recordings made of the following: the vulva is examined and any varicose veins or other abnormality noted; the condition of the vagina and the presence of any discharge or bleeding; the degree of dilatation of the cervix, together with its consistency, texture and thickness; the position of the presenting part of the baby in relation to the cervix. If the membranes have ruptured great care is taken to ascertain how closely applied the cervix is to the presenting part and also the absence of any abnormality, such as a portion of umbilical cord or a hand or foot. The position of the presenting part of the baby within the mother's pelvis is important. Any fontanelles, sutures or caput palpated through the partially dilated cervix are noted, in order that the flexion of the baby's head can be accurately assessed. Finally, the general contours of the pelvis itself are noted.

The first stage of labour

Food and labour. For some reason that is not adequately understood the stomach (that is the anatomical stomach and not the abdomen) does not function satisfactorily during labour. Any food which is eaten following the onset of labour tends to remain in the stomach and not pass to the intestine. Sooner or later such food may be vomited and although this may be uncomfortable during labour, it does not really matter from a purely medical point of view. What does matter, however, is that a general anaesthetic may be necessary at any stage of labour and if you have eaten after the onset of labour vomiting may occur either while you are going under the anaesthetic or when you are recovering from it. If you have recently had a meal the food which you vomit may be inhaled into your lungs, where it will block the tubes and can rapidly lead to severe pneumonia.

After the onset of labour it is generally agreed that you may have fluids especially if they are sweetened with a little sugar, but these are restricted when you are in established labour. At the beginning of the first stage of labour milky fluids flavoured with coffee, cocoa, Ovaltine or Horlicks may be taken. The possibility of an anaesthetic must always be considered and it is therefore important that you never overload your stomach. Most doctors allow only fluids in early labour and nothing by mouth when labour is established. Fluid is then given intravenously. This is quite painless and free from discomfort. Small doses of magnesium trisilicate, an alkaline medicine, are given every 2 hours in some obstetric units to keep the mother's stomach contents from becoming too acid and to lessen the incidence of vomiting if an anaesthetic is necessary.

Cleanliness is of greatest importance and all delivery areas should be treated as surgical theatres. Thorough scrubbing of the labour ward bed, furniture and floors follows each delivery. Personal cleanliness of staff and patients is essential for the prevention of infection. All staff with colds, sore throats or any septic lesions are relieved from duty until cleared. Women with any infections, colds or sore throats, or who have suffered from these recently, are isolated from other mothers until better. In the interests of the other mothers and babies you must always mention if you have not been well.

Position during labour. In the early stages of labour the woman is encouraged to be up and about and can relax during contractions by sitting in a chair. There is some evidence that walking around in early labour encourages the contractions to be more efficient and may even improve the descent of the presenting part in the pelvis. When labour is fully established some women find that they are more comfortable if they continue to walk around. Most women, however, prefer to lie on their sides in bed, where they can rest between contractions. Some women enjoy having their back rubbed by their husband or partner, mother, friend or midwife. Some women feel happy listening to music, or simply talking to their husband or partner between contractions. Labour is a tiring process and uses up a great deal of energy. Should analgesics be required by the woman, they may also allow her to get some rest in the earlier part of labour.

Observations. Temperature, pulse, respiration and blood pressure are recorded at hourly or half-hourly intervals during the first stage of labour. These observations may be more frequent if any deviations from normal have been noted. It is important to empty your bladder frequently during the first stage of labour and every time you pass urine it is examined. Observations are also made of the length, strength and frequency of contractions; the amount and colour of the liquor. The fetal heart is listened to either at regular intervals or continuously (see Fetal Monitoring, p. 381) by machine, and gives a good indication of the baby's welfare. Vaginal examinations may be performed during the first stage of labour every 4 to 6 hours. They are essential to assess accurately the progress of labour and the descent of the head.

The second stage of labour

Vaginal examination is made to verify the beginning of the second stage of labour and confirm that the cervix is fully dilated. There are a number of factors to indicate the beginning of the second stage: the uterine contractions become very frequent, occurring about every 2 minutes; they become very strong and expulsive in character. The membranes may rupture if they have not already done so during the first stage of labour. You will have a desire to bear down with each contraction. You may feel the anus being distended and a sensation of wanting to open the bowels.

The midwife or doctor will tell you when to bear down. Bearing down is encouraged with every uterine contraction during the second stage of labour and you will be aware of less discomfort because you are actually doing something and feel that progress is being made. The usual position for bearing down is half sitting, with your back supported by two or three pillows, grasping your legs behind the thighs and pulling upwards. You should also bring your head up with your chin onto your chest to make the bearing down more effective. Between contractions your legs should be flat so you can relax and rest. Rhythm is most important during bearing down in order to achieve the maximum push with each contraction. You should take a deep breath while the uterus is contracting, close your lips, and bear down for as long and as hard as possible. A long, strong push is more effective than a series of short ones. On the average three good pushes can be achieved in the space of one contraction. You will need plenty of words of encouragement because this is labour in the true sense of the word, requiring a lot of effort and a tremendous amount of energy.

The delivery of the baby. There are two common positions for delivering babies in this country. One is the dorsal position, the other is the left lateral position. In the dorsal position the woman lies on her back with the knees bent and widely separated. The midwife or the doctor stands on the right side of the bed and delivers the baby in this way. The advantage of the dorsal position is that it is less tiring than the left lateral position and is much easier when the woman is being delivered by a midwife on her own or at home. It is the position which is generally used when a forceps delivery is required, and then the legs will be held in special poles called 'stirrups'. It is also the position in which a breech delivery takes place. In the lateral position the woman lies on her left side, buttocks at the edge of the bed and legs slightly bent. The midwife or the obstetrician stands behind the woman's buttocks and an assistant on the opposite side of the bed raises the right leg sufficiently to take its weight and make it comfortable for the patient. The advantages of the left lateral position are that the head can be delivered very slowly and great care can be taken of the perineum.

During the actual delivery of the head you will be asked to stop bearing down and to breathe in and out very quickly. The mere fact that you are panting in and out prevents you from pushing and therefore the midwife can deliver the head very gently and slowly. This prevents lacerations occurring. As soon as the head has been delivered there is a small pause which may last for 2 or 3 minutes before the next uterine contraction which will push out the rest of the baby to complete the delivery.

As soon as the baby is born you and the midwife must look at the clock so that the exact moment of birth is recorded. The umbilical cord is clamped and cut. Most babies cry immediately after birth so that no resuscitation is necessary. The baby is usually held on your abdomen unless he requires special resuscitation with oxygen, or anything else. If the mouth and nose are blocked with fluid then gentle suction of these air passages is all that is necessary.

Alternative positions. Increasingly, in recent years, stemming from the influence of Leboyer and Odent in France, the concept of 'gentle birth' has been emphasized. There is a feeling that hospitals have become too technological in their approach, and that childbirth has lost its human position as part of the continuity of life. The bustle of hospital wards, the cold sterility of the delivery room, the uniformed attendants (who may indeed be strangers to the labouring woman), the bright lights and impersonal atmosphere have all been criticized and many hospitals now try to reach a compromise between providing more homely surroundings, yet still having facilities at hand for medical intervention, should it be required. 'Birth rooms' try to create the comfort of a woman's own bedroom, where she and her husband or partner, and children, can relax and enjoy the process of labour. Clearly this is not suitable for everyone. There are some women who feel happier or more secure in a 'hospital' environment, and there are others who have a medical need for technological monitoring.

Part of this quiet revolution in recent years (and sometimes, not so quiet!) has also resulted in women trying different ways of giving birth. Standing, squatting, sitting on a 'birth stool', kneeling on all fours, are all different positions which can result in normal birth. Indeed there is evidence from X-rays that squatting increases the size of the pelvic outlet and may therefore make birth easier. Certainly in primitive tribes today, and down through the ages, women have assumed a squatting or half-standing position when obstructed labour has occurred, as if their instincts told them that this position might help.

It is no more difficult for a midwife to deliver a baby from a squatting woman than from one who is lying down. The perineum may also be more likely to tear in this position, and the mother can actually see a bit more of the baby as it is being born.

The third stage of labour

The third stage of labour begins immediately after the birth of the baby. It is during this stage that the placenta, or afterbirth, becomes separated from the muscular wall of the uterus and is expelled, either by the mother herself or by the obstetrician or midwife looking after her. The average length of time for the third stage of labour with modern management is approximately 3 to 5 minutes. The amount of blood lost in the third stage of labour varies considerably in normal deliveries, but averages between 4 and 6 oz, some being lost before and some after the complete separation of the placenta. On completion of the third stage of labour the level of the fundus of the uterus is below the umbilicus, and the uterus, alternately contracting and relaxing, is felt to be about the size and consistency of a large cricket ball.

The modern management of the third stage of labour is based on the principle that if the uterus is stimulated to contract immediately after the birth of the baby it will expel the placenta rapidly so that the dangers of postpartum haemorrhage are minimized. As soon as the anterior shoulder of your baby has been delivered during the second stage of labour, you will be given an intramuscular injection of syntometrine (or similar substance) to stimulate uterine contractions. Immediately the cord has been clamped and divided the placenta is delivered by traction on the cord attached to the placenta, while a hand is placed on the abdomen above the symphysis pubis and below the fundus of the uterus to lift the uterus gently upwards against the direction of the cord traction. The placenta soon appears at the vulva followed by the trailing membranes. The placenta and membranes are placed in a receiver so that they can be examined immediately following their delivery.

Examination of the placenta and the umbilical cord confirms that the placenta is complete and that no part is missing; and also that the membranes are complete. Retention of even a small piece of placenta may lead to postpartum haemorrhage. The placenta is circular in shape and weighs one sixth of the baby's weight. It has two surfaces. The maternal surface is dark red in colour and has been adherent to the uterine wall. The fetal surface is nearest to the fetus while *in utero* and is greyish and covered by a shiny membrane. Both surfaces are examined carefully. There are two membranes. The chorion is the outer opaque friable membrane and the amnion is the inner tough shiny membrane. The umbilical cord measures approximately 18 to 20 in. It contains one umbilical vein and two umbilical arteries surrounded by a jelly-like substance called Wharton's jelly. The outside is covered by amnion. During examination of the cord the blood vessels are counted. If only two vessels are present instead of three, a congenital abnormality may be suspected in the baby so that he merits even more careful examination than usual.

Episiotomy

An episiotomy is the name given to the operation in which the perineum is cut and incised to facilitate the delivery of the baby's head because either the tissues of the perineum are too rigid or the vaginal entrance is too tight to allow the head to pass through without a laceration occurring. Opinions are divided not only as to whether episiotomy should be done or not, but even as to which particular type of episiotomy should be done. An episiotomy is performed after the perineum has been infiltrated with local anaesthetic. The operation itself is easily and painlessly performed and consists of incising the perineum with a pair of sharp scissors either in the mid-line or slightly obliquely just to the right or left.

There are certain conditions and circumstances where an episiotomy must be performed and these are notably when a forceps delivery is being undertaken or when a baby is being delivered as a breech. An episiotomy is also done if, in the opinion of the doctor and the midwife, the muscles of the perineum are too rigid and so strong that they are holding up the progress of the second stage of labour, or if the entrance to the vagina and the perineum are such that a laceration of the perineum is bound to occur during delivery.

The main argument concerning episiotomy is whether it should be done routinely for every delivery or not. Those in favour of a routine episiotomy argue that the baby's head is 9.5 cm in diameter and its passage over the perineum and through the vaginal entrance must inevitably lead to tearing of some muscles and overstretching to such a degree that the vaginal entrance never regains its former size and consistency. Such overstretching not only affects a woman's sex life but may later also predispose to prolapse of the vaginal walls. Whether a routine episiotomy is performed in the course of a normal delivery is a matter of individual preference of the midwife or doctor but it is probably fair to say that an increasing number are being done.

Some women are needlessly afraid of an episiotomy because of the pain they believe they may experience while this is being performed. The perineum is always injected with local anaesthetic so that the operation is painless.

Repair of the episiotomy

Since the perineum is injected with local anaesthetic before the episiotomy is performed, it remains numbed for several hours so that the repair can be done without any pain or discomfort. Should even the slightest discomfort be caused during the repair then more local anaesthetic can easily be injected.

The repair of the episiotomy is a comparatively simple procedure. The woman is placed in a rather undignified but not uncomfortable position known as the lithotomy position, lying on her back with her legs supported in stirrups or poles. The posterior wall of the vagina is gently sutured, usually using fairly fine, plain catgut, with small stitches to bring the edges of the vaginal skin together. The muscles of the perineum itself are carefully and accurately brought together and sutured by means of several individual stitches. The skin of the perineum is then sutured using several individual stitches of either fine silk or catgut. If silk or thread stitches have been put into the skin of the perineum they are removed usually on the sixth day after delivery. If catgut stitches have been inserted however, these dissolve spontaneously, although the majority of women are more comfortable if even these are removed on the sixth day. Removal of the stitches from the perineum causes no more than very minimal discomfort and the vast majority of women feel much more comfortable as soon as the skin stitches have been removed.

Repair of perineal tear or laceration

If a perineal tear or laceration occurs it requires suturing in exactly the same way as an episiotomy. The perineum is injected with local anaesthetic so that the whole of the perineum and the posterior wall of the vagina are satisfactorily numbed. The tear is sutured in the same way as an episiotomy and the removal of the stitches is exactly the same.

An episiotomy is easier to repair than a perineal tear because the edges of the incision are straight whereas the edges of a tear are frequently jagged and irregular.

25 Induction of Labour

Induction of labour is the artificial starting of labour before it begins spontaneously. The exact reason for the onset of labour is not known and, therefore, it is not possible to imitate precisely the way in which nature initiates labour. There are many reasons why a doctor may wish to induce labour before it commences spontaneously and various methods are used.

Methods used in induction of labour

Artificial rupture of the membranes

This has for many years been the most popular method of inducing labour. The membranes just inside the internal os of the cervix are perforated by gently introducing a sharp object or a pair of forceps through the cervical canal and some of the amniotic fluid can then drain away. This small procedure is easily accomplished without any pain or discomfort. The drainage of amniotic fluid from within the cavity of the uterus results in alteration of the pressure inside the uterus and it is thought that this initiates labour. In any event, labour will begin fairly soon after the membranes have been ruptured artificially and the nearer the woman is to her expected date the earlier labour will commence. When a woman is at or near term then labour starts within a few hours.

Oxytocic drugs

Oxytocic drugs are a group of drugs which have a direct action upon the uterus itself and will provoke or stimulate the uterus into rhythmic contractions and, therefore, into labour. The first of the oxytocic drugs used was Pitocin, or pituitary extract, from the pituitary gland (a small gland situated at the base of the brain). This was given by means of intravenous drip, intramuscular injection or by mouth. In recent years the use of Pitocin tablets, which are sucked to absorb the hormone from the mouth, has been replaced by the use of more reliable Syntocinon intravenous infusions.

Ergometrine (either alone or as syntometrine) is a powerful oxytocic drug but, since it makes the cervix contract as well as the uterus, it is not used for the induction of labour because during labour dilatation of the cervix is required.

Syntocinon is now the standard drug for induction of labour. The dose can be accurately measured and administered by a painless intravenous drip either directly from a bottle or through an accurate automatic pump.

Prostaglandins

Prostaglandins are so named from their original isolation from extracts of animal prostate gland. They comprise a large group of hormones found in various organs of both male and female bodies. Some hormones of this group have been found to stimulate strongly the pregnant uterus and they are now being used in many centres for the induction of labour. They are generally given as vaginal pessaries or a gel paste, and ripen the cervix as well as stimulate contractions. Intravenous infusions generally cause vomiting and diarrhoea. In some centres oral tablets are used. The advantages of prostaglandins are that the cervix is affected locally, the labour seems more natural in that the woman is not necessarily attached to a drip, and she may move about in the early stages. The baby's heart rate is usually monitored for an hour after prostaglandin usage.

Castor oil

A dose of castor oil is the well-tried and outdated method of inducing labour. Even a large dose fails unless labour is imminent, but has the side effect of producing severe colic and profuse diarrhoea usually without any sign of labour.

Oil, bath and enema. This was the traditional, though ineffective, method of inducing labour and is no longer used. The administration of a large dose of castor oil was followed after a few hours by a warm enema and then the treatment was completed by the woman having a hot bath. Not only was this ineffective, but it also resulted in the woman being exhausted, dehydrated and somewhat demoralized before labour had even begun.

There are many other methods of inducing labour that have been practised over the centuries and some of which are still practised today.

Choice of method of induction

The choice of the method of induction to be used in any particular instance will rest with the obstetrician concerned and his selection will vary from person to person according to her particular requirements. The method most frequently performed is the insertion of prostaglandin tablets or pessaries into the vagina the night before labour is due to be induced. This will ripen the cervix and will often initiate labour itself. This may be followed by artificial rupture of the membranes, which in turn is followed by the administration of one of the oxytocic drugs, usually Syntocinon, by a continuous intravenous drip. If labour has not already started following the prostaglandin, it will nearly always begin within a very short time and proceeds normally.

Indications for inducing labour

The indications for inducing labour may be either medical or social.

Medical

The medical reasons for inducing labour before it starts spontaneously may vary enormously. Pre-eclampsia, hypertension, post-maturity, placental insufficiency, diabetes, Rhesus incompatibility are just a few of the many reasons why the obstetricians may wish to induce labour.

Social

Most authorities say that there are no social indications for the induction of labour and these have long been frowned upon in Britain. By social indications one means that labour is induced for the convenience of either the patient or the doctor. The objection to this is mainly traditional and dates back to the time when induced labour was not as safe as labour which began spontaneously. The induction of labour today, however, is completely safe, providing that the woman is at or near term and everything else is completely normal. Labour can be induced by means of prosta-glandin or with Syntocinon given by a continuous drip into a vein and if this is accompanied by artificial rupture of the membranes then the onset of labour is assured.

If a woman is suffering from Rhesus incompatibility and it is known that her baby is going to need to have its blood changed as soon as it is delivered, then labour is induced so that the delivery occurs at a convenient hour during the week when the anaesthetist, the paediatrician and the laboratory are readily available. Every effort is made to ensure that such a woman is not delivered at midnight on a Saturday. This is an induction of labour done for a medical reason at a social time convenient to the doctors and the laboratory.

Now that the induction of labour is perfectly safe it is obvious that it will be used more and more frequently in order that doctors and nurses can look after their patients during the hours of daylight when they themselves are fresh and when all the ancillary services they might require are readily and easily available, rather than deliver women during the night when they themselves are tired and when the ancillary services are not so readily available. A doctor or midwife who has been up for most of the night still has to work the next day!

Labour after induction

After induction labour proceeds completely normally. An induced labour does not last any longer than a labour which commences spontaneously. An induced labour is not more painful than a labour which begins spontaneously. The chances of a normal delivery are just the same if labour has been induced as if it had begun spontaneously. Induced labour does not adversely affect the baby so long as appropriate steps are taken to ensure that labour begins within 24 hours after the membranes have been artificially ruptured.

26 Complications of Labour

Prolonged labour

Prolonged labour is by definition a labour which lasts for 24 hours or more. Modern antenatal care, together with the modern management of women in labour, has virtually eliminated a labour lasting for this length of time. The active management of labour results in normal deliveries for 85 per cent of women having their first babies, and 95 per cent of women who have had children before. This is based on the principle that the cervix dilates at a minimum rate of 1 cm per hour, and usually much faster in multigravid women. By regular vaginal examinations, delay in this dilatation can be detected early and action taken. If this is not possible, or if the remedy does not work, Caesarean section is advised much sooner than 40 years ago, when it was still an operation full of risk. Caesarean section is now a completely safe operation, and induction of labour has no risk for the mother or her baby, so that the few remaining reasons for prolonged labour can be eliminated. There are several reasons, however, why a labour lasts a little longer than one might normally expect.

Delay in labour is stated to exist when progress ceases. Progress is measured by two factors—firstly, descent of the head and secondly, dilatation of the cervix. The causes of delay in labour are:

1 Faults in the forces (abnormalities of uterine contractions).
2 Faults in the passenger (abnormal or difficult position of the baby).
3 Faults in the passage (abnormality of the pelvis, vagina, pelvic floor or perineum).

Delay in the first stage of labour

The cause of delay in the first stage of labour is most frequently inadequate or insufficient uterine contractions, so that the time factor is not important, but if delay occurs in the presence of strong regular uterine contractions the cause must be found and remedied or Caesarean section performed.

Abnormalities in the contractions

Hypotonic inertia. If the uterine contractions are weak and ineffective a state of uterine inertia is said to exist. In some instances the uterus never really seems to get going and the labour is never properly established. The uterine contractions occur at irregular intervals every 10, or even 20, minutes and are never satisfactory or really strong, as a result of which the cervix dilates very slowly and labour becomes prolonged. This condition, known as hypotonic inertia, may be treated either by rupturing the membranes artificially in the hope that this will provoke stronger contractions, more coordinated uterine activity and hence more satisfactory labour, or by giving a very small dose of Syntocinon in a continuous intravenous drip. Syntocinon provokes the uterus into normal rhythmic contractions and converts hypotonic inertia into normal activity, thus converting what is potentially a long labour into a normal labour. No reason is known why some labours develop hypotonic inertia. Both the mother and her baby are perfectly normal and eventually delivery proceeds quite normally without any ill effects to either the mother or her baby.

Hypertonic action is another type of abnormal uterine activity where the uterus contracts quite strongly and fiercely but for only a few seconds each time. This particular type of uterine action may be associated with a posterior position of the baby and may be accompanied by quite severe backache. The frequent, short, rather sharp uterine contractions are not as efficient as normal contractions and hence such a labour tends to be prolonged. Perhaps the most frequent cause of hypertonic action is fear. Modern antenatal care and instruction, together with modern management in labour, have greatly reduced the incidence of hypertonic inertia, but when it does occur it is treated either by sedation with fairly large doses of pethidine or similar analgesics, or by epidural anaesthesia, and either method may be combined with the administration of small doses of Syntocinon by continuous intravenous drip.

It must be emphasized that long labour resulting from abnormal or inefficient uterine activity is comparatively rare today.

Abnormalities in the passenger

Delay due to the baby is caused either by his size or the position of his head. Unless the baby happens to be 4 or 4.5 kg, or even more, the size does not exert very much influence on the length of labour. A big baby (say 4.5 kg) as a first baby may cause labour to be considerably prolonged. Otherwise most of the delay caused by the baby is due to his head being poorly flexed.

Under normal circumstances the whole baby is in what is known as the fetal attitude of flexion. The spine is flexed, the head is bent down so that the chin rests on the chest and the arms and legs are flexed. In this attitude the head presents its smallest or narrowest diameter to the brim of the pelvis as well as to the birth canal. If, for some reason, the head is not well flexed then the diameters of the head that are presented to the brim of the pelvis and to the birth canal are slightly increased, so that although the baby's head is absolutely normal in shape and size its position artifici-ally increases the diameters which have to pass through the pelvis. This causes a certain amount of delay.

A baby's head may be poorly flexed or actually deflexed *in utero*, especially in a woman who has had many children. If the head is not engaged in the pelvis before the onset of labour in a woman having her first baby, this is usually due to poor flexion of the head. Quite frequently, after the onset of labour, the head descends allowing normal flexion to occur, and labour proceeds normally. It is only when there is some difficulty in the proper flexion of the baby's head that labour tends to be prolonged.

Posterior position. The baby normally lies with his back towards the front of the abdomen and while in this position he can assume the correct attitude of flexion. If the back lies towards the back of the mother's abdomen, then the baby cannot lie in a properly flexed attitude and the head will be poorly flexed. It will, therefore, present a larger diameter to go through the birth canal. Such a posterior position occasionally occurs in women having their first baby and causes a rather classic series of events. The baby's head does not engage in the pelvis at the 36th week of pregnancy; it is not engaged at the onset of labour and the membranes may rupture before labour begins with the loss of a large amount of liquor; labour may be rather prolonged, but in the majority of instances the head rotates within the pelvis to allow a normal delivery to take place; finally, in the few instances where the head fails to rotate and remains in its posterior position, a forceps delivery may be necessary.

Abnormalities in the passage

The passage refers to the bony part of the pelvis, the soft tissue and the muscles of the pelvic floor.

The size of the bony pelvis is estimated at the first antenatal visit when, unless there is some contra-indication, an internal examination is performed and any obvious abnormality of the bony pelvis noted. If the baby's head has not engaged in the mother's pelvis at the 36th week of pregnancy and if it does not descend into the pelvis when she sits or stands up from a lying position, a further internal examination is performed to ascertain more accurately the internal diameters of the bony pelvis. If these are satisfactory it can be assumed with confidence that there is sufficient room in the pelvis and that the head will engage in due course. If the doctor, however, has any reason to suspect that the internal diameters of the pelvis may not be adequate then an X-ray examination may be done. If the pelvis is thought to be clinically normal the woman will be seen again at the 37th and 38th week of pregnancy and if the baby's head will still not engage within the brim of the pelvis then the doctor may consider that an X-ray of the pelvis is justified to ascertain the relative sizes of the baby's head and the pelvic brim. Usually only one film, an erect lateral picture, is taken from the side with the woman standing upright. This indicates not only the size of the baby's head and the diameters of the brim of the pelvis, but also the size and shape of the sacrum and the different angles of the birth canal through which the baby has to travel. If in the doctor's opinion the pelvis is too small then Caesarean section may be advised.

The internal size of the bony pelvis has already been proved in women who have had one baby, and provided that the previous baby was a reasonable weight and was delivered without difficulty then the pelvic measurements must be normal.

Labour may also be prolonged by the soft tissue of the pelvis. On very rare occasions the cervix is very slow to dilate, partly because it seems to become very rigid and firm, and partly because it appears to contain more fibrous tissue than usual. It is not known why this should occur, but it is a condition which may be relieved by an epidural anaesthetic.

Disproportion is a word which is commonly used, although its meaning and definition are rather uncertain. It means that there is some real or apparent discrepancy between the size of the baby's head, being the largest part of the baby, and the size of the mother's pelvic bones.

Abnormalities of the bony pelvis, which used to be known as contracted pelvis, are now comparatively rare. They do, however, occasionally occur, and are detected in the antenatal clinic so that the pelvis can be accurately measured both by internal examination and, if necessary, by X-ray. If the obstetrician considers that the pelvic bones are too small then Caesarean section will be performed. If he considers that although the pelvis is small it is satisfactory, he will allow labour to proceed normally, always with the reservation that Caesarean section will be performed if there is any undue delay or difficulty. The pelvis may be reduced in size by previous disease such as rickets.

Disproportion between the baby's head and the pelvis may be caused because a baby is too big, or because the baby's head is in the wrong position. Nature is usually very careful to ensure that small women have small babies and a woman usually has a baby of a size to fit her pelvis, regardless of the size and stature of her husband or partner. It is unusual, therefore, for a baby to be too big, but this does occasionally happen, especially in women who are diabetic or who have a diabetic tendency. The commoner cause of disproportion is because the baby's head is in the wrong position, which usually means that it is in a posterior position or is poorly flexed. A badly flexed head usually flexes itself after the onset of labour, but if it fails to do so then disproportion may occur because a larger diameter of the head presents.

It is extremely difficult to judge disproportion before the onset of labour, since it is impossible to anticipate the strength of the uterine contractions, the 'give' of the pelvis or the amount that the baby's head will flex and mould (this is the normal overlapping of the skull bones that occurs during labour and which reduces the diameter of the baby's head by as much as 1 cm). Given strong uterine contractions, with adequate flexion of the head and satisfactory moulding, there are few labours that will not be brought to a normal and satisfactory conclusion.

Delay in the second stage of labour

Progress in the second stage of labour is stated to stop when the head ceases to descend (the cervix already being fully dilated). Delay is said to occur in a first pregnancy if the baby is not delivered one hour after the onset of the second stage, or in a subsequent pregnancy after half an hour in the second stage. Most midwives and doctors agree that delay has occurred in the second stage as soon as progress ceases, which can usually be recognized in a much shorter interval of time and today the second stage of labour is allowed about half the time that was normally permitted about 20 years ago.

The causes of delay in the second stage are just the same in principle as those occurring in the first stage:

1 Inadequate uterine contractions (the forces).
2 A fetal head that is either too large or in the wrong position (the passenger).
3 The soft parts of the pelvis are too rigid (the passage).

Poor or inadequate uterine contractions may be the result of a long and tiring labour, over-sedation or over-distension of the uterus; gentle forceps delivery or ventouse extraction easily completes the second stage. If the fault is in the passenger then its position must be corrected, if necessary, and delivery by forceps or ventouse undertaken immediately. The head will be deeply engaged in the pelvis—if the head had originally failed to engage it would have caused delay in the first stage and a Caesarean section would have been performed before the start of the second stage.

Malposition of the head

Persistent posterior position. When the baby's head enters the pelvis in the posterior position it may fail to rotate through the required 180°; the head will not descend and must be gently rotated into the correct position and forceps delivery performed.

Deep transverse arrest. Sometimes the baby's head flexes and enters the pelvis in a posterior position and labour proceeds normally, but during the second stage of labour the baby's head cannot complete its rotation, so that instead of the back of the head coming to lie in front, the rotation stops halfway with the baby's head facing sideways instead of backwards. This condition is known as deep transverse arrest and no further progress will be made until the head has been gently rotated into the correct position.

Face presentation. When the baby's head is completely extended the baby is delivered face first. If the chin is pointing forward a face presentation is unlikely to cause any delay during labour, but if the chin is pointing backwards then delay is bound to occur because the baby cannot be delivered until the head has been turned so that the chin points forwards. Just as a caput, or swelling, forms over the scalp when the head is properly flexed in a vertex presentation, so a caput forms over the face when it is presenting and it becomes considerably swollen, distorted and quite bruised. This causes no permanent damage. All the swelling and bruising disappears in three or four days and the baby's face is absolutely normal.

Brow presentation results when the head is extended halfway between the normal vertex presentation and a face presentation. A brow presentation cannot be delivered because the diameters of the baby's head are too big to pass through the pelvis and the baby must be delivered by Caesarean section or flexed to become a vertex presentation, or extended into a face presentation.

The second stage may be unduly prolonged by resistance of the soft parts of the vagina, pelvic floor or perineum. This is particularly liable to happen in a woman over the age of 35 having her first baby, or in younger women who have indulged in a lot of sport and physical activity that has developed the muscles of the pelvic floor particularly well. It can always be overcome either by gentle forceps delivery or by an episiotomy.

Delay in the third stage of labour

The third stage of labour is the time between the completion of delivery of the baby and the completion of the delivery of the placenta. This should normally take between 20 and 30 minutes, but with the modern technique of giving injections of oxytocic drugs at the time of the delivery of the baby's head or anterior shoulder, the third stage should last between 2 and 5 minutes. If the placenta has not been delivered within this period of time and no haemorrhage is occurring, it is usual to wait for a short while. In approximately 3 per cent of deliveries the placenta will not deliver spontaneously and then a general anaesthetic is given and the placenta is stripped very gently off the inner aspect of the uterus.

When the placenta is retained within the body of the uterus there is always a danger that bleeding may begin and therefore a very careful and constant watch is kept on the new mother until the placenta has been safely delivered. Should any excessive bleeding occur this can always be stopped by a further injection of oxytocic drug (ergometrine or syntometrine), but the presence of undue haemorrhage is an indication for immediate manual removal of the placenta under general anaesthesia.

Fetal distress

Fetal distress is the term used when a baby is short of oxygen. There are many reasons for this but they can be broadly divided into the chronic and the acute.

The chronic, or longstanding, shortage of oxygen during pregnancy is discussed under the heading of placental insufficiency and dysmaturity. In this condition both the uterus and the baby are small and there is evidence that the placenta is inadequate.

Acute fetal distress usually occurs during labour because the uterine contractions are very frequent. When the uterus is not in labour there is no obstruction to the oxygen supply to the baby. The force of the contractions, however, obstructs the blood and oxygen supply to the placenta, but during contractions, if the placenta is healthy with good reserve, the baby will not run short of oxygen.

Acute fetal distress happens if the cord is twisted around the baby or knotted and also where haemorrhage has occurred behind the placenta. Fetal distress may also occur if the baby's head is compressed rather tightly in the pelvis.

The signs of fetal distress are passage of meconium into the liquor, changes in the baby's heart rate and excessive movements.

Meconium is the thick, green substance normally contained in the baby's rectum and passed only after delivery. When the baby lacks oxygen a reflex action causes passage of meconium into the amniotic fluid. This green-stained liquor is recognized as it drains out of the vagina and may be taken as a warning that the baby is becoming distressed. Some babies pass meconium at the onset of labour for no apparent reason. A woman should not be unduly worried if she notices meconium when the waters break because this sign is only significant when associated with an irregularity or fall in the fetal heart rate.

The fetal heart rate. The baby's normal heart rate varies between 120 and 160 beats per minute and each individual fetal heart maintains a fairly constant rate, rhythm and tone. The heart may slow during contractions but as each contraction wears off it should regain its normal rate within seconds. Rates above 160 and below 120 suggest fetal distress.

Tumulous movements

Sudden and violent movements of the baby as if it were turning over and over are an indication, especially in labour, of distress of the fetus.

Fetal monitoring

In recent years it has been appreciated that continuous recording of the fetal heart is more likely to detect early fetal distress than listening to the heart at regular intervals. Such recording is performed in many modern units using cardiograph machines which print out records of the heart rate and uterine contractions on a moving paper strip. Recordings are taken by harmless transducers strapped to the mother's abdomen though better tracings of the fetal heart are obtained using a tiny clip which attaches to the baby's scalp neither giving the baby pain nor doing it harm. If early fetal distress is detected prompt action may be taken. A normal tracing of the baby's heart rate predicts a good outcome in 99 per cent of cases. Most obstetricians feel that all high-risk pregnancies should have monitoring during labour—for example women with cardiac or renal disease, hypertension or pre-eclampsia, Rhesus disease, diabetes, placental insufficiency and where a woman has previously had a still-birth.

Fetal blood sampling

In some specialized maternity units it is possible to take a small sample of blood from the baby's head when fetal distress is suspected during labour. Examination of the oxygen content in this sample confirms or refutes the presence of fetal distress and thus enables the management of the labour to be judged more accurately.

Severe distress

The presence of severe fetal distress is an indication that delivery must take place as soon as possible. If the woman is in the first stage of labour and the cervix is not fully dilated, this will be by Caesarean section. If she is in the second stage, forceps or ventouse will be used for immediate delivery.

Maternal distress

Maternal distress is comparatively rare in modern maternity units. It may be mental or physical, of which the physical may be real or potential.

Mental distress may happen when a woman who is in labour has not been properly instructed, so that she becomes afraid and it is impossible to allay her fears. This is very uncommon today because it is nearly always due to lack of cooperation and understanding in the antenatal period. It may arise when a woman knows that her baby is dead, or if she is convinced that something has gone wrong.

Real physical distress used to happen at the end of a prolonged labour which had continued for two or three days, when a woman who had become grossly dehydrated was suffering from fever and exhaustion. Such a condition is rarely seen today, partly because long labours are not allowed and partly because dehydration is prevented by the administration of intravenous fluids.

Potential physical distress. The type of maternal distress with which the doctor and midwife are concerned today is potential rather than real. Thus, in a woman who is suffering from pre-eclampsia, cardiac disease, diabetes or a raised blood pressure, it is often thought desirable, in her best interests, to shorten the second stage of labour rather than to allow the labour to pursue its normal course or to allow her the strain or exertion of pushing during the second stage. Physical strain is anticipated and avoided.

Forceps

The exact history of the obstetric forceps is shrouded in mystery but they were probably invented by a member of the Chamberlen family about 1595 and kept as a secret within the family for about 130 years. It is quite astonishing that a discovery so important should be kept secret within one family for such a long time. The members of the family who used the forceps would only do so after everyone else had been sent out of the room and only then after the patient had been very heavily draped so that she should not see what was being done. The steel blades and handles were wrapped in leather so that no metallic sound should betray their presence.

Since 1730 many different types and shapes of obstetric forceps have been invented, each having minor and somewhat insignificant modifications. For very many years the obstetric forceps provided the only method of delivery if labour did not proceed naturally, but as Caesarean section has gradually become safer and more frequently performed, so the indications for performing the more hazardous types of forceps delivery have disappeared. The operation of 'high forceps' which carried a great risk of death or damage to the baby, as well as a risk of considerable injury to the mother, has now been completely replaced by Caesarean section. Forceps deliveries today are only undertaken when the baby's head has descended well into the pelvis or is actually in the pelvic outlet.

The modern obstetric forceps are very simple in their construction but extremely efficient. They are so made that the blades of the forceps fit

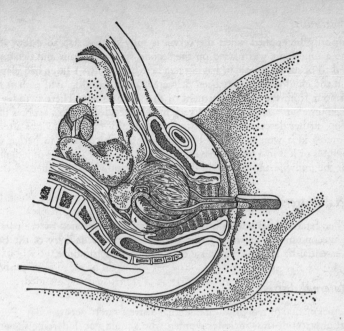

Fig 33 Forceps delivery

very accurately over the baby's head and when they are properly applied
the handles of the forceps come so neatly together that the blades cannot
possibly damage or harm the baby's head. In fact the forceps form a steel
cage round the baby's head to protect it from any injury that might occur
by pressure from the bones of the mother's pelvis. The term 'prophylactic',
or protective, forceps delivery has received a great deal of attention in the
United States, where quite a large number of babies at full term are
specifically delivered by the forceps to protect them from injury or damage.

Many midwives and obstetricians in Great Britain are in favour of
delivering premature babies by means of forceps to protect the soft and
easily damaged skull.

Indications for applying the forceps are:

1 Delay in the second stage of labour.
2 Foetal distress.
3 Maternal distress.

Delay in the second stage

In the second stage of labour the cervix is fully dilated and the only
criterion of progress is continued descent of the baby's head. Delay in the
second stage is said to occur when the head ceases to descend. The forceps

can only be applied when the cervix is fully dilated. Up to a few years ago a time limit was placed on the second stage of labour and delay was said to occur in a woman having her first baby when 1 hour had elapsed and the child had not yet been delivered, or in a multigravid patient half an hour from the commencement of the second stage. There is today no fixed time limit and forceps delivery may be decided upon as soon as there is no further descent of the baby's head, and this may be obvious after 10 minutes in a woman having her third or fourth child or in perhaps 30 minutes or less in a woman having her first baby. It is a matter of judgment for the midwife and doctor to decide in each individual instance.

Fetal distress

When fetal distress occurs in the second stage, as indicated by the passage of meconium and slowing of the heart rate, speedy delivery of the baby is essential by forceps, ventouse or possibly by episiotomy.

Maternal distress

Actual mental or real physical maternal distress rarely occurs today. Potential physical distress includes women who should not undertake the exertion of bearing down and pushing during the second stage of labour. They are relieved of this by delivery of the baby with forceps.

The conditions

Several conditions must be fulfilled before the obstetric forceps can be used.

1 The cervix must be fully dilated. It is not possible to deliver the baby by the vaginal route before full dilatation of the cervix without a considerable risk of severe injury to the mother.
2 The head must be engaged in the pelvis and there must be no obvious obstruction to delivery.
3 The membranes must be ruptured. This is really only a theoretical condition because the doctor would automatically rupture the membranes immediately before applying the forceps.
4 Uterine contractions must be present, or an oxytocic drug is given at the time of delivery. This is to ensure that the uterus contracts after delivery to prevent any severe haemorrhage.
5 The bladder must be empty and as it is extremely difficult for most women to pass urine during the second stage of labour this invariably means passing a catheter to allow the urine to drain away. It is theoretically possible for a full bladder to be injured during delivery.
6 The woman must be anaesthetized (local or general).

7 There must be a reasonable prospect of delivery (e.g. no disproportion at the vaginal outlet).

The technique of forceps delivery

Forceps delivery is performed under either general or local anaesthesia. Local anaesthesia may be an epidural, a caudal anaesthetic, or a pudendal nerve block. The woman is told that she is going to have a forceps delivery and the reasons for this decision are explained to her. If she is suffering from a raised blood pressure or from pre-eclampsia then she will probably have been told beforehand that the forceps will be applied shortly after full dilatation of the cervix. Anaesthesia is then induced. The exact position of the baby's head is confirmed. If the occiput, or the back of the baby's head, is posterior (persistent occipito-posterior position), or if the occiput is lying to one side (deep transverse arrest) then the head will be gently rotated so that the occiput comes to lie in front. Such rotation is performed either with forceps or manually. The first blade of the forceps is guided gently alongside the baby's head so that the blade passes smoothly and easily between the baby's head and the side wall of the vagina. The other blade is similarly inserted, using the fingers to ensure that it passes round the baby's head and is gently inserted between the scalp and the vaginal wall. When the forceps are correctly applied the handles fit exactly.

The baby is delivered by gently pulling the forceps. Gentle traction is exerted for 30 to 40 seconds at a time, after which it is relaxed. With each gentle pull the head descends lower in the pelvis until eventually the perineum is distended, at which stage an episiotomy is performed. The mechanism of delivery with forceps is exactly the same as for spontaneous delivery—in other words the baby's head is delivered by extending the head on the neck so that the face sweeps over the posterior vaginal wall and the perineum. As soon as the head is delivered the forceps are removed. Immediately the mouth, nose and eyes are cleaned with a sterile dry swab and the mouth and throat sucked out. If an epidural or a local anaesthetic has been administered the woman may now voluntarily deliver her baby in exactly the same way as she would do in a spontaneous vaginal delivery, because once having delivered the head the rest of the delivery is easy. Delivery is completed in exactly the same way as in a normal delivery.

Caesarean section

The history of Caesarean section is a story of almost total failure until the beginning of this century and it is really only in the last 25 years that it has become a safe operation. The incidence of Caesarean section has gradually risen during this time and although it varies from hospital to hospital it is now fairly constant at approximately 6 per cent of all deliveries. Some of these are first deliveries and some are subsequent, or repeat, Caesarean sections. The reason for this apparently high figure is that Caesarean section is now so safe that it replaces the majority of difficult or hazardous labours. High forceps delivery, internal version, difficult forceps delivery, breech delivery either of large babies or where the mother's pelvis may be too small, have all been replaced by Caesarean section.

For the woman herself, Caesarean section is just as safe as vaginal delivery and infinitely preferable to difficult or complicated vaginal delivery. For the baby, Caesarean section is certainly preferable to, and invariably safer than, a difficult vaginal delivery. The factors that have contributed towards making Caesarean section safe are:

1 Improvement in surgical technique and surgical instruments.
2 The type of operation performed today is a very much better and safer operation than those previously performed.
3 Although antibiotics are not used routinely in women who are delivered by Caesarean section it is nevertheless a fact that for many years the operation was only performed on women who had been in labour for many hours and in whom the risk of infection was therefore high. Caesarean section has become a safe operation for the mother because infection can now be prevented by the use of sterile and aseptic techniques, or be treated readily should it unfortunately happen.
4 Caesarean section is occasionally performed in women who suffer from antepartum haemorrhage and in whom, therefore, blood transfusion is essential. Even in those who do not suffer from antepartum haemorrhage the blood loss at Caesarean section is invariably greater than it is at normal delivery and the ability to replace this blood loss without any danger to the mother has made the operation much more acceptable.
5 Modern anaesthesia ensures a satisfactory oxygen supply to both the mother and her baby throughout the entire operation.
6 The rapid and great advances that have been made in the care of the new-born baby, especially of the premature baby, have meant that Caesarean section can be performed when it is urgently required to deliver premature babies.

Maternal indications for Caesarean section

It would be easy to write a long list of the instances when Caesarean section should be performed in the best interests of the mother. Such a list, however, would really be meaningless because each pregnancy is treated on its own merits and each decision to perform Caesarean section is made after careful consideration of all the factors concerned. No hard and fast rules can be laid down. As the safety of the operation improves, both the frequency of the operation and the indications for its performance continue to increase.

Perhaps the most compelling and dramatic maternal indication for Caesarean section is placenta praevia. In this condition the placenta is situated below the presenting part of the baby and the gradual process of labour inevitably results in more and more bleeding from the mother's uterus. There are, however, some degrees of placenta praevia which are better and more safely treated by vaginal delivery.

Some other maternal indications for Caesarean section may be preeclampsia, eclampsia, Caesarean section performed in a previous pregnancy for disproportion, pelvic tumours such as fibroids or ovarian cysts lying below the presenting part of the baby, previous operations upon the uterus for removal of fibroids, previous damage or injury to the uterus at either curettage or abortion. A previous history of still-birth or difficult delivery or any other obstetric catastrophe may be sufficient indication to perform Caesarean section.

Fetal indications for Caesarean section

Caesarean section may be performed if it is considered to be in the best interests of the baby, either because the baby would suffer from lack of oxygen and asphyxia if not delivered immediately, or if it is considered that vaginal delivery might injure the baby. The classic fetal indication for performing Caesarean section is fetal distress during the first stage of labour, when it is feared that the baby may either become severely short of oxygen or even die from lack of oxygen if labour is allowed to proceed to vaginal delivery. Some other fetal indications are disproportion, accidental antepartum haemorrhage (in which there has been some bleeding behind the placenta but not yet of sufficient severity to kill the baby), shoulder presentation (where the baby is lying transversely in the uterus and delivery would mean a complicated internal manoeuvre) and some instances of breech presentation. Caesarean section is certainly in the best interests of the baby if the alternative procedure is a complicated or difficult vaginal delivery.

Repeat Caesarean section

The old saying 'Once a Caesarean section always a Caesarean section' is not true today. When Caesarean section was performed in the so-called classical manner by making a vertical incision in the upper part of the uterus, then repeat Caesarean section usually had to be performed, but with the modern lower segment type of operation, delivery in a subsequent pregnancy can be normal if everything else is normal. There are several basic reasons, however, why Caesarean section should be repeated in the next and every subsequent pregnancy. if the operation was performed because of a mechanical problem caused either by the baby being too big or by the pelvis being too small, the same conditions will apply to future pregnancies; if the first Caesarean section is necessary because of previous operations on the uterus, diabetes or other constant conditions of the mother, then obviously it will be necessary in subsequent pregnancies. There are two other main reasons why Caesarean section should be repeated, although in each instance the final decision rests with the doctor. If a woman is over 30 or if the cervix failed to dilate satisfactorily during a previous attempted labour, many obstetricians consider that a repeated Caesarean section is a wise precaution. If there is any possibility that the scar of the previous operation has failed to heal satisfactorily a repeat Caesarean section is advisable. Any evidence of infection in the uterus following a Caesarean section may indicate that the uterine scar has not healed as well as might be hoped.

Many women are worried about the limitation that Caesarean section may place upon their family and they believe that once a Caesarean section has been performed their family must be limited to two. This is not true. A woman can have as many as six or eight Caesarean sections and instances have been recorded in which ten and even more have been performed. Most obstetricians consider that three Caesarean sections on any one person is a reasonable number and they will actively discourage women from having more than four children by Caesarean section.

Pregnancy after Caesarean section

The majority of obstetricians advise that a time interval of approximately one year should elapse after a Caesarean section has been performed before the woman again becomes pregnant. It should be quickly added, however, that if pregnancy occurs within 3 months of a Caesarean section this does not by itself constitute a medical reason for its termination. The uterus heals with remarkable speed and a Caesarean section scar is completely healed 3 months after operation. Nevertheless, a woman requires time to readjust after pregnancy and delivery, and this is naturally slightly prolonged after a major operation such as Caesarean section. Caesarean section has no effect on fertility and a woman will become pregnant just as easily following the operation as she did before it was performed.

Vaginal delivery of a pregnancy subsequent to a Caesarean section must always be performed in hospital. If a woman has had a previous Caesarean section she should report to her doctor and to the hospital antenatal clinic as soon as she is certain that she is pregnant. When she visits the antenatal clinic she will be treated in exactly the same way as everyone else, except that special interest will be taken in the previous operation and the reasons why it was performed, as well as in her subsequent health and progress. The method of delivery will be discussed and if repeat Caesarean section is to be performed the reasons will be explained. If vaginal delivery is planned, the doctors will always reserve the right to perform Caesarean section at any stage should the need arise. A definite decision about the method of delivery cannot be made so early in pregnancy.

As pregnancy advances a careful watch will be kept for any evidence of a recurrence of the indications for the previous operation. After the 32nd week particular attention will be paid to the scar in the uterus from the previous operation. This is situated transversely across the lower abdomen just above the level of the symphysis pubis. A vertical or a transverse incision may be present in the skin, but the doctor and midwife are not concerned with this but with the site of the uterine incision. As the uterus grows the uterine incision will stretch and may cause some discomfort. Pain or tenderness in the uterine scar may indicate that excessive stretching is taking place and although the scar normally causes a certain amount of discomfort and tenderness it is for the midwife and the obstetrician to decide whether this amount of discomfort is normal or not. As during any pregnancy, any bleeding that occurs should be immediately reported. Any undue lower abdominal pain or discomfort should also be reported.

Labour after Caesarean section

If it has been decided to allow a vaginal delivery it is unlikely that pregnancy will be permitted to go beyond term and it is possible that labour may be induced before the expected date arrives. The exact time and method of induction will depend entirely upon the obstetrician, the woman's past history and the reasons for performing the previous operation, bearing in mind that no two women are identical and each is treated as a separate individual with completely separate and unrelated problems. Once labour is established it will proceed perfectly normally. Particular attention will be paid by the midwife and doctor to any vaginal bleeding or show, to the condition of the uterine scar, to the exact type of uterine contractions and whether the uterus relaxes completely in between contractions. The labour, apart from these frequent and careful observations, will be the same as any other labour until the cervix is fully dilated.

It is usually considered advisable to allow a mother only a very short time in the second stage of labour because this stage imposes a particularly severe strain on the previous Caesarean section scar. If the second stage is easy and straightforward and the head descends without any difficulty, a normal delivery may be expected, although an episiotomy will almost certainly be performed. If there is any delay or difficulty in the second stage, so that the woman is not delivered after about 20 minutes, then forceps or ventouse delivery will be conducted under general or local anaesthesia. After a vaginal delivery the third stage of labour and the puerperium will be completely normal.

Subsequent deliveries, even having achieved one vaginal delivery following Caesarean section, must be conducted in hospital. The same care and meticulous attention to detail are always bestowed even on a fifth or sixth baby following the original Caesarean section. The obstetrician always reserves the right to perform a repeat Caesarean section should he consider it necessary. If any mechanical problem develops, or should the cervix fail to dilate satisfactorily, or the baby's head get itself into the wrong position, then Caesarean section may be repeated.

Rupture of a previous Caesarean section scar

Rupture of a previous classical (vertical) Caesarean section scar is stated to have occurred after approximately 4 per cent of operations. This is a remarkably fine achievement when one considers that most classical Caesarean sections were performed under conditions vastly different from those which exist today.

Rupture of a lower segment Caesarean section scar is stated to occur in 0.5 per cent of operations (1 in every 200). Even so, these figures are approximately 20 years old-and surgical technique and the management of the operation have advanced greatly since then. The present day figure is more likely to be 0.1 per cent (1 in every 1,000) and the majority of obstetricians and midwives have never seen a lower uterine segment Caesarean scar rupture. Rupture usually results when labour begins in a woman in whom Caesarean section was previously performed because of disproportion between the baby's head and the bones of the pelvis. The disproportion naturally recurs so that an undue strain is eventually placed upon the previous scar, resulting first in overstretching, and then in rupture.

Much care is devoted during pregnancy and in labour to the condition of the uterine scar. If undue stretching or thinning of the scar is detected, repeat Caesarean section will be recommended long before rupture occurs.

Technique of Caesarean section

Caesarean section is a comparatively simple operation. The woman's abdomen is shaved and, providing it is not an emergency operation, she should have nothing to eat or drink for 6 hours before it is due to begin. Premedication consists of an injection to reduce secretions from the throat and lungs as well as an antacid or similar drug given orally. Sedatives that might cross the placenta and affect the baby are not usually given. A woman having a Caesarean section is thus fully conscious and aware of everything that is going on when she is taken to the operating theatre. A special pre-heated incubator is in the operating theatre, a special anaesthetic is prepared, oxygen and the resuscitation equipment for the baby are available. Besides the normal theatre staff, a midwife is present to take care of the immediate requirements of the new-born baby, as well as a paediatrician. Blood will have been taken to confirm the mother's blood group and also to cross-match blood should a transfusion be required. In many hospitals nowadays the obstetrician may agree to a woman's request to stay awake during the operation. Here epidural anaesthesia numbs the lower half of the body so no sensation is felt. The mother cannot see the operation but will be able to hear the baby's first cry, see him immediately after delivery and even hold him before he is wrapped up.

The operation is not begun until the patient has been completely anaesthetized. The incision made in the skin of the abdominal wall may be vertical (up and down in the mid-line below the umbilicus) or it may be transverse (known as a Pfannenstiel incision) extending from side to side across the lower abdomen so that, when the pubic hair regrows, the scar will be almost completely covered and virtually invisible. The muscles of the lower abdominal wall are gently separated and the abdominal cavity opened. The uterus and abdominal organs are inspected to make sure that everything is satisfactory. The bladder is then dissected free from the lower part of the anterior surface of the uterus. A transverse incision is made in the lower uterine segment extending across the uterus from right to left to divide completely the muscular wall of the uterus. The membranes are thus exposed and incised. The baby's head is delivered and immediately his mouth, nose and eyes are wiped clean with a sterile swab and the mouth and nose sucked out to remove any fluid or mucus that happens to have collected there. Delivery of the baby is then completed by gently lifting him out of the uterus and he is immediately held upside down while his mouth and throat are again aspirated. The baby will breathe or cry almost immediately. The umbilical cord is clamped in two places and divided between the clamps. The baby is handed to the midwife for further resuscitation, if necessary, and examination by the paediatrician. As soon as the baby is delivered an injection of either ergometrine or syntometrine is given to the mother by the anaesthetist and as soon as the uterus contracts (about 40 seconds after the injection) the placenta is delivered through the uterine incision.

The incision in the firmly contracted uterus is now repaired with catgut using either two or three layers of stitches. The bladder is then stitched back over the lower uterine segment, so that the incision in the uterus is completely covered. Both Fallopian tubes and both ovaries are inspected. If everything is normal the anterior abdominal wall is sutured with catgut in four distinct layers, using different stitches for each separate layer. The incision in the skin is then closed either with individual stitches or with skin clips.

From beginning to end the operation takes between 45 minutes to one hour. The first part of the operation, that is up to delivery of the baby, usually takes about 10 minutes and the remainder of the time is spent in carefully suturing the incisions that have been made. If urgency demands it can be done in half this time.

When a Caesarean section is repeated it is performed in almost exactly the same way. The same scar is used as on previous occasions, so that any woman who has had two, three or even four Caesarean sections has only one scar. The same scar in the uterus is used as at the previous operation so that the uterine wall is not weakened by several different incisions.

Convalescence

On waking up following Caesarean section there will naturally be pain in the operation scar. An injection of morphine or pethidine (or similar analgesic) is given to the mother to relieve this discomfort and after another sleep she will wake up feeling much better. Within a few hours of operation she will be encouraged to start drinking and to sit up. She will at first find that movements cause discomfort in the abdominal scar, but will nevertheless be encouraged to move her legs and feet as much as possible, as movement is essential for the circulation. She will also be encouraged to cough up any phlegm or sputum from her throat or chest.

The days of abdominal binders and huge dressings have long since gone, and the incision will be covered with only a small piece of gauze strapping, or there may be no dressing at all because it will have been sprayed with a special transparent, plastic skin-like dressing. The carefully inserted stitches are sufficiently strong not to need supporting by a binder or by large dressings. If the operation has been performed in the morning the mother will probably be encouraged to get out of bed in the afternoon or evening to pass urine. This is generally easier than using a bed pan. On the day after operation she will be encouraged to get up to wash her hands and face and to clean her teeth, but the midwife will give her a blanket bath in bed. She will now be drinking a normal amount and will be having a light diet, and on the second day after operation she should be taking a full diet, sitting up, getting out of bed for the toilet and bathroom, as well as holding and starting to breast-feed her baby.

Wind pains may cause discomfort on the second or third day after operation. These are completely normal and will disappear quite quickly, or as soon as wind is passed from the rectum or when the bowels are open. A mild purgative is taken on the second evening after operation and on the third morning either a suppository or an enema is given.

The stitches or clips are removed from the abdominal skin on the fifth, sixth or seventh day according to the preference of the surgeon, and thereafter the woman is allowed in the bath or shower once or even twice a day. She will be allowed out of hospital on the eighth or tenth day after operation.

Vacuum extraction

Vacuum extraction, or the ventouse, is a method of delivery frequently used as an alternative to delivery by forceps. Its principle is very simple

When the cervix is fully dilated and the baby is ready to be delivered, a small metal cup is passed gently into the vagina and placed against the baby's head. The cup is connected to a special vacuum apparatus and a vacuum is created within the metal cup which makes it adhere to the baby's scalp. Gentle traction is then exerted upon the cup which in turn causes the baby's head to descend in the pelvis and to be gradually delivered.

The ventouse has become very popular in Scandinavian countries and is being used more frequently in Great Britain where it can take the place of a simple forceps delivery, especially in association with epidural anaesthesia. The indications for using vacuum extraction are when there is delay in the second stage of labour and where an easy delivery is anticipated. Occasionally the ventouse may be used before the end of the first stage of labour in order to help dilatation of the cervix if labour is becoming unduly prolonged.

There are no real complications to the use of the ventouse. When the vacuum is applied to the metal cup to make it adherent to the baby's scalp, the tissues of the scalp are sucked into the cup so that when the baby is delivered he has a swelling on his head which is the exact size of the cup that has been applied. The swelling is filled with tissue fluid and disappears within a few hours of delivery.

Postpartum haemorrhage

Postpartum haemorrhage is the technical term for bleeding after delivery of the baby. Almost every woman is afraid of haemorrhage. One of the first things that young doctors and midwives are taught is to control bleeding from the uterus after delivery of the baby. This used to be quite a difficult procedure, but now it is extremely simple. The uterus obeys a very simple rule. If it is completely empty it will contract and when it has contracted it will neither bleed nor, under normal circumstances, will it become infected. In certain instances, however, the uterus fails to contract properly and therefore postpartum haemorrhage occurs. Postpartum haemorrhage should not now cause any fear because drugs are readily available that will make the uterus contract and satisfactorily control even the most profuse bleeding.

Causes of postpartum haemorrhage

The relaxed uterus. Occasionally, even after a normal delivery, the uterus does not contract satisfactorily and bleeding continues unless or until the uterus is made to contract into a hard ball. It will contract if it is gently massaged or if an injection of ergometrine or syntometrine (Syntocinon with ergometrine) is given either into a muscle or into a vein. As soon as the uterus contracts it will stop bleeding. The uterus fails to contract because it is tired, usually as a result of a prolonged labour or because of overdistension by twins or polyhydramnios, or as a result of anaesthetic drugs or sedative drugs given during labour.

The modern practice is to give an injection of either ergometrine, Syntocinon or syntometrine as soon as the baby's head is crowned or as soon as the shoulders are delivered, so that the uterus contracts satisfactorily very soon after the baby has been delivered. There is then no danger that the uterus will fail to contract properly or that undue bleeding will occur. Even if an injection has not been given while the baby is being delivered, a lazy uterus can easily be made to contract satisfactorily within 30 to 40 seconds of an injection of ergometrine or syntometrine into a vein.

Retained placenta. Occasionally the placenta may not be delivered normally during the third stage. If the uterus is not empty there is always a possibility that haemorrhage may occur. In this instance an injection of ergometrine or syntometrine is given to ensure that the uterus contracts satisfactorily, first in an attempt to expel the placenta and secondly to prevent any haemorrhage. If the placenta still remains within the uterus it is removed by a simple operation known as 'manual removal of the placenta'. The newly delivered woman is anaesthetized and the placenta is very gently stripped away from its attachment to the inner surface of the uterus.

Fibroids or any similar tumours in the uterus will not usually prevent the uterus from contracting satisfactorily after delivery. Occasionally a very large fibroid may make haemorrhage likely because it hinders uterine contraction. Instances of such large fibroids are extremely rare but when they are present any bleeding can be stopped by giving repeated injections of ergometrine or Syntocinon.

Injuries to the cervix. On rare occasions, if labour has been particularly rapid and forceful, or if the baby is unduly big, a tear or laceration may damage the cervix. Small lacerations frequently happen but these are of no significance. A large laceration in the very vascular cervix, however, can cause quite severe haemorrhage. Bleeding from a small laceration of the cervix stops within a few minutes after delivery. If a large laceration is present then one or two small catgut stitches may be inserted into the cervix to repair the injury and stop the bleeding.

Lacerations of the perineum and episiotomy. A small amount of bleeding may come from lacerations of the perineum or from the site where an episiotomy has been performed. The bleeding from these injuries is usually quite small but occasionally it may be increased because of the presence of varicose veins or other large vessels in the perineum. Treatment is quite easy. Simple pressure will stop any bleeding until the injuries can be satisfactorily repaired by suturing.

27 Breech Delivery

Breech presentation

A description of breech presentation together with the details of external cephalic version is given in Chapter 23. There are so many different reasons for breech presentation that it is impossible to generalize as to whether delivery should be vaginal or by a lower segment Caesarean section. Breech presentation may occur in the presence of a low lying placenta or uterine fibroids or congenital uterine abnormalities. It is particularly common in premature infants and in the second of twins. Any attempt to give a comprehensive review of breech delivery, or even of the part that breech presentation plays in the whole of midwifery, would be doomed to failure.

A baby is perfectly free to move in the uterus and it undoubtedly turns over and over on many occasions until about the end of the 28th or 29th week of pregnancy when it becomes stable in the breech presentation with the head in the fundus of the uterus. Between the 30th and 34th weeks of pregnancy the baby usually turns round to present by the head, but about 3 to 4 per cent fail to do so and remain as breech presentations. When a breech persists, an external cephalic version may be performed. Nevertheless a certain number of babies arrive at term or labour with the breech presenting.

In normal circumstances where the baby is a normal size and the mother's pelvis is adequate, a breech labour is no more difficult or longer than any other labour, and there are no increased difficulties after the delivery. The real problem in breech presentation is not the breech delivery of the small baby through a normal pelvis, but a mechanical problem concerning the delivery of a large baby, or of a normal baby with an extended head, or when the mother's pelvis is small. Any factor that slows the delivery may lead to lack of oxygen. Any factor that forces the delivery to be hurried may cause injury to the baby.

The head is the largest part of the baby. When the head presents it is the first part of the baby to descend through the cervix and also through the pelvic cavity. The head will mould and flex, thus reducing its diameter by more than 1 cm, and its passage through both the cervix and the pelvic cavity, which takes several hours, is accomplished in slow, gradual and very easy stages. In a breech presentation the head does not have time to mould and flexion is always incomplete resulting in the presentation of much larger head diameters. Furthermore, the baby's pelvis is smaller than the head so that the largest part of the baby has to be delivered at the end of the labour. The head has to travel the entire distance from above the brim of the pelvis to the outside world in approximately 7 minutes or less because as soon as the head enters the pelvic brim the umbilical cord is squeezed between the bones of the head and the pelvis and the baby's oxygen supply is cut off. If delivery is too slow, taking more than 7 minutes, then the baby will suffer from lack of oxygen.

It is a very simple mechanical problem. If the baby's head is normal in size and the mother's pelvis is normal in size, the baby's head may travel through the pelvis quite easily and naturally without any trouble. If, however, the baby's head happens to be slightly larger than normal, or is not well flexed, or if the mother's pelvis happens to be a little smaller than usual, it will take too long for the head to be delivered in its own time and, on the other hand, if the baby's head is delivered too quickly it may be injured.

The answer to the problem of breech delivery is that every instance, every woman and her baby, are judged on their own merits. Various precautions are taken to ascertain whether mechanical difficulties are likely to arise during a vaginal delivery and if the obstetrician is satisfied that there will be none, the breech delivery is allowed to proceed normally. When a woman has already had a good-sized baby it is known that she has a 'favourable pelvis' and therefore the risk from breech delivery is minimal. On the other hand there are many obstetricians who believe that a Caesarean section is the most convenient and safest method of delivery, and this should be accepted philosophically without any feeling of having been 'robbed of the delights of childbirth'.

Breech labour

Labour begins in breech presentation exactly as it does in a cephalic presentation. However, should the membranes rupture spontaneously before the onset of labour the woman is immediately admitted to hospital without waiting for uterine contractions to begin.

Labour proceeds normally and the first stage of labour lasts the usual length of time. At the onset of the second stage the woman is placed in the lithotomy position. During the second stage the breech descends slowly through the pelvis. The mother is usually told *not* to push, letting the breech descend under the power of uterine contractions alone. Spontaneous descent indicates that the remainder of the delivery will be smooth, straightforward and satisfactory. If the breech does not descend spontaneously through the pelvis it may be decided, even at this very late stage, to perform Caesarean section.

The passage of meconium by the baby in a breech labour may not be a sign of fetal distress, as it usually is in cephalic presentation. The baby's anus and lower bowel are being squeezed continuously throughout labour so that the meconium is forced out automatically.

When the baby's buttocks distend the perineum an episiotomy is performed. Uterine contractions will then proceed to deliver the baby's buttocks, legs and abdomen as far as the umbilicus when the doctor gently pulls down a short loop of umbilical cord to prevent tension on it during delivery when its upper part will be trapped between the baby's head and the mother's pelvis. The baby's arms and shoulders are then delivered. The modern method of completing the delivery is by forceps so that the baby's head can be delivered steadily and gently without any hurry and without any possibility of damage or injury. A local anaesthetic is usually given before this is done.

After the baby's head has been delivered, the cord is divided in the usual way and the third stage of labour is conducted quite normally.

Breech extraction

Breech extraction is the delivery of a breech baby by applying traction and pulling on the lower limbs. This is not now performed except in very special circumstances and usually only when a second twin happens to present in a difficult manner.

28 The Puerperium

For 9 months the body has been gradually adapting itself to the very complex condition of pregnancy. There have been extensive physical changes, not only in the uterus, the vagina and the breasts, but also throughout the whole body (see Chapter 6) and these culminated finally in labour and delivery. Extensive and very far reaching emotional changes have also been occurring. The safe arrival of the baby may have brought massive relief to the tensions and fears with which his arrival had been anticipated, but the mother must still undergo a slow and gradual psychological change which takes several months to complete. This is entirely normal and accompanies the physical changes that occur during pregnancy and which must now be reversed in order to return the body to normal. While the majority of the physical changes are rapid and dramatic, it is nevertheless several months before the body returns to its normal non-pregnant state. This is particularly applicable during breast-feeding.

The puerperium is defined as being the first 4 weeks after the delivery of a baby, but for the purposes of this narrative we are only really interested in the first few days after delivery, during which most of the dramatic changes occur. After the end of the first week return to normality is very slow and completely automatic providing certain very basic rules, which are detailed later, are obeyed.

Physical changes

The uterus and vagina

Immediately following delivery it will be noted with some astonishment that the abdomen has become completely flat. It may seem quite extraordinary that an enormous pregnant lump has disappeared in only a few minutes, but careful examination of the abdomen will reveal that there is, in fact, a small swelling just below the umbilicus. This is the uterus, which has now contracted down following the expulsion of the baby and the placenta. It will be firm and hard, partly because this is the normal response of the uterus after delivery and partly because an injection has been given to make it contract. Contraction of the uterus is essential, because without it excessive bleeding occurs from the place at which the placenta was attached.

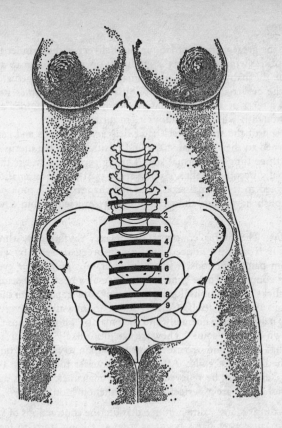

Fig. 34   The height of the uterus in the puerperium (in days)

If a hand is gently run over the abdomen it is possible to feel the firm, hard, round, smooth swelling of the uterus, which may feel slightly tender. This is completely normal and indeed the uterine contractions may continue to be so powerful that some uterine cramps may be felt rather like period pains. This discomfort is perfectly normal.

The return of the uterus to its normal state is known as involution. The total involution of the uterus takes approximately 2 months, although the vast majority of the changes occur within the first 2 weeks. Immediately after delivery the top of the uterus reaches almost to the umbilicus. As each day passes the top of the uterus will get lower and lower, until after about 7 days it will no longer be possible to feel it in the abdomen. Another interesting fact is that when the bladder is full it will push the uterus upwards and to one side, usually the right, and the uterus will resume its normal position in the mid-line after the bladder has been emptied.

One of the great marvels of labour and delivery is the manner in which the neck of the womb or cervix is gradually opened in order to allow the passage of the baby without any damage occurring. Immediately after delivery the cervix is open and patulous. It rapidly resumes its former shape and after 2 or 3 days will have re-formed and refashioned a cervical canal, although it will still be about 1 cm dilated.

At the end of the second week after delivery the uterus and cervix will have returned to their normal shape and position, but the uterus will still be about three times its normal size. During the next 4 weeks the uterus will gradually become smaller, so that at the post-natal examination it will have returned to its normal size. Thus the changes which took 9 months to accomplish have been almost completely reversed within 6 weeks of delivery.

After-pains. The uterus contracts and relaxes rhythmically throughout life. This is frequently noticed in the non-pregnant state by girls who suffer from painful periods, when uterine cramps may occur every time the uterus contracts. These contractions have also been appreciated as the Braxton Hicks' contractions during pregnancy, quite apart from the uterine contractions of labour itself. Contractions continue after delivery so that the uterus may involute normally and they may occasionally cause discomfort, known as 'after-pains'. They are far more likely to affect a woman who has had her second or subsequent baby than to affect a woman who has just had her first child. After-pains may last for as long as several days and can usually be relieved by simple analgesics, such as aspirin or paracetamol. They are a perfectly normal phenomenon.

Breast-feeding. Many women notice that uterine contractions of sufficient severity to cause after-pains begin as soon as a baby starts to feed at the breast. This is perfectly normal since stimulation of the breasts provokes contractions of the uterus. Breast-feeding a baby, therefore, will not only make the uterus contract but will help in the normal process of involution of the uterus.

The lochia

The lochia is the vaginal discharge after delivery. Immediately following delivery the lochia is bright red and the amount is noted by the nurse. The quantity of bleeding for the first few hours after delivery will be about as much as a normal period, or even slightly more. Occasionally a few small blood clots are passed. The lochia remains red for the first two or three days and then gradually changes to a reddish brown, and by the fourth or fifth day the lochia will be brown. The colour and the amount of lochia are noted and recorded by the midwife. The lochia continues to be brownish, or pinkish brown, for several days but when the mother gets up and starts to be more active, doing her household duties or the shopping, the colour changes and may for a few hours again become red. This is quite normal, and the colour will change back to pink or brown within a few hours, or at most within a few days. The lochia continues as a yellowish brown or pinkish loss with occasional interludes of bright red until it ceases altogether. There is no standard duration of bleeding following delivery. In some women the lochia dries up altogether after about 14 days, whereas in others it may continue for as long as 6 weeks. The average is about 21 days. Frequently, and especially if the baby is not breast-fed, the lochia finishes after the first period which may come approximately 4 weeks after delivery, when the loss suddenly becomes heavier and brighter for several days.

The amount and the colour of the lochia indicate the degree of involution of the uterus. The more rapidly the uterus involutes the more rapidly will the lochia become brown and cease altogether. Breast-feeding helps the uterus to involute more rapidly and the lochia will therefore dry up more quickly in a woman who is breast-feeding than in a woman who is artificially feeding her baby.

Not only will the midwife make a note of the amount and colour of the lochia, but she will also note any offensive smell that may be associated with it. This may be of no significance but may indicate that there is some mild form of infection in the uterus.

The breasts

The changes in the breasts during pregnancy are discussed in Chapter 6 and the care of the breasts in Chapter 15. Any woman wishing to breast-feed her baby should be adequately prepared by the time her baby arrives.

There will be no sudden or dramatic change in the breasts or in their condition immediately after delivery. A woman who has been wearing breast shells during her pregnancy should continue to wear them after delivery. The breasts and nipples show very little change during the first 24 hours after delivery, and although the baby may be suckled at the breast for a short time he is unlikely to get anything except a few drops of colostrum, which is the yellow fluid secreted by the breasts before the actual milk is formed.

During the second day after delivery the breasts may begin to 'fill'. They become firmer and heavier and it is at this stage that satisfactory support with a good brassiere is essential. On the third day the milk will usually 'come in'. This means that the breasts start to produce milk in reasonable amounts. They may become quite firm and even tender and certainly increase considerably in size. The routine varies in different hospitals but the baby is usually put to the breast twice on the first day and three times on the second day. He is put to the breast every 4 hours on the third day and as he sucks off the milk so the breasts soften and become less tender, only to refill and again become firm in readiness for the next feed.

The law of supply and demand applies to breast-milk as it does to most other things in the world and the breasts soon become accustomed to producing and supplying the amount of milk that the baby requires. In other words, the more he sucks and removes, the more are the breasts stimulated to produce more milk. On the fourth or fifth day the discomfort disappears from the breasts and they become slightly smaller and quite soft immediately after feeding, only becoming firm again in time for the next feed. This recurrent change in the condition of the breasts continues throughout breast-feeding.

Circulation

One of the less obvious changes that takes place after delivery is in the circulation. The normal circulating blood volume is about 5 litres and during pregnancy this increases by about 30 per cent in order to supply the demands of the uterus and of the growing baby. Since this demand ceases on delivery, the circulating volume returns to normal over the next 2 or 3 days and is accompanied by passing quite large quantities of urine.

Weight

At the time of delivery and during the first 2 or 3 days immediately afterwards a woman automatically loses a certain amount of weight. The amount is usually about 6.4 kg, consisting of: baby—3.2 kg, placenta—.68 kg, liquor—1.1 kg, and extra circulating blood volume—1.4 kg. If she does not breast-feed her baby a woman loses a further .91 kg as the breasts gradually return to their normal size. One further kilogram is lost as the uterus gradually involutes during the first 2 weeks following delivery. Thus a woman who is not breast-feeding loses approximately 7.5 kg automatically after delivery.

If a woman has gained weight in excess of this amount during her pregnancy this is either fluid (which is also lost during the first few days after delivery), or it is fat, in which case it is there to stay until she goes onto a rigid diet. In other words, if a woman has gained only 8 or 9 kg during her pregnancy then she will, after her delivery, return to her pre-pregnant weight and rapidly regain her figure.

Emotional reaction

A mother's reactions following delivery are extremely complex. They vary from individual to individual and it is impossible to predict a pattern for any one person. Reactions after delivery depend upon basic psychological make-up, together with the fears and anxieties that have been present during pregnancy and the manner in which these have been answered by the doctors and midwives. They are also affected by labour and by the presence or absence of a husband both during labour and at the time of delivery. There are, however, several basic emotional reactions common to almost every woman who is safely delivered of a normal baby. Although these reactions may vary with the second, third or subsequent baby they nevertheless remain basically the same.

A woman's first reaction on hearing that her baby is safely delivered, and especially on hearing him cry, is usually one of extreme relief that he has arrived safely and that he is normal. This emotion of relief is associated with an immense release of tension, and while it sounds very simple when written on paper it is the most profound and one of the most deeply moving emotions that a woman ever experiences. This lasts for only a very short time and is superseded by one of thanks and appreciation. Thoughts of gratitude that pass through the mind immediately after the sense of relief are also very profound and very real. They may encompass an immense scope ranging from gratitude to God, to people who have helped and who are held dear, to whoever has been responsible for the delivery, to a husband or partner (more especially if he has been present during the delivery), to an immense gratitude to the new baby for having arrived safely. The depth of this sensation also passes very quickly.

When a mother first holds her baby she is usually filled with a sensation of wonder and disbelief that she has been able to grow this baby within her body and that he is now being held in her arms, alive and healthy, while a few moments previously he was still inside her uterus. This wonder verges on disbelief and is tinged with a certain amount of awe and reverence that nature should be able to accomplish such a feat. If it is her first baby she may also be rather apprehensive and perhaps a little shy and embarrassed because she does not know how to hold him properly. If it is her second or subsequent baby she will compare him with her previous children, but will still marvel at the wonderful manner in which this new child has been created and delivered. She will probably search for some resemblance to her husband or partner or herself and even if there is none she will imagine it. As a mother holds her new baby in her arms she also experiences a sensation of emotional and physical fulfilment that here at last is what she has been waiting to see and she is also emotionally fulfilled by producing a child for the man she loves.

All these emotions, feelings and sensations which pass through her mind, or which she experiences during the first few minutes after her delivery, gradually subside and are replaced by much more gentle emotions of thankfulness and peace.

Not all mothers react in this way; some feel detached from or even dislike the new baby, especially if they have been given a lot of drugs or an anaesthetic. These apparently inappropriate emotions are quite normal and need not give rise to anxiety or depression because they are only temporary

During the next day or two when she is becoming acquainted with her new baby, especially if it is her first baby, a mother may well feel inadequate and incompetent at handling and looking after her new charge. This is a perfectly normal experience and she should be comforted with the knowledge that even the most experienced midwife or doctor goes through the same sensation of inadequacy when presented with her own first child. As mothers they are no more capable than anyone else. All a new mother needs is a little time and practice and then she is able to handle and look after her baby just as well as anyone else has looked after theirs.

You will, of course, feel anxiety at various times. Anxiety first of all as to whether your baby is normal, whether he has the right number of fingers and toes and whether he looks reasonably presentable. Later you may become anxious about any small aspect of either your child's behaviour or your own progress that may cause you the slightest concern. Usually such anxieties are without any real foundation and can be easily relieved by asking your midwife or doctor. It is surprising how often a new mother becomes anxious about a particular problem which, deep down inside, she knows to be completely irrelevant but because she fails to ask she is never reassured and her anxiety continues. If a mother has a worry she must ask about it; if it has a basis it will be dealt with and if it has no basis she will be reassured. Either way, she can only benefit by asking.

Puerperal blues

It is said that every new mother should experience 'the blues'. This is a period of fairly acute depression which starts for no apparent reason and disappears for no reason. It usually lasts for 12 to 24 hours generally between the third and the sixth day after delivery. She may feel rather miserable and will certainly burst into tears at the slightest provocation, or even without provocation. Most midwives and doctors consider that an attack of 'the blues' is almost essential to relieve tension after delivery. If a woman does not experience this so acutely she will almost certainly have a good cry for no apparent reason.

Care of the mother

Cleanliness

Cleanliness is of the utmost importance, especially as it helps to prevent infection in the mother and her baby. Soon after delivery the mother is gently washed or sponged down, her bedclothes are changed, and she puts on a clean nightdress. She will have been given a sterile maternity sanitary towel. This attitude towards cleanliness should permeate the whole of the puerperium. The midwife adopts similar principles in the care of the baby. She makes sure that the clothes in which he is first wrapped are clean and that his cot is clean and tidy.

Apart from general cleanliness there are three particular ways of observing cleanliness in order to prevent infection. Firstly in handling the baby; everyone should wash their hands before doing anything to him such as picking him up, changing his nappy or giving him a feed. Always ensure that his clothes are clean and, if he is being artificially fed, that his bottles, teats and milk have been properly sterilized. Secondly, in breast-feeding, the breasts should always be carefully washed and dried before and after feeding so that the nipples are absolutely clean prior to a feed. Thirdly, the vulva; keeping the vulval area clean prevents vaginal and uterine infection and the routine adopted varies from hospital to hospital and from midwife to midwife. Generally speaking only sterilized or surgically clean maternity pads should be used. In some maternity units the vulval area is washed with an antiseptic solution three times each day, as well as after micturition or defaecation, for the first 3 or 4 days after delivery. In others, antiseptic washing is restricted to twice on the first day, and thereafter only when a large number of stitches have been necessary. Other units use bidets. The sanitary pad may be held in place with a sanitary belt or with a bandage tied round the waist, but probably the most satisfactory and efficient method is to wear disposable paper pants.

Temperature, pulse and respiration

After delivery, either before or immediately after the mother has been washed and tidied, her temperature is taken and her pulse rate and blood pressure recorded. Thereafter if everything proceeds satisfactorily the temperature and pulse rate are recorded daily for the first 10 days, or for as long as she remains in hospital. Slight movements in the temperature or pulse rate may occur frequently but these are not generally of any significance. A mother who is breast-feeding may have engorged breasts on the third or fourth day after delivery, causing the temperature to rise to 99° or 99.5°F (38°C) and the pulse to about 100.

Observations on the lochia

Observations on the lochia are recorded daily by the midwife, including the colour and the amount, as well as any offensive smell. She may also measure and record the height of the uterine fundus each day to ensure that involution is normal. This is done after the bladder has been emptied, because a full bladder pushes the uterus upwards and to one side. Many doctors and midwives no longer consider that the height of the uterine fundus is significant, because it is affected not only by a full bladder but also by the presence of faeces in the bowel, and the fact that not everyone's uterus involutes at exactly the same rate. More important than the actual height of the uterus is pain or tenderness. Immediately after delivery the uterus may be quite tender and painful because of the strong contractions which follow the administration of the oxytocic drugs. During the next day or so there may be slight tenderness on one side at the site of the attachment of the placenta. Apart from this, however, tenderness should gradually diminish with each succeeding day and if it increases or pain begins, it should be reported to the midwife or doctor.

Bathing

There is a great deal of prejudice and tradition involved in the care of a woman during her pregnancy and shortly after delivery; bathing after delivery is one of the major areas of disagreement. It used to be believed that bath water entered the vagina and thereby gained access to the uterine cavity, so causing infection within the uterus itself. This is now known to be untrue, and there is no reason why a woman should not bath as soon after delivery as she can comfortably do so; similarly she may have a shower as soon as she wishes. The fact that she is bleeding is no reason for avoiding a bath, although for the first day or two it should not be too hot. The skin is very active during the puerperium and a daily bath or shower is necessary; twice daily is even better if the facilities are available.

Lactation

Lactation begins early in the puerperium. For the last few weeks of pregnancy and immediately after delivery the breasts contain a thick, milk-like substance called colostrum; during the third and fourth days the amount of milk will steadily increase until lactation is established. The baby is usually put to the breasts twice on the first day and three times on the second day and thereafter every 4 hours, except during the night, and spends longer at the breast on each succeeding day as more milk becomes available.

Before each feed the nipples should be cleaned. It is important to get into a comfortable position for feeding and it is equally important that the baby is held comfortably and feels secure. The midwife will guide and help with the feeding regime and is a valuable source of information concerning breast-feeding. On the second or third day after confinement the breasts feel rather tender, heavy and uncomfortable, but this disappears as the baby gets hungry and takes more milk from the breast. Breast-feeding is the best and the most natural way to feed a baby; while he is being fed he also receives comfort and assurance.

The bladder

Most women will have either emptied their bladder during labour or will have been catheterized so that immediately after delivery the bladder is empty. It is the modern practice to allow women who feel quite fit and well up to the lavatory or the commode as soon as they wish after delivery and to encourage them to pass urine within an hour of delivery, although they may not wish to do so for 5 or 6 hours. It is much easier to pass urine on the lavatory than when perched precariously on a bed pan. After passing urine for the first time there is no reason why a mother should not go to the toilet perfectly normally as often as she wishes.

Occasionally, especially after a long and difficult labour or a forceps delivery, a woman may be unable to pass water because of bruising around the base of the bladder. When this happens a small catheter is passed into the bladder and may be left draining continuously for 1 or perhaps 2 days after which she will be able to pass water normally. If an in-dwelling catheter is used an antibiotic will be given to prevent any infection developing in the bladder.

The bowels

Women have a tendency to become constipated during the puerperium because a lot of fluid is lost from the body in the urine, through perspiration and in the milk. Constipation can cause discomfort and perineal stitches may lead to a natural reluctance to exert any pressure in the area. The bowels will need less artificial stimulation if the diet contains sufficient roughage and a lot of fluid. Senokot is a useful laxative if dietary measures are not satisfactory.

Sutures. Perineal stitches are often necessary and consist of catgut or synthetic material. Both are rapidly absorbed and do not need to be removed, though this may be done to increase comfort and allow a woman to move about much more and empty her bladder and bowels more easily. It is important to keep the stitch line clean and as dry as possible to promote quick healing.

Convalescence

It is quite natural that tremendous excitement should follow the delivery of a new baby when everyone wants to visit to offer congratulations and good wishes, and much as one may wish to see them, most women find visitors extremely tiring. If it were possible to limit the visits to one minute or two minutes each, then quite a number could come, but when someone has travelled a long distance it does seem rather unfair to say that they can only stay for a few minutes, especially if they consider themselves to be a favourite aunt or best friend. The easiest way out of this situation is to restrict visitors to husband or partner and immediate family for the first two or three days when a woman really needs to settle down after the excitement of pregnancy and delivery. After this most women feel more able to cope with the disturbance that visitors and their children inevitably bring with them. When a woman has had her baby at home, it is extremely difficult to restrict visitors. Those who have been in hospital or who have had a baby know how tiring even the best intentioned visitors can become if they overstay their welcome, so everyone should bear in mind that while the new mother will be delighted to see her friends, they need only stay for a short while even if she, out of courtesy, presses them to stay longer.

Since most hospitals now have 'open visiting' your husband or partner can usually visit you at any time except when the ward is closed at feeding times or during the resting hours. If you already have children, ask the sister in charge when they may visit you.

Rest

Rest, which does not necessarily mean sleep, is most important. After a normal delivery a woman is not an invalid, but she must rest to allow her body to readjust after the pregnancy and confinement. Most of the first day should be spent in bed, except to get up to go to the lavatory or pick up the baby. From the second day onwards she may get up for meals as well, but when there is nothing definite to do she should rest in bed, and this regime should be continued for the first week. It is certainly true that a normal mother may feel like doing more and she may feel as though she ought to be doing more, but it cannot be too strongly emphasized that the body requires rest to readjust and the more she rushes about the longer will it take to return to normal. An adequate amount of sleep is essential, so she should settle down and try to sleep as soon as the ten o'clock feed is over. For the first few days a new mother may be spared having to get up in the night to give her baby a night feed, especially if she is in hospital, but she will be woken at six o'clock for the first morning feed.

'Rooming in' or keeping your baby by your bed is practised by many hospitals. You can pick him up when he cries, even at night, but if he is particularly noisy at night he may be put in the nursery for one or two nights.

It is surprising how quickly the night passes and 7 hours' sleep are not really sufficient. Most midwives insist on their patients resting during some part of the day. The best advantage should be taken of this time for relaxation and sleep, because not only is it beneficial to the woman herself but, if she is well rested, it also helps her baby.

For some strange reason most mothers do not sleep well on the first night after delivery. After a long and tiring labour it would seem that a woman should feel so tired that nothing could keep her awake, but even in these instances the excitement of delivery and the new arrival seems to overcome tiredness. Thereafter she usually sleeps well and it is of paramount importance that she has adequate sleep. Any woman suffering from insomnia or waking during the night should report this to her midwife. The necessity for an adequate amount of sleep cannot be too strongly emphasized.

It is a very mistaken belief that rest in hospital for 5 or even 7 days after delivery is something in the nature of a light-hearted holiday; nothing could be further from the truth and having a baby at home is certainly not a holiday unless there is a great deal of help in the house. Rest after delivery is even more important than it was during pregnancy. It is really surprising how the day is occupied so that there is, in fact, very little opportunity to relax and a certain amount of time must, therefore, be set aside each day for a formal rest period which should, if possible, be for 2 hours. Relaxation taught during pregnancy is for use during labour, but it is just as important that the resting time after delivery should provide as much relaxation as possible. The longer the rest and the better the relaxation during these days the more easily will a woman cope with the many problems which are bound to crop up from time to time.

During pregnancy everyone is enthusiastic about looking after the pregnant woman, and her husband is actively encouraged to do so. After delivery, however, people are frequently more interested in the new baby or busy congratulating the father as well as being full of guidance and advice concerning how to divide time, love and energy in looking after two people instead of one. They all seem to forget that the mother has also to look after herself. A complete book could be written on how a mother should look after herself after having a baby, not only for the next few days or even the next few months, but also the next few years, and this, like so many things in life, is far from easy but extremely important.

Just as time must be found to rest and relax, so must time be found to wash, bath, put on make-up, comb your hair, put on a clean nightgown, see that the bedclothes are tidy, that flowers are properly arranged, that the baby is clean and that his cot is tidy as well as a thousand other little jobs that can only be accomplished if a simple straightforward plan is made to organize the day's work early in the morning.

Diet

The traditional treatment in Britain for a woman who has just had a baby is a nice cup of tea, and this should herald a return to a normal unrestricted diet. After having a baby a woman may start eating a normal diet as soon as she feels like it. Good eating habits are essential during the puerperium, particularly as a nursing mother requires a wholesome diet to build up her strength and enable her to produce sufficient breast-milk. This refers to the kind of food that is eaten, not the quantity. Regular meals of protein, fruit and vegetables are better than snacks consisting mainly of carbohydrate which is fattening. As some women are anaemic at this time, foods rich in iron should be included in the diet, though iron supplements should be continued after leaving hospital especially if there is any sign of anaemia.

The diet in the puerperium should contain:

Proteins. Good sources of protein are meat, fish, cheese and eggs. All cuts of meat, bacon, ham and poultry are equally good. White fish should be included. An egg every day is a cheap source of protein.

Calcium. Milk provides protein as well as calcium, used in milky drinks, puddings, soups and cereals. A piece of cheese three or four times a week helps to supplement the calcium in milk and also provides protein.

Vitamins and minerals. Good sources of iron are liver, kidney and heart. These should be eaten once or twice a week as well as other meats, eggs and green vegetables, especially spinach.

Vegetables. At least two helpings of vegetables or salad a day should be eaten. Potatoes and high carbohydrate vegetables should be limited.

Fruit. Fresh fruit should be eaten at least once a day. Oranges, grapefruit and tomatoes are excellent sources of vitamin C which helps to keep the skin and gums healthy and to give vitality.

Cereals. Foods such as bread, breakfast cereals, rice and semolina are all necessary to increase the bulk and provide variety. Too much of these foods, however, leads to unnecessary increase in weight.

Fluid. If you are breast-feeding your baby you should drink plenty of fluid, at least 1 litre a day, of which at least a half should be milk.

When the bowels have returned to normal the mother should take the iron and vitamin tablets she was taking during pregnancy and should continue to take these for 3 months after delivery.

Position

Following delivery a woman is encouraged to move about as soon as possible and free movement of the legs is essential while still in bed. After a normal delivery she usually remains in bed for the first six hours, and is then allowed up to the bath and toilet. Her position in bed does not matter; she may lie on either side, whichever is more comfortable, or sit up. For many years it has been the custom for women to lie on their tummy for an hour a day to prevent the uterus becoming retroverted. Lying on the abdomen for an hour's relaxation is to be encouraged but it has no influence on the position of the uterus.

Abdominal distension

Immediately after delivery the abdomen is flat. It must be remembered, however, that during pregnancy the abdominal muscles have been stretched and it takes them a little time to return to normal. For the first few days after delivery a woman looks as though she is about 20 weeks pregnant. This abdominal enlargement is caused by gaseous distension within the intestine, associated with the slack abdominal muscles. If too much weight has been gained during pregnancy there may also be some extra fat.

The return to normal of the abdominal outline depends on the weight gained and the return to normal of the abdominal muscles. This may take up to several months. If a mother practises postnatal exercises her muscles will recover more quickly and she will regain her figure sooner. There is no need to wear an abdominal support immediately after delivery unless one was worn before or during pregnancy. An abdominal support, however, does not strengthen the muscles but rather weakens them, because once they come to rely on the support they gradually become weaker and weaker.

Ambulation

Nowadays women are allowed out of bed as soon as they wish after their delivery. Over the centuries fads and fancies have changed but there is certainly nothing new in early ambulation after delivery. In many parts of the world it is common practice for women to have their babies and immediately return to their daily tasks. It is generally believed in this country that a certain amount of rest is beneficial to a new mother. The accent, however, is on rest rather than confinement to bed, and after a normal delivery a mother may get up as soon as she wishes to go to the lavatory and attend to her baby. If she has had a prolonged or difficult labour the midwife or doctor may decide that she should stay in bed for 24 hours, but if she is fit and well enough, she will be allowed to get up. It is a matter for individual decision and no firm rules are laid down. When a woman gets up she must always put on slippers, which should be properly constructed with the same height of heel as that normally worn during the day time and not casual slippers without heels. She should not walk around barefoot.

Blood tests

A routine blood test is usually taken on about the fourth or fifth day after delivery to ensure that the mother is not suffering from puerperal anaemia, even if the delivery was absolutely normal and the blood count has been satisfactory throughout the pregnancy.

Examination on discharge

It is the routine in many hospitals for a woman to be examined by the house surgeon immediately before discharge. This includes a pelvic examination to assess the condition of the perineum and to be certain that the sutures are healing satisfactorily. It also checks that the cervix is closing properly and the uterus is involuting normally. There may also be a more complete examination, with examination of the breasts and the abdomen, to note the degree of uterine involution. The blood pressure is recorded and blood taken for a further haemoglobin estimation.

Many hospitals no longer have discharge examinations, reserving most of the points until the postnatal examination 6 weeks after delivery. It is important to attend the postnatal clinic, especially if an examination was not performed before discharge from hospital.

Advice on leaving hospital

After a normal delivery and a stay in hospital of approximately 7 days, a woman needs some advice on what she is allowed to do when she gets home.

She should continue with more or less the same routine that has been established in hospital; this is particularly important for her baby. She may walk up and down stairs, but should obviously do no more climbing than is essential. She should rest in the afternoon and, if possible, try to get 2 hours' sleep, and should certainly go back to bed after the 6 a.m. feed for a further rest. If her husband or partner can be persuaded to get breakfast, so much the better. She should get someone to do the shopping for 2 weeks after which she can go out and do it herself, but should avoid carrying heavy parcels or doing heavy household chores for about 4 weeks after delivery.

When organizing the daily routine always leave a few spare minutes for going to the lavatory otherwise you will find that you are too busy to go when the need is felt, or alternatively you will rush and strain because there is insufficient time. Both are equally bad. The former eventually leads to constipation and straining, and the latter causes discomfort and will strain the muscles of the pelvic floor, eventually predisposing to prolapse and piles.

A mother should not drive a car until 3 weeks after delivery because judgment is often impaired. The exact date when a job can be resumed depends on the exact nature of the work, but it is most inadvisable to return to work before 6 weeks after confinement. It is inadvisable to take a new baby visiting until he is at least 4 weeks old, unless there is some very special occasion, or to subject him to the risk of infection (e.g. aunt's common cold).

Postnatal exercises

Postnatal exercises are even more important than antenatal exercises. In the antenatal period a woman is taught how to relax her muscles but after delivery she has to make certain that any muscles which might have been stretched or bruised during delivery are encouraged to return to normal as soon as possible. This refers in particular to the muscles of the back, the abdomen and the pelvic floor. Details of postnatal exercises are given below. They fall into three groups:

1 The care of the back.
2 The care of the abdomen.
3 The care of the pelvic floor.

The muscles in the back must not be allowed to get slack. Correct posture and sitting in the correct position is one of the best ways of ensuring that they are maintained in the new strength they have developed during pregnancy.

The muscles in the anterior abdominal wall return to normal providing too much weight has not been gained and that the proper exercises are performed regularly.

The muscles of the pelvic floor are not only the most important but the most difficult to return to normal because in the first few days after delivery, and especially if stitches have been inserted, they may be too sore and bruised for the mother to feel like starting pelvic floor exercises. It is so easy, therefore, to forget them, but they must be done not once or twice a day but many times each day. The muscles of the pelvic floor can be tightened up and pelvic floor exercises repeated while feeding the baby, washing up or doing almost anything. Details of special pelvic floor exercises will be given by your midwife or physiotherapist.

The postnatal exercises below restore the tone of the abdominal and pelvic floor muscles which have become overstretched during pregnancy and labour, stimulate the circulation and encourage good posture.

a Lie on the back with knees slightly bent and the feet flat on the bed. Draw the abdominal muscles in firmly, then raise the head. Hold the position for a few seconds while breathing naturally, then lower the head slowly. Repeat 10 times.
b Lie on the bed with one knee bent. Draw the abdominal muscles in firmly. Lengthen and straighten the leg by sliding the heel towards the foot of the bed, then draw it upwards from the waist to shorten the straight leg. Repeat 5 times with each leg.
c Lie on the back with knees bent and feet flat on the bed. Draw the abdominal muscles in firmly, then reach across the body to place one hand on the opposite side of the bed on a level with the hips. Return to starting position. Repeat 5 times each way.

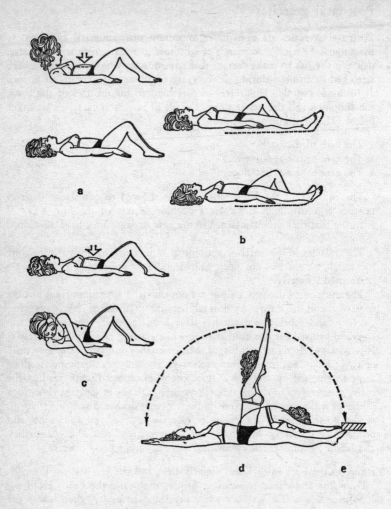

Fig 35 Postnatal exercises

d Lie flat on the floor on the back with the feet tucked under the edge of a heavy piece of furniture. Cross arms on chest. Raise up slowly to a sitting position and slowly lie back. Keep the back very straight. Repeat 10 times.

e When (d) can be done easily repeat with the arms fully extended above the head. Repeat 10 times.

German measles (rubella) immunization

Where antenatal testing, available in most hospitals, has shown a mother to be 'susceptible to rubella' this means that she has never built up immunity to the disease by developing it, being in contact with it or by being immunized. To prevent the possibility of contracting the illness during a future pregnancy, immunization should be offered in the first few days of the puerperium. Should such an injection be accepted, the mother *must not* get pregnant for at least three months, and adequate contraceptive advice is usually offered at the same time. Rubella is further discussed in Chapter 11, page 172–3.

29 Complications of the Puerperium

Women who have just had a baby may suffer from any incidental disease or illness which has nothing to do with their pregnancy or delivery. Occasionally women get infectious diseases such as mumps, measles, German measles, influenza, simple colds or bronchitis and may even develop surgical emergencies such as acute appendicitis. If a mother develops an infectious disease it is most unlikely that her baby will suffer from it, since new-born babies have not only a transmitted but also a natural immunity which lasts for several weeks after birth.

Puerperal pyrexia

A puerperal pyrexia is defined as a rise in temperature on one or more occasions during the first 28 days after a woman has been delivered. It used to be a statutory requirement for a puerperal pyrexia to be notified to the local medical officer of health. This was a legacy dating back 40 or 50 years to the time when puerperal pyrexia was very much feared as a disease which killed quite a large number of newly delivered mothers. Up to nearly 50 years ago, if a vicious infection gained access to the uterus it was uncontrollable because no satisfactory treatment existed and it could spread from one woman to another with alarming speed. The control and cure of puerperal infection began in 1935 with the introduction of the first sulphonamides, and as better sulphonamides and subsequently antibiotics were introduced puerperal fever became controllable. It is today a preventable disease. The organism most feared was the haemolytic streptococcus, which was eventually conquered by the use of penicillin, to which it is nearly always sensitive. Puerperal pyrexia today is a condition that is treated with respect, but it is no longer feared or notified, because the bacteria that cause puerperal pyrexia are easily controlled by modern antibiotics.

Up to 1935 many women dared not have their babies in hospital because of the risk of contracting puerperal fever by cross infection. This argument is still put forward by some people for preferring home to hospital confinement. The incidence, however, of all types of puerperal pyrexia today is less than 4 per cent and even then the infection is usually in the urinary tract. Severe infections of the uterus are extremely rare, so much so that it is difficult today to appreciate the severity of puerperal fever that existed only a few decades ago.

The reasons for the reduction in puerperal infection are many and a full appreciation of their extent can only be achieved if one considers all the preventive measures as well as those used in the early treatment of the condition. Samples of urine are taken during pregnancy to detect those women in whom a urinary tract infection is liable to occur. These infections are treated vigorously in the antenatal period. Swabs are taken of any vaginal discharge and the organisms cultured so that they can be eliminated before the onset of labour. The care of breasts and instruction given to facilitate breast-feeding during the antenatal period render them less liable to infection. The prevention of anaemia and the correction of many other minor abnormalities or deficiencies during pregnancy all help to avoid puerperal infection.

Sexual intercourse, however, which has long been blamed as a major factor in causing infection during pregnancy and after delivery, is in no way responsible. Normal sexual intercourse can continue right up to the onset of labour in a normal pregnancy without any risk of infection.

Rigid antiseptic measures taken during labour and delivery also help to eliminate infection. The cleansing of the vulva, the use of antiseptic creams and lotions during examinations, the avoidance of catheterization if possible, the use of sterile instruments and towels, as well as the extensive measures taken to ensure that infection should not be passed from the midwife or doctor to the patient, are just a few of the aspects in the care of the pregnant woman which have gone such a long way towards the control of infection. Last, and probably most important, is that when an infection does begin the organism can be rapidly cultured, isolated and killed with an antibiotic before it has had time to cause damage to the woman herself or be transmitted to another person.

Uterine infection

Infection in the uterus used to be the classic cause of puerperal fever and a uterine infection caused by the haemolytic streptococcus was a dreaded disease before the introduction of sulphonamides and penicillin. Today this particular infection is not only rare but controllable. It is nevertheless true that uterine infections do occasionally happen to women who are looked after by the most modern and up-to-date techniques.

The uterus may become infected by a variety of bacteria: the signs and symptoms vary according to the organism concerned and the severity of the infection. The first sign is usually that the lochia becomes slightly offensive, perhaps more profuse and brighter in colour than previously. The uterus may be slightly tender or the woman may become aware of lower abdominal discomfort which is more marked on one side than on the other. The temperature and probably the pulse are slightly raised. There is nothing very sinister or serious about any of these symptoms, but they will be noted by the midwife, who will suspect that there is an infection if the uterus is slightly tender on palpation and movement. A swab is taken from the vagina and sent to the laboratory for bacteriological culture and isolation of the organism to find its antibiotic sensitivities. The doctor is notified and the woman examined and given an antibiotic to control the infection.

One of the commonest causes of a uterine infection is the presence within the uterus of some products of conception, such as a small portion of the placenta which failed to be delivered with the majority of the placenta during the third stage of labour. Any foreign body in the uterine cavity forms an ideal culture for bacteria and the possibility of some retained products of conception must always be considered, especially if the infection is accompanied by some vaginal bleeding.

Perineal infection

The perineum can only become infected after a perineal laceration or an episiotomy, when an infection may begin in the stitch line or in the deeper layers of the perineum. This may be first noticed because of considerable discomfort in the perineum. Infection in the superficial stitches does not have any lasting ill effect, and is relieved when the stitches are removed on the fifth or sixth day. It clears up very quickly indeed but sometimes there is a slight discharge for several days or even weeks after the stitches have been removed.

If the infection is deep seated it forms a small abscess in the deeper layers of the perineum, which discharges through a small hole in the stitch line. This continues for several days before the abscess heals, which it does quite spontaneously and naturally.

When the infection has been extensive the perineal wound breaks down and will then need resuturing after the infection has been controlled by giving an oral antibiotic and warm saline baths two or three times daily. On about the tenth day after delivery the infection should be sufficiently controlled to permit resuturing, which is done under general anaesthesia in hospital. If the infection is less severe and the perineal wound breaks down only partially, it may be left to heal on its own during the following two or three weeks.

Breast infection

Infections of the breast are very rare during pregnancy but, unfortunately they are more frequent after delivery and during lactation Breast infection must not be confused with engorgement. The breasts normally become engorged on the third or fourth day after delivery, when it may be associated with a slight rise in temperature but there is no infection present. Breast infection, or acute mastitis, occurs in a localized part of the breast being the result of infection gaining access to a part of the breast itself. Breast infections are usually, but not always, preceded by a crack in the nipple and it is for this reason that cracked or sore nipples are treated with such respect.

A baby who is sucking normally at the breast will seldom cause a break in the skin of the nipple. This results because the baby has been chewing rather than sucking the nipple. It is of paramount importance, therefore, to make sure that the nipple is always placed well inside the baby's mouth where he cannot 'chew' it.

A cracked nipple is painful and requires expert attention and treatment. Since it causes pain the mother does not allow the baby to feed satisfactorily, which results in the breast becoming engorged and tender. The milk must be expressed by hand or by a breast pump and the nipple rested until it has completely healed, which usually takes 24 to 36 hours, after which normal breast-feeding can be resumed. If the crack becomes infected bacteria gain access to neighbouring milk ducts where they grow and flourish and then infect the tissue of the breast itself unless the breast is properly emptied. The first sign that infection has entered the breast is usually a sharp rise in temperature, with a rise in pulse rate and tenderness, frequently in the outer part of the breast. This may be accompanied by a flushing or reddening of the skin over the affected part of the breast, which will be tender to touch and also rather engorged. Treatment with a wide spectrum antibiotic such as ampicillin may arrest the infection so that the reddening of the skin disappears, the soreness goes and the breast gradually returns to normal, providing it is satisfactorily emptied by manual expression or breast pump.

Sometimes the inflammation does not subside; the temperature continues to rise and an abscess forms in the deeper tissues of the breast. When this happens breast feeding is stopped and lactation suppressed. A specimen of milk is collected from the nipple and sent to the laboratory so that the organism concerned can be cultured and tested against various antibiotics. Once an abscess has formed, however, it is unlikely that it will be cured by antibiotics alone. The area of the breast in which it has formed becomes extremely reddened, firm or even hard and very tender. Eventually, when the centre of the abscess liquefies, it can be opened and drained under a general anaesthetic. A breast abscess is not only extremely disappointing for the mother (because breast-feeding has to be discontinued) but is also a very painful and demoralizing experience. Inflammation of the breast is much more common following a first pregnancy and is very unusual once a woman has breast-fed one child.

Breast abscesses were once relatively common but are now much less so, because modern antenatal instruction teaches a woman to breast-feed her baby correctly, and because modern treatment with both antibiotics and breast expression is very effective.

Cracked nipples usually develop on about the ninth or tenth day and the midwife is nearly always able to treat the condition so that breast-feeding can be resumed satisfactorily. Inflammation of the breast causing flushing or redness of the skin also happens at about the tenth day. Immediate treatment by antibiotics and satisfactory emptying of the breast usually cures the infection and breast-feeding can be resumed. Inflammation of the breast also tends to occur during the fourth week after delivery, when the mother is usually unaware that a crack has developed in the nipple and the first thing she realizes is that the breast is painful and tender. This should be reported immediately, and if it is treated early an abscess can be avoided.

Once a woman has had a breast abscess most obstetricians consider that breast-feeding should not be attempted in a subsequent pregnancy. Every case is considered on its own merits, however, and there are instances where satisfactory breast-feeding has been accomplished after an abscess has been previously operated on and drained.

Infections of the urinary tract

Infections of the urinary tract (pyelonephritis and cystitis) are now much less common than they used to be because the majority of potential infections are eliminated during the antenatal period. A certain number of women do have bacteria in their urine during pregnancy and if anything happens to disturb the function of their urinary tract they are always liable to develop an infection. Women who develop a urinary tract infection during pregnancy are treated in the antenatal clinic or may even require admission to hospital for efficient therapy. Occasionally a urinary tract infection may develop after delivery.

There are two main varieties: cystitis, in which the symptoms are localized to the bladder itself, and pyelonephritis, where the symptoms involve the kidney and the person feels more ill.

Cystitis may develop as a result of catheterization during a prolonged or difficult labour, or may follow a forceps delivery or even a Caesarean section. Pain and discomfort on micturition are often accompanied by an urgency and desire to pass urine at frequent intervals. All these symptoms indicate an inflammation in the bladder itself. Cystitis alone does not usually cause much rise in temperature, but the symptoms can be very annoying. The urine is cultured and the infection is treated by a wide spectrum antibiotic and usually subsides within 24 hours.

Pyelonephritis develops when the organisms extend up from the bladder towards the kidney. There is usually a rapid rise in temperature which may be accompanied by a rise in the pulse rate, although the pulse itself may remain surprisingly normal. There is pain not only in the region of the bladder, but also over one or other kidney, with quite severe discomfort in the loin which may radiate downwards to the groin. The sudden rise in temperature may be associated with a rigor (shivering attacks) and sweating. The condition starts quite suddenly and is equally dramatic in its relief when the appropriate antibiotic is given. A mid-stream specimen of urine is sent to the laboratory for culture and the organism tested to find the most efficient antibiotic, but meanwhile treatment with a wide spectrum antibiotic is usually started.

Uterine haemorrhage

Bleeding which occurs immediately after delivery of the baby is known as primary postpartum haemorrhage. A secondary postpartum haemorrhage is one that occurs more than 24 hours after completion of delivery. The lochia, which is bright red blood for the first two or three days, then becomes pinkish and later brown, and may become red again as a result of exercise or a return to household chores. Excessive bleeding occasionally occurs and may be the result of infection (when the bleeding is not usually severe and does not generally require any specific treatment other than for the infection itself) or retention of a small piece of placenta, known as a cotyledon. If the bleeding becomes more serious and the woman starts to pass clots then the presence of a retained cotyledon is always considered.

Subinvolution

Subinvolution follows a low grade infection inside the uterus so that the uterus does not involute, or return to its normal size, properly. Because the involution is not satisfactory there is a tendency to excessive bleeding. When the infection is treated, normal involution ensues and bleeding ceases.

Retained products

Although the placenta is carefully inspected at delivery it sometimes happens that small fragments, retained within the uterus, are too small to be detected as missing. Retained products of conception may result in the sudden onset of brisk bleeding often associated with the passage of clots. This usually starts about the tenth day after delivery.

If bleeding suddenly begins the midwife or doctor must be notified immediately. The treatment follows two principles. Firstly, the administration of ergometrine, Syntocinon or syntometrine, which contains both ergometrine and Syntocinon, will make the uterus contract and stop bleeding for at least 3 to 4 hours, and secondly, admission of the woman to hospital where (under a general anaesthetic) a gentle curettage operation is performed to remove the remaining cotyledon. Once an injection has been given to make the uterus contract, the bleeding will cease and from then on everything will be under control. If much blood has been lost a blood transfusion may be necessary even before a general anaesthetic is given. When the offending cotyledon has been removed from the uterus, there will be no further haemorrhage and the uterus will continue to involute normally.

Anaemia

Anaemia is due to a reduction either in the amount of blood in the body or in the haemoglobin level. The quantity of blood in the body is assessed by measuring the level of haemoglobin either in gm per 100 ml or as a percentage; 100 per cent is equivalent to 14 gm (i.e. 1 gm ≡ 7 per cent).

Antenatal care ensures that normal haemoglobin levels are maintained throughout pregnancy. If anaemia is allowed to develop in the antenatal period then it will almost certainly be present after delivery; therefore, the best insurance against postpartum anaemia is adequate antenatal care. In this respect anaemia is no different from most of the other complications of pregnancy.

An excessive blood loss at or immediately after delivery may also result in anaemia in the puerperium. The average quantity of blood lost at delivery varies from about 75–250 ml and this amount is unlikely to affect the level of haemoglobin adversely. However, if this amount of blood loss is exceeded, or if a woman loses a half litre or even 1 litre of blood, then postpartum anaemia is likely to develop.

Postpartum haemorrhage is now comparatively rare, although some instances are unavoidable. The loss of 1 litre of blood at the time of the delivery is usually an indication for an immediate blood transfusion to replace the blood loss and therefore prevent anaemia. A blood transfusion immediately after delivery is a precaution taken when blood loss has been greater than expected. This may happen during complicated deliveries, or Caesarean section. It does not mean that anything has gone wrong and it should give no cause for alarm. If a woman has in fact lost a half-litre or even a litre of blood at Caesarean section it is much better that this should be replaced so that she is fit and healthy in the puerperium rather than anaemic and likely to suffer from the associated weakness, lethargy and susceptibility to infection. Anaemia also makes lactation less efficient.

Unsuspected anaemia

The midwife and doctor know all the haemoglobin levels during pregnancy and will therefore be aware of any tendency to anaemia. They will thus be warned to look out for any anaemia that might develop after delivery. Unsuspected anaemia may be the result of this tendency and an excessive blood loss at delivery, for example, in a woman whose haemoglobin level has been just within the normal range during the latter part of pregnancy, that is about 74 or 75 per cent (or 11 g), and who loses slightly more than the expected amount of blood at delivery (about 300 or even 400 ml).

Symptoms of anaemia

These are all rather indefinite. The complexion is pale and has a rather pasty appearance. Excessive tiredness associated with adequate sleep, impatience, shortness of breath, irritability and lethargy as well as a feeling that every-thing is too much trouble, are all minor symptoms of anaemia. The nails, lips and also the inner aspect of the lower eyelid are a pale colour. The pulse rate may remain persistently high, over 100 per minute, and this in itself is one of the most significant of all recordings in the puerperium.

The natural prevention of anaemia

The total amount of blood normally circulating in the female body is approximately 5 litres. This amount is gradually increased in pregnancy by about 30 per cent to a total of 6.5 litres. This initially results in some dilution of the blood but if adequate iron and vitamins and a good diet are taken during the antenatal period then the haemoglobin level should be 80 per cent or higher when labour begins.

During the first three days after delivery the total circulating blood volume gradually returns to normal, which means that it is reduced by 1.5 litres to its usual non-pregnant level of 5 litres. This reduction in the circulating blood is accomplished by removing some of the serum from the bloodstream itself, leaving the red cells and the other blood constit-uents, which means there is some concentration of these factors and the haemoglobin level therefore rises. This is nature's way of compensating automatically for the amount of blood lost during delivery and for the blood lost in the lochia during the postpartum days. Some women can lose almost half a litre of blood at delivery and yet on the fourth postpartum day have a haemoglobin level higher than before the onset of labour.

Blood tests after delivery

Blood is usually taken on the third or fourth day after delivery for a haemoglobin estimation. If there is mild anaemia extra iron and vitamin tablets are given. If there is severe anaemia a blood transfusion may be considered necessary. If so there is no cause for alarm, because it is much better to be fit and well after receiving a transfusion than to have to struggle along for the several weeks, or even months, that it may require to raise a very low haemoglobin level to normal.

All women who have recently had a baby should continue to take their iron and vitamin tablets for at least 3 months after delivery.

Venous thrombosis

Superficial venous thrombosis

Varicose veins do sometimes develop during pregnancy and tend to become more severe with each subsequent pregnancy, although they regress somewhat after delivery. Comparatively severe varicose veins are always liable to become inflamed after delivery and this is known as superficial phlebitis, or superficial thrombosis. The superficial varicose vein, usually on the inner side of the thigh or on the inner side of the calf, becomes slightly inflamed and then extremely tender. The vein itself can be felt as a firm, rather hard, very tender, cord-like structure lying immediately beneath the skin. The inflammation may extend along the vein for several inches and may be extremely painful on standing or walking. If this sort of inflammation should occur in the region of a varicose vein it should be reported to the midwife or doctor, who usually arranges for the leg to be bandaged and rested as much as possible until the inflammation has subsided. There is no specific or dramatic cure for superficial phlebitis or thrombosis and the painful swelling may continue for several days. The only real consolation is that the phlebitis results in obliteration and cure of the affected varicose vein. Above all, there is no need to worry about superficial thrombosis, because it never causes any real harm and although the terms 'thrombosis' and 'phlebitis' can conjure up in most people's minds pictures of terrible complications, no serious complications or disasters ever follow a superficial thrombosis. It is merely a rather painful and annoying, but quite safe, complication of childbirth.

Deep venous thrombosis

A deep venous thrombosis is a condition where the veins in the centre of the leg become thrombosed. This may or may not be associated with superficial varicose veins but is very seldom associated with a superficial thrombosis or superficial phlebitis. Deep venous thrombosis is unlikely when newly delivered mothers get up on the day after delivery and wear proper bedroom slippers with 1-inch heels. The worst type of shoes to wear after delivery are those without a heel or with just a strap across the front of the foot so that the toes have to be curled up to keep the slipper in place.

The condition usually starts on about the fifth day following delivery and the first thing noticed is a tightness in the middle of the calf in one leg. There is a certain discomfort or even pain on walking, and the calf is tender, especially between the two parts of the main muscle. There may be some swelling or oedema of the foot, or the ankle itself and even the calf of the leg may feel thickened and swollen. Pain may be felt in the back of the leg if the foot is forcibly pushed upwards, which is why there is pain on walking or on leaning forward.

Deep venous thrombosis used to be considered a potentially dangerous condition since it was feared that a blood clot could be dislodged from the thrombosed vein in the calf and could circulate back to become lodged either in the heart or the lungs—a condition known as a pulmonary embolus, which is not only painful but can also be very serious.

A woman who develops a deep venous thrombosis is usually instructed to rest in bed as much as possible. A crepe bandage is put on the foot and the leg to above the knee. A simple antibiotic such as penicillin or ampicillin may be administered. In some hospitals heparin is given by injection every 6 hours, or as a continuous intravenous drip to reduce the coagulation time of the blood. The heparin usually relieves the pain in the leg within a few hours. After 24 hours a slower acting anticoagulant drug, such as dicoumarin, is given for 7 to 10 days or even longer. If such thrombosis can be shown, by tests, to extend above the knee, anticoagulant therapy may be continued for three months.

White leg

White leg is now extremely rare. It is a serious complication of pregnancy in which there is a thrombosis of the main femoral vein which drains most of the blood from the leg. The thrombosis occurs in the groin and in the outer side of the pelvis and its onset is usually quite sudden causing quite severe bursting-like pain in the whole leg, especially in the thigh and the calf. The whole leg rapidly becomes very swollen, right up to the groin, and the skin becomes tender; the swelling of the leg makes it become pale and white—hence the term white leg. There is continuous aching, nagging, bursting, heavy discomfort in the leg.

White leg is nearly always caused by an infection in the pelvis, invariably the uterus, which may follow a prolonged and difficult labour. The leg is treated by bandaging, to give some relief from discomfort, and the administration of antibiotics and anticoagulant drugs.

Pulmonary embolus

Pulmonary embolus is a condition in which a blood clot moves from one of the veins in the leg or pelvis, travels along the great vessels to the heart and is transmitted to the lungs, where it lodges and obstructs the blood supply. The part of the lung obstructed by the clot cannot obtain any blood supply and collapses. The patient experiences sudden and severe pain, usually in the lower part of the chest. Occasionally, if the diaphragm itself is affected, pain is felt either in the upper abdomen or in the shoulder. The onset of this severe pain is accompanied by shortness of breath and a feeling of faintness and tightness in the chest. The pain itself is sharp and knife-like usually causing a considerable amount of distress. It is worse on breathing or coughing, and is severe on taking a deep breath. A small amount of blood-stained sputum may be coughed up.

The treatment of pulmonary embolus is complete bed-rest, sedation and the administration of drugs to relieve the pain. Although opinion is divided concerning the administration of anticoagulant drugs most women will be given heparin for several days and then warfarin which is usually continued for several weeks or even months.

Pulmonary emboli are much less common than they used to be. Careful antenatal care, the treatment of anaemia and pelvic infection, adequate supervision in labour and the elimination of destructive or complicated obstetric procedures and extensive lacerations, are all factors which have helped to reduce its incidence. The more frequent use of intravenous injections, or drips, of dextrose or saline prevent dehydration which has always been a cause of pulmonary embolus.

Anticoagulants and breast-feeding

If anticoagulant therapy is given orally it is usually considered inappropriate to breast-feeding, some of the drug reaching the baby via the milk and possibly thinning its blood. This effect is usually minimal but the continuance of feeding will necessitate repeated blood tests on the baby and possible injections to restore its blood to normal.

Puerperal depression

Some emotional disturbance, together with the 'postpartum blues', is present in varying degrees in almost every woman who has had a baby. It used to be believed that there was a special type of mental illness known as puerperal psychosis which particularly affected women after childbirth. In actual fact there is no such condition, but some women who are liable to mental illness may become emotionally unstable, and pregnancy, delivery, the puerperium and responsibility of the new baby may impose an unreasonable strain upon them, leading to the onset of mental illness. There is nothing specific about pregnancy or delivery which causes a woman to develop a mental illness. Any other stress, strain or emotional disturbance of similar severity may quite easily provoke mental illness in such a person.

The treatment of puerperal psychosis is exactly the same as the treatment of any other mental illness: expert advice, reassurance, treatment with the appropriate drugs and perhaps rest in hospital. The doctor usually arranges for a psychiatrist to be consulted, because he is the ideal person to know exactly what dose or which type of drug should be administered in each instance. The prognosis of puerperal psychosis is similar to that of any other mental illness, with the exception that the new-born baby imposes an additional strain upon the newly delivered mother.

When one considers the stresses and strains of pregnancy, labour and the puerperium it is rather surprising that puerperal psychosis is not more frequent. The anxieties of pregnancy, fears of the unknown, perhaps lack of sleep, concern as to whether the baby will be normal, whether the delivery will be easy, and then, when delivery has been completed, the progress of the baby (more especially the anxiety which may arise over breast-feeding) could impose an intolerable burden on any woman. The best intentioned of relatives and friends often add a very considerable strain.

Puerperal depression is frequently underestimated. It can occasionally be severe, prolonged and very distressing especially because few doctors understand its depressing effect upon the mother and the fact that it may continue for several months, or even as long as one year. It is sometimes very difficult for a woman to persuade those around her or even her doctor that she is miserable and depressed. The treatment is difficult and must be judged on an individual basis but it must include a lot of sympathy and support.

30 Twins

The incidence of twin pregnancy is approximately 1 in every 80 pregnancies in Great Britain. Some races are more likely to have twin pregnancies than others; they are more common in some African races than in this country, and less frequent among the Chinese. Twins are relatively uncommon in women who are under 20 or over 40, occurring most frequently in women who are in their thirties, and then in women who are in their twenties. It is certainly true that the bigger the family the greater the likelihood of twins, but the incidence of twins probably has nothing to do with the number of babies a woman has actually had—it is just a simple fact that the more babies she has the more likely is she to catch up with the inevitable 1 pregnancy in every 80 that happens to be twins.

Twinning is certainly an inherited characteristic and may be inherited by both men and women, although it is more likely to be handed down by a daughter than by a son. Nevertheless, if there is twinning in either family there is a possibility of having a twin pregnancy. It tends to skip generations; it is quite common for grandmother and granddaughter to have twin pregnancies, whereas mother had a succession of single pregnancies.

The perinatal mortality for twin babies is four or five times higher than for singleton pregnancies, partly because of the high incidence of premature labour and also because of an increased incidence of other complications of pregnancy.

Types of twinning

Twins may be identical or non-identical.

Identical twins

Identical twins are formed when a single egg is fertilized by a single sperm which instead of proceeding to form a single baby divides into separate halves very early in its development so that it proceeds to develop into two separate babies within the same pregnancy sac. These babies will be identical, or uniovular twins since they have exactly the same genetic structure and the same chromosomes. While developing in the uterus they each have their own amniotic cavity, but there is a single placenta in which the blood of their circulations mix—although the circulation of the babies is completely separated from that of the mother. They are always the same sex; they will have the same features, the same colour hair, the same physical characteristics and exactly the same blood groups. In their relationship one twin will assume authority and become dominant, but to the outside world they will be similar and identical.

Siamese twins, or conjoined twins, are a uniovular (one egg) twin pregnancy which started to divide but in which the division was incomplete, so that as the babies developed they were not completely separated. Such babies may be joined by the head, the trunk or the limbs. Attempts to separate them are occasionally successful. The incidence of conjoined twins is very rare indeed.

Non-identical twins

Non-identical twins develop from the fertilization of two separate eggs by two separate sperms. The two separate pregnancies proceed side by side. They implant in the uterus almost without exception at the same time but at different sites so that each has its own placenta. There is therefore no mixing or communication of blood between the twins. They may or may not be of the same sex: half the sets of non-identical twins will be of the same sex and half will not. They will certainly not have the same characteristics and they may not be of the same blood group. These are known as dissimilar, non-identical or binovular twins.

The difference between uniovular and binovular twins can be recognized at delivery by examination of the placenta. If two placentae are present then obviously the twins are binovular (dissimilar), but if only one placenta is present this is carefully examined to ensure that it is in fact a single placenta with a single chorion and two amniotic cavities, having the mixed circulation of a uniovular, identical twin pregnancy. Occasionally the two placentae of binovular twins lie side by side and appear to be one. Careful examination, however, shows there are two which are actually separate.

Causes

The exact cause of twin pregnancy is not known. A binovular pregnancy occurs when there is fertilization of two separate ova. An ejaculation may consist of at least three or four hundred million sperms, so the presence of two or more sperms in the region of the ovary at the time of ovulation is readily accepted. In fact, many authorities believe that several sperms must necessarily be present around the ovum before any single sperm can penetrate it. The fertilization of a single ovum by two sperms is not possible because the total number of chromosomes within such a cell would then be 23 from the ovum and 23 from each sperm; such a cell could not survive. The inheritance of twin pregnancy through the male side of the family can only depend on the division at a very early stage of a single fertilized ovum, that is, uniovular twins. The production of more than one ovum in each menstrual cycle is unusual and depends only on the female.

Modern fertility drugs have been developed to provoke ovulation and they occasionally lead to the formation of more than one ovum in each menstrual cycle, resulting in multiple pregnancies. When the exact characteristics of these drugs are better understood, the control of ovulation will be more accurately achieved and multiple pregnancies will occur less frequently.

Superfecundation is the fertilization of two separate ova at different acts of sexual intercourse. During the Middle Ages a twin pregnancy was always considered the result of superfecundation and was interpreted to mean that a woman had intercourse after she knew that she was pregnant. Such an act was considered indecent and the poor creatures were sometimes stoned to death. Although incidents of superfecundation have been proved both medically and legally, it is virtually impossible unless two separate acts of sexual intercourse occur very close together, and two ova have been released at ovulation. Once pregnancy has been established the circulating hormones automatically suppress further ovulation.

Diagnosis of twin pregnancy

The diagnosis of a twin pregnancy should be simple. It ought to be obvious that two babies are present; that the uterus is larger than it would be for one baby and that there are two of everything including two fetal hearts Before ultrasound about 5 per cent of twin pregnancies reached delivery before the discovery of the second baby—usually to the equal embarrassment of the midwife and doctor as well as the mother.

The following factors may make the midwife or doctor consider the possibility of twin pregnancy.

Excessive nausea and vomiting may be associated with a multiple pregnancy, especially if the symptoms continue beyond the 13th or 14th week.

The uterus is consistently larger than the dates suggest. Pelvic examination is performed at the first visit to the doctor or the antenatal clinic and the presence of any fibroids or tumours is noted. If the uterus is subsequently noticed to be larger than the dates it is essential to know that a previous pelvic examination has been performed to exclude any other pelvic mass. In early pregnancy the commonest reason for the uterus being larger than the dates would suggest is the very simple fact that it is sitting higher in the abdomen than it normally does.

Fetal movements are felt in a twin pregnancy at the same time as they would be felt in a single pregnancy. As pregnancy advances, however, excessive movements may lead the mother to consider the possibility of twin pregnancy.

Two fetal hearts. It used to be very difficult to confirm the presence of a twin pregnancy by listening to the fetal hearts through the ordinary fetal stethoscope, but electronic aids will detect the presence of two fetal hearts as early as the 14th week.

Acute hydramnios usually accompanies a uniovular twin pregnancy. During the 24th week there is a rapid and dramatic enlargement in the size of the uterus. This may be so sudden that it causes considerable pain and discomfort, and the abdominal girth may increase from about 70 cm to more than 112 cm within a few days. Acute hydramnios only occurs in uniovular (identical) twin pregnancies because the circulation of one twin becomes so dominant that the second twin is forced to produce a large quantity of amniotic fluid to prevent itself from getting heart failure. In binovular twins there is a separate circulation serving each twin so that this does not occur.

Many fetal parts. The midwife's or doctor's suspicion is aroused if an excessive number of fetal parts are felt within the abdomen, especially if two heads are palpated.

Small baby. If a baby's head is easily palpable and is rather small for the size of the uterus or for the duration of the pregnancy, then the presence of a twin pregnancy is always considered.

Pre-eclampsia does not usually occur until after the 32nd week of pregnancy, but a raised blood pressure or excessive weight gain before the 28th week is associated with twin pregnancy.

Two babies. The presence of a twin pregnancy is established if the midwife or doctor is absolutely certain that two babies are palpable within the uterus, or if a fetal-heart-detecting machine can positively identify two fetal hearts.

Ultrasound. The routine use of ultrasound scan in early pregnancy ensures that the diagnosis is made before any of the above physical signs arouse suspicion. Twins can be diagnosed by scan as early as the end of the 6th week of pregnancy and the examination can always be used to confirm any suspicions.

X-rays. The X-ray is not justified because ultrasound ought to be available.

Duration of pregnancy

The average duration of a twin pregnancy is 36 to 38 weeks, but the incidence of prematurity in twin pregnancy is becoming less.

Abortion in early pregnancy does not appear to be more common in twin pregnancy than single pregnancy. Hydramnios, anaemia and pre-eclampsia predispose to premature labour of which the incidence is fairly high at about the 32nd week of pregnancy. If a twin pregnancy can safely negotiate these hazards, then there is no reason why it should not proceed to 38 weeks or to term.

Complications

There are many complications which may occur in a twin pregnancy, some being minimal and of no real significance, but others are serious.

Nausea. There may be an increase in the amount of nausea during the first 3 months of pregnancy and this can continue beyond the end of the 14th week, when it is normally expected to stop.

Vomiting. Similarly, vomiting may be more severe in twin pregnancy and may continue beyond the 14th week.

Anaemia is particularly liable to occur in a twin pregnancy, especially iron deficiency and megaloblastic anaemia due to folic acid deficiency, since there are the demands of two babies instead of one.

Acute hydramnios may occur at the 24th week of pregnancy; this is indicative of a uniovular, or identical, twin pregnancy. The uterus may enlarge quite suddenly and dramatically, sufficient to cause considerable discomfort and even abdominal pain.

Pre-eclampsia is more liable to develop in twin pregnancies than in single pregnancy, but what is more important is that it is liable to develop at an earlier stage of pregnancy.

Oedema may occur partly due to pre-eclampsia but also because the presence of the large uterus causes some obstruction to the return of blood from the legs.

Excessive weight gain during a twin pregnancy is associated with pre-eclampsia, oedema and fluid retention.

Premature labour is more likely in a twin pregnancy than in a single one, partly because of the greater likelihood of pre-eclampsia and partly because of the over-distension of the uterus.

Abdominal discomfort and shortness of breath may be caused by the over-distended uterus as it pushes up against the diaphragm, especially when a woman is sitting down so that her uterus is compressed against her chest.

Piles and varicose veins are more frequent because of the increased level of circulating progesterone which causes dilatation of the blood vessels, and also because of the obstruction in circulation resulting from the over-distended uterus.

Heartburn and indigestion may also become frequent because of the pressure of the distended uterus on the stomach.

Very rarely one twin dies at an early stage of the pregnancy but the amount of hormone produced by the other is sufficient to prevent abortion and for the pregnancy to continue to term when one normal baby and one dead baby are delivered.

Care of twin pregnancy

A twin pregnancy requires special care for several reasons:

1 To avoid anaemia.
2 To avoid pre-eclampsia.
3 To prevent premature labour.
4 To alleviate many of the minor symptoms which can be annoying.

Anaemia can be prevented by making absolutely certain that good, satisfactory meals are eaten, and that iron and vitamin tablets are taken as instructed together with an extra supply of folic acid. The blood is tested more frequently than if only one baby is expected.

Pre-eclampsia can be prevented by rigid control of weight gain and by reducing salt intake. Throughout the whole of pregnancy weight gain should be no more than 13 kg and any swelling of the feet and ankles should be discussed with the doctor. Plenty of rest is also important.

Premature labour is avoided if the mother has no anaemia or pre-eclampsia and has rested sufficiently. Many obstetricians are recommending hospital rest for 3 or 4 weeks to help prevent prematurity. Many of the minor symptoms will not occur if care is taken to rest as much as possible and not to become anaemic, or to gain too much weight. Elastic supporting stockings may be necessary; some special cream or suppositories if haemorrhoids are troublesome, and an extra supply of alkali for severe indigestion or heartburn.

Labour

The most serious complication of twin labour is prematurity. If premature labour begins, intravenous salbutamol or other drugs may be given to prevent it continuing. Labour may be longer because the muscle fibres in the over-distended uterus are not as efficient as usual. This does not mean that the labour is harder or more difficult, but only that the uterine contractions are not so powerful.

Abnormal positions of one or both of the babies may give rise to complications. The commonest position for the babies is for each baby to arrive head first. However, breech presentation does occur in about 40 per cent of all the babies delivered as twins. Postpartum haemorrhage is more likely following a twin pregnancy because the overdistended uterus has difficulty in contracting and because the area of the placental site is twice as large as normal.

Twin labour must always be in hospital.

If premature labour persists, analgesic drugs may be given though epidural anaesthesia is preferable so that respiratory depressant drugs do not get to the premature baby. Care is taken in the delivery of the premature twins so that they are not injured. This may mean that the babies are delivered by forceps for their own protection, and an episiotomy is always performed. Resuscitation equipment and incubators are ready to receive the babies as soon as they are delivered. Twin babies who are premature have exactly the same chance of progressing normally as do single babies of the same maturity and weight. Twin babies, however, are very often smaller and so the risk is slightly greater.

If labour is at term the management of the first stage is the same as for a single pregnancy, except that two fetal hearts are listened to instead of one. The mother may require more sedation because labour may be slightly prolonged. The second stage of labour is conducted absolutely normally if the first baby is presenting head first as it usually does. He is delivered in the usual manner, the cord is clamped and divided and the uterus is immediately palpated to ascertain the position of the second baby. If the second twin is presenting head first then no action need be taken. Uterine contractions recommence after a few minutes and the head descends into the pelvis, the membranes are artificially ruptured and the baby is delivered quite naturally and normally. During delivery of the second baby an injection of ergometrine or syntometrine is given to ensure that the uterus contracts properly.

The third stage of labour is exactly the same as for a single pregnancy.

If the second baby is presenting as a breech, it is delivered as a breech baby. When the second baby is lying across the abdomen with neither the breech nor the head ready to engage in the pelvis, external cephalic version is usually attempted. The baby is gently rotated so that his head presents over the brim of the pelvis and the baby can then be delivered, head first, in the normal manner. Occasionally, however, if uterine contractions start almost immediately after the first baby has been delivered, it may be impossible to turn the second twin, and an internal version is performed. The woman is given a general anaesthetic and after appropriate cleaning and draping the membranes are artificially ruptured. One of the baby's feet is gently grasped between two fingers and the foot is gently pulled down through the cervix. This turns the baby into a breech presentation and gentle pulling on the foot results in delivery of the leg, then of the buttocks, following which the rest of the baby is delivered as a breech presentation. The third stage is normal.

Weight and size of babies

Uniovular, or identical, twins are seldom the same size because even in the uterus one twin becomes dominant and grows more quickly than his brother or sister. After delivery, however, the smaller twin soon makes up the lost ground and two or three months later they will both be the same weight. Binovular, or non-identical, twins are naturally of different sizes and the larger twin nearly always remains larger. The weight of the twin depends on many factors and if premature they will naturally be small. The average weight of twins delivered at term is approximately 2.5 kg which is perfectly normal.

The puerperium

A twin puerperium is not liable to complications that are any different from the puerperium after a single pregnancy, always accepting that a woman who has become anaemic or had a postpartum haemorrhage or a prolonged labour, which are more common in a twin pregnancy, is liable to develop anaemia or infection during the puerperium.

Care of twin babies does not differ in any way from that of a single baby. If the babies are premature their management is exactly the same as for any single baby weighing less than 2.5 kg. The decision as to whether the babies are to be breast-fed or bottle-fed is very much an individual problem and should be discussed with the midwife or doctor. As two babies have to be fed instead of one increased attention must be given to the feeding schedule and as much rest as possible taken.

31 Multiple Pregnancy

The development of three or more babies in the uterus as a multiple pregnancy is treated separately from twin pregnancy because the use of the fertility drug in recent years has greatly increased the number of multiple births. Several years ago the production of quads or even triplets was worthy of a place on the front page of the newspaper. Today, however, less than five or six babies do not attract much publicity. In any case, publicity in childbirth is something which most people would rather avoid.

Why do multiple births occur?

Multiple births occur for exactly the same reason as do twins. Either one egg divides into two or more at a very early stage in its development, or more than one egg is produced. When more than two babies are present both these factors can occur together. In triplets two babies may be identical, that is arising from a single ovum, and the third non-identical, arising from a completely different ovum. The non-identical baby has its own placenta whereas the identical babies share a placenta. It is possible for the three babies to be identical and to share a single placenta and for their circulations to mix as they do in identical twins.

The production of an ovum from each ovary, or the early division of the fertilized egg, seems to be an inherited factor since twinning tends to run in families. Until recently very little was known about ovulation and its mechanism; however, it is now known that the ovaries are stimulated to ovulate by follicle stimulating hormone which is produced normally by the pituitary gland. If follicle stimulating hormone is given artificially to a woman it will promote the formation of follicles within the ovaries and, however careful the doctors may be, the ovaries occasionally become hypersensitive and produce more than one follicle and more than one ovum. They may sometimes produce five, six or even more eggs, all of which may be fertilized, and hence a large number of fetuses begin to develop.

Development

Just as twins may develop at an unequal rate, so may triplets or quadruplets develop so that they are different sizes. It is also possible for one baby, or perhaps even more than one baby, to die in the uterus while the others continue to grow normally.

Multiple pregnancy is not usually diagnosed until after the 20th week when the uterus may be noticed to be particularly large for the dates and there may be an excessive amount of movement 'all over the place'. Nowadays it is possible to confirm the presence of a multiple pregnancy, which has been clinically suspected, by using an ultrasound scan. In nearly every instance the signs and symptoms all point to a twin pregnancy and there is general consternation when three or more babies are discovered. A multiple pregnancy is undoubtedly more difficult to handle than a single pregnancy. There is a greater incidence of pre-eclampsia, raised blood pressure, oedema, anaemia, excessive weight gain and, of course, premature labour, which is a hazard of every multiple pregnancy.

During a multiple pregnancy very special attention is paid to the blood count and to iron and vitamin supplements. Diet must be very carefully controlled to prevent too much gain in weight, but if quads are expected it is almost impossible to avoid an excessive weight gain unless the woman adheres very rigidly to a light diet containing protein, vegetables and fruit. Rest and relaxation are the other main factors that are of paramount importance in a multiple pregnancy. However difficult it may be, an adequate amount of rest is absolutely essential, since this is the only real way in which premature labour can be avoided.

One of the most troublesome things about a multiple pregnancy is the abdominal enlargement. The uterus and the abdomen get bigger and bigger so that not only does moving around tend to be clumsy, awkward and quite an effort, but breathing also becomes difficult. It is extremely difficult to breathe when lying down flat, so that even when she goes to sleep a woman should sit in a semi-upright position, propped up with plenty of pillows or against a special foam-rubber backrest.

Because multiple babies tend to be premature it is essential that everything should be prepared for their arrival long before the expected date. There is an old-fashioned superstition that too much preparation should not be made, but a certain amount of work and preparation must be undertaken. This is especially important since it may be necessary to go into hospital for rest when the abdomen becomes too uncomfortable or it is difficult to manage satisfactorily at home. When a woman is feeling particularly uncomfortable towards the end of a multiple pregnancy she may also suffer from fairly severe indigestion and heartburn and will find that small, frequent meals are a great help.

Labour

The main problem with triplets and quads is to keep them in the uterus sufficiently long to enable them to grow large enough. They invariably arrive early and labour is usually easy, smooth and straightforward. Labour begins in exactly the same way as any other labour. The first baby is nearly always a head presentation. It is usually much smaller than a single baby so that the cervix does not have so far to dilate, but as the over-distended uterus will not contract as efficiently as a uterus containing only one baby, labour is usually about the same length as a singleton labour. When the first baby has been delivered, uterine contractions cease for a short time. The doctor carefully ascertains the position of the second baby and may manoeuvre it into the correct position if it is lying obliquely or transversely. If contractions have not commenced in 10 or perhaps 20 minutes, he may very gently break the bag of water surrounding the baby so that its head can descend into the pelvis, and then with one or two expulsive contractions the next baby is delivered. The third baby follows in exactly the same way.

It is an almost invariable rule in the delivery of multiple pregnancies that an episiotomy is performed to protect the babies' heads and not because there is insufficient room. This is done under a local anaesthetic usually just as the first baby is being delivered.

The babies are always smaller than usual but the actual size is relatively unimportant. The really important factor is maturity. For instance, a 2.2 kg baby who is 37 weeks mature is much stronger and fitter and will get on much better than a 3.2 kg baby who is only 34 weeks mature. Therefore if babies are sufficiently mature, their size is of secondary importance. The babies are resuscitated in the normal manner and nearly always put into incubators. The practice of putting all small babies into incubators is rapidly increasing. This is because it is much easier to look after and nurse them in an incubator where their whole condition can be seen at a glance and where they are kept at the correct temperature and humidity, and not necessarily because they require oxygen or some other form of high-powered treatment.

32 Postnatal Clinic

The postnatal clinic, together with the postnatal examination, must be regarded as part and parcel of the overall management of a pregnancy. The anatomical and physiological changes that take place in the body throughout pregnancy do not return to normal at the moment of delivery, or even within the 7 or 10 days that are generally considered the usual resting period after confinement. It takes several days or weeks for some of the functions of the body to return to normal whereas other physiological processes may take up to 6 months. After discharge from hospital a return to normal life should be as gradual as possible and an adequate amount of rest and sleep must be taken, which is more easily said than done with a new baby in the house. No firm rules can be laid down regarding activity or progress after delivery, since these depend on how the pregnancy progressed and the ease of delivery. The doctor or midwife will readily offer instruction and advice on what can or should not be done, and will thereby help to plan your future activities.

An essential part of postnatal adjustment is attendance at the postnatal clinic. Its importance cannot be overemphasized. The postnatal clinic is usually visited 6 weeks after delivery. If the baby is delivered in hospital an appointment is given before discharge; if the baby is delivered at home the doctor arranges an appointment. This appointment should be delayed sufficiently to allow all uterine bleeding to cease but it should not coincide with the first menstrual period and should be sufficiently early for contraception to be discussed before the mother can possibly become pregnant again.

A baby delivered in hospital is examined by the paediatrician during his stay and before he leaves hospital. An appointment is made for the baby to attend the paediatric clinic, usually on the same day as the mother's postnatal appointment. A report is sent by the hospital to the general practitioner, so that he has full details of the confinement, of the health and condition of the baby, and how he is being fed, and can quickly help the mother with the many small points and problems that often arise as the days go by.

Every birth is notified to the local authority and a Community Health Visitor, who is a highly trained nurse with additional training in baby care, visits every mother at home, shortly after her return from hospital, to help either with practical matters concerning the care of the baby or any problems. She can also advise on the facilities offered by the local authority and on the ever recurring feeding problems of a new-born baby.

When a baby is delivered at home, the midwife and doctor are available to answer any questions, solve any problems that may arise, and give advice about the facilities provided by the local authority. The doctor will have examined the baby shortly after birth and usually re-examines him on about the 10th day. An appointment should be made to see the doctor for a postnatal examination 6 weeks after delivery, when he also examines the baby and will discuss any problems concerning his management or feeding.

Postnatal examination

After being checked into the clinic by a midwife or the clinic clerk, the woman undresses and produces a specimen of urine for routine testing. Her weight is recorded and if the rules regarding weight gain during pregnancy were obeyed she should have returned to her non-pregnant weight, although if she is still breast-feeding her baby an extra pound or two may be justifiable.

The value of a postnatal clinic falls roughly into three categories:

1 Immediate advice.
2 Medical examination.
3 Long-term advice.

Immediate advice

The history of the pregnancy and confinement are available at the postnatal clinic.

A woman now discusses with her doctor what has happened since she left hospital. He will enquire about the lochia and will want to know if it has been red or brown and for how long it remained so. If she is breast-feeding he will want to know if any vaginal bleeding persists; and if she is not breast-feeding he will ask if she has had an actual menstrual period. This may be difficult to distinguish but is usually recognizable by the relatively sudden onset of a heavier flow for no particular reason starting about the 28th day after delivery. A period does not occur during complete breast-feeding.

The doctor must know about any pelvic or perineal discomfort and the amount and colour of any vaginal discharge. If the mother had an episiotomy and stitches at the time of delivery she must tell the doctor if her perineum is comfortable. If she had haemorrhoids at any time during pregnancy or at the time of delivery, she should tell the doctor what has happened to them and if the bowel habit has returned to normal.

Anal fissure. One of the most unpleasant things that can happen to a woman after her delivery is the development of an anal fissure. This is a small crack in the skin just inside the margin of the anus, usually associated with piles, which is first noticed several days after delivery because opening the bowels is very painful. It causes intense pain at the time of defaecation, passes off after a few minutes and then causes no discomfort until the bowels are opened again. This should not be confused with the discomfort caused by piles or stitches. The pain at defaecation caused by an anal fissure often persists for many weeks if not treated. The treatment consists of passing a dilator, well lubricated with local anaesthetic ointment, into the anus twice daily; this soon cures the condition.

The bladder. Frequency of micturition is a common complaint during pregnancy, but shortly after delivery it should return to normal. However, in a number of women some frequency of micturition may continue for a few weeks after delivery and in others (especially after a difficult labour) there may be some difficulty in holding urine, especially on coughing or sneezing. Leakage of urine, known as stress incontinence, may begin during pregnancy and continue after delivery, or it may occur for the first time after delivery. Its cause is weakness of the muscles in the pelvic floor and the greater the leakage, the weaker the muscles. The pelvic floor returns to normal and the bladder symptoms are cured if postnatal exercises are regularly and consistently performed. This cannot be emphasized too strongly.

Weight. If extra weight has been put on during pregnancy it is very difficult to lose in the immediate postpartum period, but if a woman is overweight she should discuss an appropriate diet with the doctor, or arrangements can be made to see a dietician. There is only one way of losing weight and that is to restrict calorie, or food, intake. Usually, it is much better to do this voluntarily than to depend on so-called slimming pills or injections which artificially control the appetite.

Sexual intercourse is discussed, and if it has been resumed the doctor should be told of any pain, discomfort or lack of satisfaction.

If the postnatal examination is held in hospital, details of the baby's feeding are discussed with the paediatrician. Enquiries are made about the condition of the breasts, regardless of whether the mother is breast-feeding or not.

During the few days before attending the postnatal clinic it is wise to write a list of questions to ask the doctor or midwife, and take this to the clinic. It is surprising how quickly even the most obvious questions are frequently forgotten.

Menstruation

The majority of doctors and midwives will advise women that external sanitary towels should be used until after the end of the first period and certainly until all continuous vaginal loss has ceased. There is always a fear that internal tampons may predispose to infection, especially if they are not changed frequently, although this has never been proved. Internal tampons must not be used until permission is obtained from the doctor and generally, if everything is normal and the loss is minimal, there is no reason why a woman should not begin to use internal sanitary protection about 3 weeks after delivery.

Breast-feeding. Bleeding stops more quickly in the woman who is breast-feeding her baby than in a woman who is not. If lactation has been established and full lactation is being continued, the uterus returns to its normal size more quickly than in the absence of breast-feeding. Rapid involution results in an early cessation of blood loss but it is impossible to forecast the exact duration of loss or its amount. When a mother is breast-feeding her baby it is most unusual, once the normal lochia has ceased, for there to be any bleeding until breast-feeding is partially or completely discontinued. The process of lactation causes the normal menstrual periods to be suppressed. If weaning is sudden a period may come in only a few days or not until 4 weeks or even more have passed, and if weaning is slow a period may come before breast-feeding has completely stopped, or may not arrive until several weeks later.

When a mother is not breast-feeding uterine bleeding frequently continues for up to 4 weeks, and may even go on for as long as 6 weeks after delivery; some women finish after about 2 weeks. Probably the commonest pattern is for bleeding to continue as a brownish discharge, which occasionally becomes pinkish or bright red when work or exercise is increased, until about the 28th day after delivery, when the first actual period may begin. This period is usually longer and heavier than a normal period, frequently lasting 7 or more days, but when it ends there is no further postpartum loss.

The exact timing of the first period after delivery is completely uncertain, and varies according to whether breast-feeding is being undertaken or not. In the absence of breast-feeding the first period may occur on or about the 28th day, but it may be delayed until up to 3 or even 4 months after delivery. Many instances are recorded where women have not had their first period until up to 6 or even 9 months after delivery. If there is undue delay a doctor should certainly be consulted, but a delay is rarely of any significance.

Contraception

Contraception should be discussed with the doctor. This is explained in Chapter 43.

Medical examination

The medical examination at the postnatal clinic is a very straightforward routine examination. The urine is examined. The blood pressure is recorded and compared with the blood pressure at the commencement of pregnancy, noting any rise that happened during pregnancy. The breasts are examined to ensure either that lactation is proceeding satisfactorily or that the breasts have returned to normal following the suppression of lactation. The abdomen is examined to ensure that there is no abnormality and that the muscles of the abdominal wall have regained their strength. A woman may be asked to cross her hands on her chest and sit upright while the doctor gently lays a hand on the abdomen to make sure that the muscles are strong and that the separation between them in the mid-line has closed spontaneously. This separation, known as divarication, happens during pregnancy, especially in the presence of twin pregnancy, and can only be corrected by careful and religious postnatal exercising. The legs are examined for the presence of varicose veins. A specimen of blood may be taken to exclude anaemia.

An internal examination is performed, special care being taken to observe the presence of haemorrhoids or anal fissure. The perineum is examined to ensure that it has healed satisfactorily. Gentle vaginal examination confirms that internal stitches have healed satisfactorily, that the vaginal walls have returned to normal, that the cervix is healthy and that the uterus has involuted to its normal size, shape and position. No one would pretend that the reproductive pelvic organs have really returned to their normal physiological state as early as 6 weeks after delivery, but the majority of the changes have taken place and the experienced doctor soon knows if everything is satisfactory. A cervical smear may be taken for routine cytology.

If a diaphragm (Dutch cap) or intrauterine device (coil) is to be used as a contraceptive it is fitted at this postnatal examination.

Any other special points which have arisen during the course of pregnancy or upon which the doctor's advice is sought, or which may require examination, are dealt with at this time. If haemorrhoids, piles or pain on defaecation have been a feature of the pregnancy or delivery, the rectum will be examined.

Long-term advice

The majority of gynaecologists consider that the body does not return to its non-pregnant state until about 6 months after delivery or until 3 months after the cessation of lactation. A full discussion with the doctor about future health is an essential part of the postnatal visit. Iron and vitamins should be continued for at least 3 months after delivery, and longer if so instructed. A woman should discuss lactation with her doctor, how long she should continue to feed her baby and what she should do when she wants to discontinue breast-feeding. He will also advise on postnatal exercises, which should normally be continued for several months after delivery.

Sexual intercourse may be recommended as soon after delivery as desired. Obviously the presence of stitches in the perineum will make sexual intercourse painful or uncomfortable until the perineum has healed completely. It will usually heal in 5 or 6 days but the soreness will persist for 2 or 3 weeks and it is unwise to attempt intercourse before the soreness has disappeared. The majority of women will obviously wait until all vaginal bleeding has ceased before sexual intercourse is recommenced, but there is no medical reason why intercourse should be deferred until all bleeding has stopped. It may not be socially and aesthetically acceptable, but so far as is known no possible harm can ensue if intercourse begins while some vaginal bleeding is still present.

Pregnancy. It is extremely rare for a woman to ovulate sooner than 7 weeks after her confinement. It is, therefore, extremely rare for conception to occur before 8 weeks after delivery even if lactation is suppressed at the time of delivery (i.e. the mother is not breast-feeding) and no contraceptive precautions are taken. It is also extremely rare for ovulation to begin while full lactation is present. If the baby is fully breast-fed, therefore, pregnancy is most unlikely. As soon as the baby is weaned or a few breast-feeds are discontinued, ovulation may begin and if no contraceptive precautions are taken, the mother may become pregnant. It follows that pregnancy is extremely rare before the sixth week after delivery (or the attendance at the postnatal clinic) or during the course of a full lactation. A discussion on contraception is an essential part of the attendance at the postnatal clinic. Methods of contraception are discussed in Chapter 43.

High-level antibodies

On very rare occasions a woman has a very high level of antibodies in her blood during pregnancy. Antibodies are created in response to the introduction into the body of almost any foreign matter or bacteria, such as German measles or the Rhesus factor. The majority of tests performed in the laboratory for the presence of antibodies are done on a small amount of serum that has been taken from another patient who has developed a high level of antibodies against the same factor. Serum containing such a high level of antibody is comparatively rare and is difficult to obtain but is essential if the satisfactory testing of other patients is to continue. If, therefore, a woman has a high level of antibody to a particular factor in her blood, she may be asked after her confinement to donate some of her blood so that it can be used for testing other women. Please do not think that such a request is made because someone in a laboratory wants to do some experimental work. It is hoped that anyone will readily acquiesce to giving some blood for this purpose. The actual donation of blood is completely painless and is indeed very little different from the many blood tests that were taken during pregnancy.

Genetic counselling

Those who consider that they have a problem associated with heredity or genetics can obtain advice from their family doctor. The science of genetics, however, is very modern and highly specialized. If there is an unusual or complicated problem he will probably refer to a genetic specialist. For those who are particularly interested in heredity and genetics, *Human Heredity* by Dr C. O. Carter (Penguin, 1970) is to be recommended.

The science of genetics can offer considerable help to those who have some abnormality in their family or to anyone who has a handicapped baby and needs to know the possibility of the abnormality recurring. It is commonly believed that a marriage between related people (cousins or half-cousins) is more likely to produce congenital abnormality than that between people who are not related. A discussion with a genetic counsellor will help to make sure that the couple are not exposed to an undue risk. The most up-to-date and extensive information may be able to tell them the mathematical chances of any trait being handed to their child; whether a particular disease is capable of being transmitted or when precautions or preventive steps should be taken because an abnormality is possible or likely. Whether the couple accept the advice is up to them once they have been presented with the available facts. Even the genetic expert is not able to answer all questions, but he can at least guide and help many people to reach a sensible and constructive answer to their problems.

Queen Victoria inherited the genes of haemophilia, which is a rare disease that prevents clotting of blood. The disease itself does not occur in girls, although it is transmitted solely by the female. The disease only affects boys, but is not transmitted by them. This particular disease has caused considerable trouble in the families of Queen Victoria's ancestors but fortunately she transmitted only normal genes to Edward VII so that haemophilia died out of Britain's Royal Family. This example illustrates

445

how genetic counselling may help to explain the hereditary nature of some disease, or how it is possible in some circumstances to explain why a disease is likely or unlikely to be transmitted to the offspring of a particular couple.

Some genes are dominant and will prevail in any circumstances over their opposite number, while others are recessive and will not produce their particular trait unless matched by a similar gene in the other chromosome of its partner. This means that some inherited traits pass from father or mother to all the children, while others only occur on rare occasions. It also explains why some hereditary factors skip a generation, which may happen when a potentially dangerous but recessive gene is dominated by a dominant but otherwise normal gene.

Mental illness is frequently considered to be hereditary and, although this may be true in certain circumstances, it must be borne in mind that 1 in every 25 members of the population suffers from some sort of mental illness at some stage in their life and an even greater number suffer from a 'mental breakdown'. It therefore follows that some of the genes concerned with mental instability must be present in nearly every family. Epilepsy, on the other hand, contrary to popular belief, is not usually hereditary, save in less than 2 per cent of people who suffer from it. Consultation with a genetic expert may easily reassure a couple who are seriously worried because there is epilepsy in their families. Diabetes may, under certain circumstances, also be hereditary, although not all instances are, and an expert can give a couple a statistical answer as to the likelihood of their children developing diabetes, based on the incidence of diabetes in their families.

Mongolism, hydrocephaly, hare lip, cleft palate, club foot, are some of the conditions in which a genetic specialist may be of particular help. It is possible today for scientists to detect abnormalities in chromosomes. A small amount of blood is taken from a vein of both the woman and her husband and after the chromosomes in the white blood cells have been examined, a more accurate opinion can be given of the possibility of abnormality occurring in their offspring.

The science of genetics is one in which knowledge is accumulated only by slow and painstaking investigation. It is made up of a mixture of common sense, complex statistics and highly complicated scientific investigations.

33 Permanent Effects of Pregnancy

The majority of the permanent adverse effects of pregnancy are only caused because women do not take sufficient care of themselves during pregnancy or do not report abnormal symptoms to their medical advisers at the earliest available opportunity.

This chapter details some possible permanent effects of what would be considered by many people a normal pregnancy. At first sight this is a long and tragic list but in fact most effects can be avoided.

Weight

The control of weight gain during pregnancy has been stressed throughout this book. The weight gain associated with pregnancy alone is 18 lb and any weight gain in excess of this is caused in the majority of instances by the deposition of fat and subsequent retention of fluid. Retention of excess water is a very unusual phenomenon in a woman who has not already gained an excessive amount of weight. Excessive weight gain leads not only to problems during pregnancy itself but also to tiredness, lassitude and other minor difficulties after delivery.

It used to be said that every woman was allowed to gain one stone per baby. What a tragic comment. Any woman who has gained an excessive amount of weight in pregnancy and who finds herself to be overweight after delivery and puerperium should go on a reducing diet as soon as possible so that she returns to her original weight, regardless of whether she is breast-feeding or not. Many women who have gained extra weight argue that they will go on a diet when they have finished breast-feeding, but after 6 or 9 months they have become so used to the extra weight that they no longer have the desire to lose it or the determination to adhere to a diet. It is quite possible to continue satisfactory breast-feeding while gradually losing weight. A crash diet during breast-feeding is not recommended. Tablets or injections intended to make people lose weight are never advisable and are most definitely contra-indicated during breast-feeding.

Anaemia

Anaemia may be a permanent effect of pregnancy only if it started during the antenatal period or if there was excessive bleeding at delivery or shortly afterwards. Any woman who becomes anaemic during pregnancy is treated; if she loses too much blood following delivery this is corrected by a blood transfusion or by giving her extra iron. Apart from some rare diseases, therefore, there is no reason why anaemia should persist after the completion of the puerperium, and to ensure against it mothers should continue taking their iron pills for at least 3 months after delivery. If a woman considers she is anaemic she should report to her doctor for a blood test. In any event a blood test is nearly always taken at the postnatal clinic and any tendency to anaemia treated. One of the hazards of not attending the postnatal clinic is that such a tendency may never be discovered and will develop without treatment.

The bowels

Constipation is a relatively common symptom during pregnancy. A large number of women suffer from mild constipation before pregnancy and when they become pregnant this gets worse so that they resort to purgatives of ever-increasing strength. This is entirely unnecessary. The control of the bowels during pregnancy should be dealt with as far as possible by the adjustment of diet and fluid intake and if purgatives are required they should be used as sparingly as is necessary to open the bowels regularly once a day. As soon as a woman returns to her normal life and diet her bowels should return to normal. If she has developed the habit of taking a purgative during her pregnancy she must stop as soon as possible or she may find that she has to continue taking it for an indefinite period, or occasionally for the remainder of her life.

Skin

Pregnancy does not have any adverse effect on the skin except in women whose skin is normally dry and becomes excessively so during pregnancy. They must take special care to keep their skin well oiled throughout pregnancy and it will then return to normal afterwards. A certain coarseness may develop in the skin of women who gain an excessive amount of weight and do not lose it soon after delivery. Intertrigo, an inflammation in skin creases which occurs in women who are overweight, may be permanently present in those who fail to lose weight.

Hair

Quite a high percentage of women complain that their hair becomes unmanageable during pregnancy and occasionally thinner, more brittle and tends to break easily. Providing it is carefully looked after during pregnancy it will return to normal afterwards.

Teeth

The care of the teeth during pregnancy depends on the care of the gums and oral hygiene. Any dental caries that starts during pregnancy will progress afterwards until it has been satisfactorily treated. Gingivitis should be treated in pregnancy. It causes the gums to recede away from the teeth so that even after delivery the tender and vulnerable part of the tooth is exposed to the ordinary bacteria in the mouth.

Stretch marks

Stretch marks may occur on the breasts in early pregnancy as a result of rapid breast enlargement. On the rest of the body, however, stretch marks are the direct result of excess weight gain or of excessive uterine enlargement caused by the presence of too much water or a twin pregnancy. Once they have appeared they will never completely disappear. The marks on the breasts become pale quite quickly after delivery and almost invisible after several months. The marks on the abdomen and thighs, however, take much longer to disappear and always remain as silvery, thin tissue-paper-like scars. Once a stretch mark has occurred nothing further can be done about it although, if the abdomen has been particularly stretched by multiple pregnancy or excessive fluid, plastic repair can help.

Varicose veins

There is always a tendency for varicose veins to appear during pregnancy. They tend to disappear quite rapidly after delivery. During each subsequent pregnancy, however, the varicose veins gradually become worse and, each time, it takes the legs longer to return to normal, until eventually permanent varicosities remain. Although improvement may well continue for as long as 6 months any varicose veins still present 1 month after delivery are unlikely to disappear completely. Permanent varicose veins can be treated either by injections or by surgical removal.

Piles or haemorrhoids

Piles or haemorrhoids may develop during pregnancy but are far more likely to occur at the time of delivery. They may cause a great deal of pain or discomfort for the first few days of the puerperium. Piles usually settle down quite quickly after delivery but, rather like varicose veins, they tend to become worse with each subsequent pregnancy until eventually they become permanent. If the symptoms are still present at the time of the visit to the postnatal clinic they should be discussed with the doctor. Treatment for persistent piles is not usually advised until several months after delivery when they can usually be corrected by a simple injection.

The breasts

The breasts become larger and heavier during pregnancy and require more support since they do not contain any muscle tissue and, once allowed to sag or stretch, there is nothing that can be done to make them return to their former shape. Adequate support, therefore, throughout pregnancy and lactation is absolutely essential.

A great deal of argument rages concerning the effect of breast-feeding on the shape, texture and size of the breasts. While it is certainly true that some women can breast-feed their babies without any subsequent effect on their breasts, the majority do find that it results in permanent alteration in the shape and size of the breasts themselves.

The pigmentation that appears on the areola of the breasts at about the 14th week of pregnancy is usually permanent, unlike pigmentation that occurs elsewhere on the body during pregnancy.

Feet

If too much standing and tiredness are avoided and sensible shoes worn during pregnancy, there will be no permanent effect on the feet. The ligaments become softer during pregnancy and if the feet are not satisfactorily supported the arches may flatten with resulting foot strain, aching feet and eventually flat feet.

Posture

It is very difficult to maintain good posture throughout an entire pregnancy and unless particular care is taken to regain normal posture after delivery and to perform postnatal exercises, backache and other associated symptoms may eventually develop.

The bladder

The bladder is particularly vulnerable during pregnancy, and after delivery some women suffer from its inadequate control or actual lack of control resulting in leakage of urine on coughing, sneezing or on exercise. Frequency of micturition gradually subsides over a few days or a few weeks. Weakness or lack of control can only be restored by the religious performance of postnatal exercises, especially those that involve the muscles of the pelvic floor.

The perineum

If stitches have been inserted in the perineum they will be sore for a few days after delivery and the perineum will be tender for several weeks. Normally the discomfort gradually disappears but occasionally small areas of tenderness persist. These symptoms may make postnatal exercises uncomfortable so that they are not performed properly and the muscles do not return to normal. Weakness of the muscles of the perineum can have an effect on sexual intercourse. Any discomfort should be mentioned to the doctor at the postnatal clinic.

The cervix

After delivery the cervix resumes its normal shape but it is invariably a little larger and the canal slightly wider. The external cervical os, which before pregnancy was circular, becomes oval across the cervical entrance. This may be the only sign that a woman has had a baby when there have been no stitches or stretch marks.

Approximately 75 per cent of all pregnant women develop ulcers or erosions on the cervix and these are the main cause of the vaginal discharge which is normally present throughout pregnancy. About 50 per cent heal spontaneously. An internal examination is performed at the postnatal clinic both to take a cancer test from the cervix and to ensure that any erosions have healed. These occasionally become infected and the simple inflammation persists after delivery causing a continuous yellowish, sometimes offensive, vaginal discharge. If this happens then the cervical erosion ought to be treated. Although a persistent cervical erosion may not cause any symptoms, the doctor may decide that it is unlikely to heal on its own and should be treated.

The uterus

After a pregnancy the uterus is slightly larger even when completely involuted. This cannot be noticed but it does allow more room for an intrauterine contraceptive device which is therefore less likely to cause bleeding or pain in a woman who has had a baby than in one who has not.

Most doctors maintain that every uterus becomes mildly infected at the time of delivery but in a few instances the body is unable to deal with the infection and the uterus remains tender and bleeding continues after delivery for rather longer than usual. The lochia will be redder than normal and the first period heavier than usual. Occasionally periods continue to be heavy and prolonged over several months. The doctor should be consulted about these symptoms.

Periods

After having a baby a woman's menstrual pattern changes. The cycle usually becomes more regular. The pattern of the menstrual flow may change and the number of days may be different but the total loss should be about the same. A girl who suffered from the classic spasmodic type of pain on the first day of her period will find that this does not occur after she has had a baby. Unfortunately a few women do develop a slightly different kind of period pain after pregnancy.

34 The Normal Baby

The normal baby is one that is born at term, fully mature and is capable of leading an independent existence. Every infant must make certain essential adjustments after birth, for example to establish breathing, maintain a normal regular temperature and to start feeding and begin the actions of digestion. These and many other processes have, until birth, been performed almost automatically by the placenta, uterus and the mother.

The paediatrician

The paediatrician is a doctor who has specialized in looking after children, especially new-born babies. All doctors and midwives are trained to look after and take care of new-born babies, but the paediatrician has made this his speciality. There are no dividing lines between the relative responsibility of the doctor or midwife for a new-born baby: they work as a team in the best interests of both the mother and her baby. In some hospitals the paediatrician has charge of the medical supervision of the baby from the moment it is delivered, whereas in others he may only supervise the treatment of either premature or sick babies. The paediatrician, however, cannot possibly watch over the details of the day to day welfare of every baby. His usual role is to examine the new-born infant and then reassure the mother that everything is normal and satisfactory, as well as to supervise the investigation and treatment of any baby who requires special care or who becomes ill.

The first breath of life

The first breath of life is a most miraculous moment for everyone present at the birth. A healthy baby breathes very soon after birth.

Probably the most exciting experience you will ever have is hearing your own baby cry for the first time. It is one of the most astonishing feats of nature that a baby, who has been living inside the uterus, dependent on his mother for all his needs, should, when he emerges into the outside world, be capable of a completely independent existence. In the uterus he has relied upon the placenta to extract oxygen from his mother's bloodstream, but as soon as he is delivered he must immediately start to use his own lungs to obtain oxygen from the air. This extraordinary phenomenon in which a baby breathes for the first time is accompanied by extensive and rapid changes in his lungs as well as in the whole of his circulatory system.

While inside the uterus a baby is surrounded by amniotic fluid which he swallows and probably inhales. This inhalation probably helps to develop his lungs and respiratory passages. The baby's lungs are in a collapsed state while he is in the uterus, but the finer air passages contain a fluid secreted by the lungs themselves, containing a special material called surfactant. It is the presence of surfactant that enables the lungs to expand easily immediately after delivery.

This first breath on which the infant's life depends is brought about by the response of the respiratory centre in the brain to a variety of impulses that it receives from the physical contact that the body makes with its surroundings, and from the many changes that rapidly follow within the body itself as a result of the dramatic alteration in the baby's circulation. The exact cause of the initiation of respiration is not known. A newly delivered baby, however, is subjected to so many new and different stimuli such as a sudden fall in oxygen levels after the umbilical cord has been clamped, handling, change of temperature, noise, and suction of the mouth and nasal passages, that it is not surprising that these provoke him into breathing for the first time.

A baby does not breathe as soon as his mouth is delivered. An interval which varies from a few seconds to 2 or 3 minutes usually elapses between delivery of the mouth and the first breath which is taken by a spontaneous expansion of the chest, accompanied by a tightening of the diaphragm. This results in the inhalation of approximately 50 cm^3 of air, which immediately opens up all the respiratory passages in the lungs as far as the tiny tubes, or alveoli, which have been previously filled with surfactant and are therefore easily expanded. The oxygen from the air inhaled is absorbed into the bloodstream. The first breath is frequently followed by coughing or spluttering as the baby expels any remaining moisture from his trachea and bronchi. Any fluid left in the lungs will be rapidly absorbed into the bloodstream. Breathing is usually irregular for a short while and most babies will begin to cry as soon as regular breathing has been established.

Babies make strange noises and your baby will be no exception. He may remain quiet for long periods and then start to make the strange snuffling noise with each breath that is so characteristic of a young baby. Babies also cough, sneeze and hiccough all of which are part of their normal development. In fact a baby may sneeze quite often and at the slightest provocation. This should cause no concern because it seems to be a normal reaction and it does not mean that your baby has caught a cold.

The umbilical cord

When the baby is newly delivered the umbilical cord is wet and slippery and pulsating. As soon as the baby's air passages have been gently sucked out to remove mucus and liquid, and he has started to breathe properly, he is laid down on the bed and a clamp is placed on the umbilical cord about 15 cm from his umbilicus. Another clamp is placed on the cord about 7.5 cm closer to his mother, and the cord is then divided between these two clamps. The baby is now a separate entity, totally and completely free from the placenta and uterus that have looked after him so well for the previous nine months. There is some disagreement, but most authorities believe that the umbilical cord should be clamped and divided as soon as the baby is breathing normally.

Cry

A baby may make his first cry a few seconds or a few minutes after birth. Some new-born babies cry almost as soon as the head is delivered whereas others take several minutes and only cry after normal breathing has been established. The doctor or midwife recognize different types of cry, the characteristics of which vary according to the maturity and general condition of the baby. The first cry of some babies is more in the nature of a whimper, which after being repeated several times gradually assumes the full force of a normal cry. Other babies will cough and splutter for a few moments, or even minutes, before they cry normally.

A baby who is crying normally becomes so tense and angry and red that it is difficult to believe that this is a normal process. The child takes in a big breath, after which his whole body tenses, his face grimaces and becomes bright red, he opens his mouth wide and literally screams, demonstrating all the characteristics of supreme bad temper.

It is probably at this moment above all others that you would wish to console and cuddle your new baby to comfort him as well as to protect him from the things that have made him so angry. This is a normal response and a very natural one but your baby's anger is only assumed. The vigorous type of crying indicates a completely healthy baby and is welcome because not only does it ensure that the normal changes have taken place in the baby's circulation which are essential for his natural transformation from intrauterine life to existence in the outside world, but it also completes the full expansion of the lungs, ensures that his breathing will be normal and diminishes the chance of breathing difficulties or infection later on.

Colour

Do not expect a bright pink, freshly shampooed baby at the moment of your delivery.

While the baby is still inside the uterus his skin is a pale pink. At the time of delivery, however, most babies are a pinkish-blue or even purple colour. The bluish discoloration, known as cyanosis, is caused by a temporary lack of oxygen at the time of birth. It causes the baby no harm and as soon as he is breathing his colour will change to pink; first the lips, then the skin around the mouth, then the body to be followed very quickly by the rest of the face. The arms and legs do not change colour until after the body has become completely pink. Last of all are the hands and feet, which remain pale bluish colour for several minutes or occasionally several hours.

Very occasionally babies are born in a slightly shocked condition and their colour is pale, or even white. A baby that is white at the time of delivery is not necessarily ill but he will require more careful handling and more resuscitation than a baby that is blue or pink. The white colour is known as white asphyxia, and the blue colour as blue asphyxia.

The first sight of a new-born baby is a strange experience. The bluish, or even purple, colour of the skin is partly covered by a greasy white substance known as vernix. If you put your hand in a bowl of water and leave it there for 20 or 30 minutes the skin becomes white and sodden and slightly wrinkled. This change in the skin after immersion in water is frequently noticed after a day's washing. The baby who has been living in liquid for the past nine months requires some protection to prevent his skin becoming sodden and therefore damaged. The greasy vernix secreted by the skin is evenly spread over the whole body, and satisfactorily protects the skin and preserves it in its beautiful natural state. The presence of this vernix is one reason why a new-born baby is so slippery and difficult to handle.

The baby is also covered in very fine hair, known as lanugo. This very fine down-like hair covers the whole body except for the palms of the hands and the soles of the feet.

Very frequently a new-born baby will have some blood smeared over his face, head or body. It is quite normal for a small amount of bleeding to occur from the vagina as the head descends before it is delivered. An episiotomy, or even the smallest laceration of the perineum, also causes bleeding. Do not be alarmed, therefore, if you see that there is some blood on your baby as soon as he is delivered. Nurse will soon wipe it away and you will find that your baby is unharmed.

Tone

The tone of a new-born baby is the amount of muscular activity. A baby that is born limp and floppy has very little or no muscle tone, whereas one that is vigorous and tense has a high degree of tone. Most babies are born with a high degree of muscular tone and although they do not move excessively for the first few moments after delivery, their muscles can be felt to be tense and rigid. Muscle tone at delivery is quite important, for it is an indication of the baby's general condition. A baby with good tone is always a fit baby. A baby lacking in good tone may still be fit and healthy, although it may take him longer to establish normal breathing than a baby that has good tone. A limp, or flaccid, baby will require more resuscitation than normally.

Resuscitation

New-born babies sometimes require a certain amount of resuscitation immediately after their delivery. This is normally a very simple procedure designed to ensure that the upper air passages are freed from mucus and liquor and that the baby does not inhale liquor and mucus into his lungs when he takes his first breath.

As soon as a baby is delivered, therefore, he is tilted upside-down by the doctor or midwife holding his feet or ankles and placed on your tummy. An adult held upside-down will rapidly become very uncomfortable, or even unconscious, but the baby is quite used to it because he has in fact been lying with his head downwards in the uterus for the past several weeks, and he does not come to any harm. As soon as possible the midwife will suck the mucus and liquor out of his mouth, nose and throat, using a special pre-sterilized 'mucus extractor', one end of which she places in her mouth and the other end in the baby's mouth. As she sucks, mucus and liquor are aspirated from the baby's mouth and throat into a mucus trap. Aspiration, or suction, of the nostrils is one of the most vigorous stimulants of breathing and crying. After the baby has taken his first few breaths, or even his first cry, he usually coughs and splutters bringing up quite a lot of mucus and liquor that has previously been present in his lungs and trachea. This is also sucked out immediately.

If everything has been normal and you are fit and well you will be given your baby to cuddle as soon as he has been wrapped and before he is placed in his cot. This is a most exciting moment and should not be missed by any new mother. Do not be afraid to hold your baby tightly; you cannot hurt him. Do not be afraid to kiss your baby, touch him or hold his hand; you cannot harm him nor can you give him any infection. It may be difficult for you to appreciate that only a few seconds previously this baby was actually inside your abdomen and now he is a living, screaming infant, perfectly capable of an independent existence so long as you provide him with plenty of food, love and care.

Occasionally a baby takes a few minutes to breathe properly and even longer to begin crying normally. He is then wrapped up and placed in his cot with the head tilted slightly downwards. He is watched carefully by the midwife so that any mucus can be aspirated as soon as it appears in his mouth. A small amount of oxygen may be administered by means of a small face mask. The administration of oxygen to a new-born baby does not necessarily mean that there is anything wrong. It is considered to be more in the nature of helpful than essential and is a simple precaution to ensure that the baby receives an adequate supply of oxygen. The concentration of oxygen is certainly not sufficiently high to cause him any harm and in any event it is only continued for a few minutes. The great thing to realize is that this is a precautionary measure and does not mean that there is anything wrong with the baby.

Intubation

On very rare occasions babies have difficulty with their breathing and regular spontaneous respirations do not begin even after the mouth and throat have been aspirated. The baby then becomes pale and limp. Generally speaking the actual process of delivery, followed by the aspiration of the mouth and nose, provides sufficient stimulation to establish normal breathing in most babies. Further mild forms of stimulation are, however, practised by most people. These include massage of the back, movements of the arms, movements of the legs, gentle slapping of the back, flicking the soles of the feet and blowing on the abdomen and chest, but it is doubtful if they really exert any beneficial effect because they nearly always coincide with the onset of spontaneous breathing anyway.

Sometimes even these extra stimuli fail to provoke normal or satisfactory breathing. The baby becomes limp and gradually changes from the blue asphyxia of birth to a rather pale greyish colour. His tone is entirely limp. If after 5 minutes there is no indication that breathing is going to begin, then intubation is frequently performed. A special instrument, known as a laryngoscope, is introduced into the baby's mouth, with a small light at its far end, which enables the doctor to look down the baby's throat and see the vocal cords and the entrance into the trachea or lungs. A small tube is passed down the mouth and throat and in between the vocal cords into the trachea. The laryngoscope is then withdrawn and artificial respiration commenced either by breathing down the tube or connecting it to a special low pressure supply of oxygen. By this means the baby is supplied with oxygen until normal breathing begins. The tube is then removed from the throat and shortly afterwards the baby will begin to cry. The delay in normal spontaneous breathing varies but so long as the baby is adequately supplied with oxygen he will come to no harm.

Artificial respiration

If there are no facilities for intubation various methods of artificial respiration may be performed on the baby, such as movements of his arms, gradual squeezing of his chest or flexing of his body. All these methods cause expansion and contraction of the rib cage and therefore the suction of air into the lungs followed by its expulsion. They are satisfactory although not as efficient as intubation.

Artificial respiration may also be achieved by a special mask which fits over the baby's nose and mouth and is connected to a low pressure supply of oxygen. The pressure of oxygen and the amount allowed into the baby's lungs are very carefully controlled.

Mouth-to-mouth breathing ('kiss of life')

Another method of maintaining a good oxygen supply to the baby is by mouth-to-mouth respiration. This is now a well recognized method of resuscitation in adults as well as new-born babies. The baby's nose and mouth should be covered by a thin piece of gauze and then the midwife covers the nose and mouth with her own lips and gently breathes into the baby's mouth. At the same time she watches the baby's chest expanding as air enters the lungs. Mouth-to-mouth resuscitation of a baby is a highly skilled procedure because only a small amount of air is required at a relatively low pressure to expand the small lungs. Repeated breaths will be needed to maintain a good oxygen supply until normal breathing begins.

All these methods of artificial respiration are only very rarely required and then only when a baby fails to breathe spontaneously.

Physical adjustment

Temperature

When your baby is delivered his temperature will be exactly the same as yours, that is approximately 98°F (36.6°C). It is most important that your baby should not be allowed to become cold. You yourself know how easily you become cold if you stand about without drying yourself after getting out of the bath, especially if you happen to be standing in a draught or cold wind. Exactly the same applies to your baby, only more so. After birth a baby is wet as well as greasy and if the room is cold, or if there is a draught, his temperature will drop rapidly as the water evaporates quickly from his skin. Everyone looking after you will be very conscious that your baby should not be allowed to get cold and it is for this reason that the baby is wrapped in a clean or sterile sheet as soon as the cord has been divided. You will notice that the wrapping is placed in such a way that his arms and legs, and even his head, are included, so that only his face is visible. You must not be surprised, therefore, when you are shown your baby for the first time if the face is all that you can see, because the midwife will have carefully wrapped him to prevent any loss of heat. You may ask to see your baby's head as well as his arms and body, but do not ask to have your baby entirely exposed until after he has had a short while to adapt himself to his new surroundings.

The speed with which a new-born baby loses heat and therefore lowers his temperature is one of the main principles governing his management shortly after he is born. The fact that a baby has great difficulty in raising his temperature to normal once it has been allowed to fall is also of paramount importance. It is for this reason that the delivery room should be warm (about 72°F, 22°C), and that the baby is placed in a cot that has been previously warmed. A cold baby is not a well baby. A cold baby is lethargic, he does not breathe well, does not cry well and requires frequent observation until his temperature has been gradually raised to normal. If an incubator is available he can be placed in it until his temperature returns to normal.

Many hospital maternity units place each new-born into an incubator for the first few hours after delivery. This is entirely precautionary because it enables the nurse to observe the baby more closely in a carefully controlled environment where the temperature and humidity are meticulously regulated. Oxygen can also be administered if this is necessary.

Regulation of heat

A new baby not only loses heat rapidly but has great difficulty in maintaining his body temperature. This is one of the three main principles governing the care of the new-born baby:

1 Control of temperature.
2 Freedom from infection.
3 Satisfactory food intake.

The management of a new-born baby must include careful control of his temperature because even after it has stabilized he still requires a fairly even environment so that he can maintain a normal temperature. For this reason the nursery should be kept warm—approximately 72°F (22°C)—and the baby should be wrapped in warm clothes but not sufficient to make him sweat or perspire. He should not lie naked for longer than is necessary, and should be bathed in warm water and dried immediately afterwards.

Babies who become cold are liable to develop infections; they do not feed satisfactorily and they therefore lose weight. Babies who are overheated perspire and develop sweat rashes; they become irritable and do not feed properly. Generally speaking, overheating a baby is almost as bad as allowing him to become cold.

Pulse rate

The speed of a baby's heart inside the uterus varies between 120 and 160 beats per minute in normal conditions. The average rate is approximately 140 and although changes do occur it remains remarkably constant. At the moment of delivery it is about 120. The rate gradually falls until the first breath is taken. This usually happens before the pulse has fallen below 100. The baby's heart rate remains between 110 and 120 for the first 6 to 10 hours of life. The pulse gradually slows during the first 3 or 4 days to between 80 and 100 beats per minute, where it stays for the first few months of life.

Respiration

A new baby, having established normal respiration, cries quite violently for a period of time which may last from 5 minutes to half an hour and this is perfectly normal. When the baby stops crying he usually settles down and goes to sleep and it is then that his normal breathing pattern begins. The rate of breathing is from 40 to 50 breaths per minute with an occasional deep sighing breath. If your baby happens to be in an incubator you will notice that most of the effort in breathing is abdominal and not in the chest. The abdomen moves up and down with each breath and the chest moves relatively little.

If there is any difficulty in breathing, or if any chest infection occurs, then the rate of breathing will increase to above 60. Each breath becomes more shallow and the baby appears to be having difficulty in breathing.

An 'expiratory grunt' is a small grunting noise which a baby makes as he breathes out. It is common and is a normal phenomenon in many babies for the first hour or two of life but if it continues beyond this period of time it may indicate some difficulty in breathing. An expiratory grunt is particularly common in premature babies.

Reaction to infection

A new-born baby has a very limited resistance to infection, and therefore has to be protected from all types of infection. This is one of the reasons why delivery is conducted under aseptic conditions and why such great care is taken to see that no infection enters the baby at the time of resuscitation and during the first few hours of life. Anyone who has a cold or other type of infection should not be allowed near a new-born baby. While clothes need not be sterile they should be freshly washed and clean. If the baby is breast-fed the breasts and nipples should be washed before feeding, and if the baby is bottle-fed the bottle and teats, as well as the milk, must be sterilized. Care should be taken during bathing or washing the baby to make sure that no infection is introduced by means of dirty water or infected hands. The umbilical cord and the umbilicus need special attention until the cord is detached and the umbilicus is clean and dry. Antibiotics in carefully calculated doses can be administered to a new-born baby quite safely to combat any infection which may develop.

All new-born babies have some immunity transferred to them from their mothers while they are still in the uterus. Antibodies against certain diseases in the mother's circulation cross the placenta to confer a temporary immunity from their appropriate diseases which will last for a few months. This is the reason why a young baby rarely develops ordinary infectious diseases from which his mother has suffered and to which she has gained an immunity, such as measles or German measles. The efficiency of this secondary immunity, however, gradually diminishes as the antibodies are destroyed and because the infant has no means of replacing them unless or until he eventually develops the appropriate disease himself.

Changes in the circulation at birth

Changes which occur in the baby's circulation at birth are the result of expansion of the chest. While in the uterus the fetus obtains oxygen and nutrition from the mother via the complicated mechanism of the umbilical cord and the waste products are excreted in the same way. The special type of fetal circulation which is needed to meet the requirements of the fetus while still in the uterus must be capable of sudden and dramatic

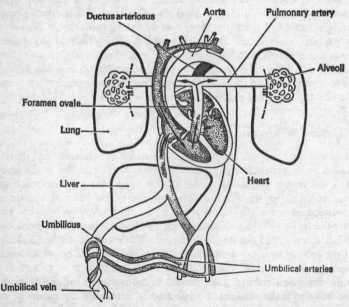

Fig 36   The baby's circulation after birth

change at the moment of birth because when the baby becomes an independent individual his source of oxygen changes completely. The heart is mature enough to function satisfactorily but certain alterations must occur at the moment of birth to convert the fetal circulation into the adult type of circulation.

The mechanism of the first breath of life is the result of an elastic recoil in the lungs causing the baby to suck in air and then to cough or breathe out. When this happens the lungs expand, the blood supply to the lungs is increased so that the blood which has been passing through a temporary structure, the ductus arteriosis, to the main artery in the body, the aorta, now flows through the pulmonary arteries to the lungs where it can obtain oxygen. The increased flow of blood to the lungs together with chest expansion alters the pressures in the heart chambers and this is responsible for closing the temporary hole in the heart, the foramen ovale. The adult type of circulation is now established. The ductus arteriosus and the foramen ovale close completely. If either of them persist it forms a congenital abnormality in the heart.

Digestion

The normal infant is able to feed within a few moments of birth. The sucking reflex is highly developed at this stage and the infant will readily suck at any object placed in the mouth. No active sign of hunger is apparent within the first few days of life. The infant is able to breathe between each act of swallowing and may even swallow a certain amount of air with each feed.

Feeds are swallowed and passed down into the stomach where the process of digestion begins and is continued throughout the intestines. Occasional regurgitation occurs after feeds and if this is small in amount it may be regarded as normal.

The best and most easily digested nutrient for the baby is breast milk. Colostrum, a yellow-coloured fluid, is secreted by the breasts in late pregnancy and for the first 2 or 3 days following the birth of the baby and is then replaced by milk. Breast milk is suited to the baby's needs and digestion.

Examination of the new-born baby

Immediately after delivery and as soon as the baby is breathing and crying satisfactorily he is placed in his cot so that attention can be devoted to the mother during the completion of the third stage of labour. The baby usually continues to cry, which is a sign that he is doing well, and if he is quiet frequent glances ensure that everything is all right. After the completion of labour about half an hour will be required while the mother is bathed or washed, tidied up, puts on a clean nightdress and combs her hair. It is most important that you should make yourself presentable as soon as possible after delivery and it is surprising what a clean nightie does for the morale. As soon as you have been cleaned and tidied the midwife will turn her attention to your baby. She will unwrap the clothes while still leaving him in his cot and inspect him for any evidence of congenital abnormality.

A preliminary inspection of a baby takes only a few seconds in the hands of the experienced midwife or doctor. It is done routinely and so automatically that unless you are very observant you may not even notice that it has been undertaken. Such a rapid examination done by a skilled person might even be performed at the time the umbilical cord is divided and before the baby is wrapped up and put in his cot, so that when you are told that your baby is normal you can rest assured that a very rapid and yet thorough examination has already been undertaken.

The midwife will examine his head and will show you the degree of 'moulding'.

Moulding is caused by the gentle pressure exerted by the uterus and the vaginal walls upon the baby's head as it passes through the pelvis during labour. The pressure causes the bones of the skull to overlap in such a way that the actual diameter of the head is diminished by as much as 1 cm and this gives it an elongated and abnormal appearance. This is a normal phenomenon and your baby's head will return to its normal round shape within 24 to 48 hours of delivery. Some babies' heads are moulded more than others and the degree of moulding usually varies with the length of labour, being more noticeable when the labour is long and more difficult. It must be emphasized that moulding does not damage the baby's head, his brain or his intellect. Babies that are delivered by Caesarean section or as breech deliveries do not have any skull moulding and their heads are normal and round in appearance.

Caput succedaneum. A caput succedaneum is a swelling of the scalp caused by pressure of the baby's head on the dilating cervix during the first stage of labour. The caput is situated on one side and varies in size according to the duration of labour. A caput is quite normal and does not indicate any abnormality. It is caused by a collection of fluid within the layers of the scalp and gradually disappears in the first 12 to 24 hours after delivery.

Cephalhaematoma. A cephalhaematoma may be present on one side of a baby's head, or very occasionally on both sides. It may be recognized as a fairly large, circular, fluctuating, cyst-like swelling measuring about 4 cm in diameter and about 1 cm thick. It is nearly always the result of a rather difficult labour and is caused by pressure of the baby's head against the posterior part of the mother's pelvis. It is in actual fact a collection of blood beneath the scalp, rather like a large bruise. A cephalhaematoma does not require any treatment. The cystic swelling gradually reduces in size as the blood contained within it is slowly absorbed. The process of absorption may take up to 6 months, but when complete it will leave a perfectly normal head.

Examination of the baby by the paediatrician

There is seldom anything wrong with a baby who is a good colour and who is crying normally. If the preliminary examination by the midwife reveals any abnormality the house surgeon or paediatrician will be notified or the doctor will be informed if the confinement is at home.

If you have had your baby in hospital he will be seen and examined by the doctor, usually the paediatrician, within 24 hours of delivery or before if indicated. The paediatrician has a similar routine in his examination to that of the midwife. He inspects the head and examines it for the presence of moulding, for caput and for cephalhaematoma. He feels the skull bones and the fontanelles (soft spots). He examines the ears and the baby's eyes. The nose is inspected and the mouth opened by gentle pressure on the chin. The gums and palate are inspected for any evidence of congenital abnormality. The neck is examined for any cysts or swellings.

Examination of the chest includes listening to the baby's heart with a stethoscope and listening to the lungs to make sure that they are properly expanded and working normally. Many babies have a heart murmur for the first 2 or 3 days of life. If someone happens to mention that your baby does have a murmur in his heart, do not be worried because the vast majority disappear quite spontaneously and very quickly.

Abdominal examination includes palpation of the liver and spleen, both of which are slightly enlarged in the new-born baby, as well as an inspection to make sure no ruptures are present. If the child is male the scrotum is inspected to see if the testicles have descended and the penis examined to make sure that the urinary passage is normal and to decide whether circumcision is medically advisable. If the child is female the vulva is inspected and the amount of white mucus at the vaginal entrance noted.

The pulsation of the blood vessels is felt in the groins. The legs are especially tested to ensure that there is no congenital dislocation of the hip. Examination of the feet excludes any form of club foot abnormality and examination of the arms excludes any form of paralysis. Finally the baby is turned over and the spine and anus inspected. The paediatrician also notes the normal reflexes of the baby.

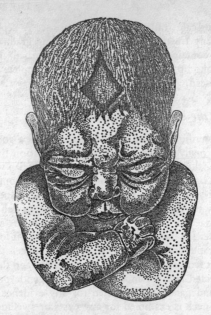

Fig. 37 A baby's head showing the position of the anterior fontanelle in the top of the skull

Weight

The average weight of a baby at the time of birth is 7 lb (3.3 kg) but there are large variations. A loss in weight usually takes place during the first 3 or 4 days following birth due to the fact that feeding is not established and that the contents of the bowels have been expelled. The weight loss at this time is usually about 4 to 6 oz (120–180 g). One or two days of stable weight is followed on the sixth day by a weight increase which averages 6 oz (180 g) per week.

Length

The average length of the baby at term is 19 to 20 in (49.5–52 cm), but once more large variations are sometimes seen.

The reflexes

The new-born infant has a large number of normal reflexes. Certain movements are unmistakably protective in function. For example the eyelids close tightly when touched and if the nose of the new-born baby is lightly held between the finger and thumb he tries to remove them by striking out with his hands. Only a few reflexes, however, are really important:

The grasp reflex. If pressure is applied to the palm of a baby's hand he will automatically clench his fist. In the majority of babies this reflex is so powerful that they can be lifted by their fingers if an adult's thumbs are pressed gently into the baby's palms.

The sucking reflex. Pressure in the baby's mouth, on the palate just inside the upper margin of the gum, provokes quite strong and rapid sucking which continues for some time.

The Moro reflex. The Moro reflex is most frequently used as a test of a baby's general condition and the normality of his central nervous system. The baby is undressed and left lying quietly on his back. After a few moments a loud noise, such as a handclap close to the baby, or any violent movement causes him to immediately throw out his legs and arms with the fingers extended, then slowly to draw his arms into his body with the fingers clenched and to bend his knees up to his abdomen—rather as though he were stretching out to grasp something and then hugging it towards himself. Both sides of the baby's body respond simultaneously and equally.

The swallowing reflex is present from birth and swallowing food is automatic for the normal infant.

The rooting reflex. If the baby's jaw is touched he opens his mouth for food and turns his head in the same direction, as he would react by searching for his mother's breast.

The walking reflex. When the infant is held under the arms and his feet touch a firm surface he shows active walking movements.

The umbilical cord

The umbilical cord gradually shrivels up and separates within the first 5 to 7 days of life. The cord can easily become infected and must be kept clean and dry, for which daily care is essential. Separation can best be achieved by cleansing the umbilical area with spirit and dusting with a sterile antiseptic cord powder. Binders should not be used as they only restrict breathing and prevent the cord from drying. A cord kept damp by a binder may become more easily infected. The umbilicus is treated in the same way after the cord has shrivelled and separated because there is still a slight risk of infection.

The skin

The skin of a new-born baby is soft, delicate and can be easily damaged It should always be kept clean and dry Daily bathing with a good reliable baby soap is all that is necessary, paying particular attention to the deep folds under the chin, the arms and in the groin. These areas in particular should be thoroughly dried. The area surrounding the buttocks should be protected by zinc and castor oil ointment or petroleum jelly.

Quite a large number of maternity hospitals do not bath babies every day. A baby is bathed, washed, cleaned and dried at birth. Thereafter the skin is oiled or cleansed once or twice daily. Water is used only on the nappy area to remove stains.

The nails

At birth the nails in the normal mature infant reach to the ends of the fingers. They are very soft and easily damaged if the baby grasps anything rough. They become quite firm in 2 to 3 days when the baby may scratch his face, but he will never damage or injure his eyes. It is difficult and unnecessary to cut a new-born baby's nails. If he scratches his face the edges of the nails can be removed and his hands should be kept in cotton mittens. Infection of the nail folds may be caused by sucking the fingers but this can also be prevented by putting cotton mittens on his hands for a few days.

The eyes

Examination of the eyes of a new-born baby is a highly skilled task. The eyelids should never be forcefully separated and although expert paediatricians can do this gently, the easiest way of making a baby open his eyes is to hold him above your head so that he is looking down at you and you are looking up into his face. His eyes will then open.

All babies are born with blue eyes, or to be more precise the white part of the eye of a new-born baby is white, the iris is blue and the pupil is black. If a baby is going to develop brown eyes the blue gradually changes to brown, sometimes within a few hours of birth. Generally speaking, however, the change does not begin until after a few days or even a few weeks. Both eyes usually change colour simultaneously.

Haemorrhages. There are occasionally small haemorrhages in a baby's eye at birth and these can be recognized as reddish triangular marks in the white part of the eye. The base of the triangle is towards the iris and the point towards the outer part of the eye. Another type of haemorrhage appears in the outer part of the eye and seems to spread from the back of the eye towards the pupil. These bruises are the result of delivery, do not require any treatment and disappear spontaneously. They do not cause any damage to the eye or the baby's sight.

The pupils. The pupil is the black part in the centre of the eye. It is circular and should be equal in both eyes. In the baby's eyes the pupils are usually quite widely open, so that the baby appears to have dark eyes. If a light is shone into his eyes the pupils contract until they become quite small. Both pupils contract equally and, when the light is removed, they will enlarge again equally and together.

The sight. A new-born baby cannot see. He can differentiate light from dark. He responds to a bright light shone in his eyes, but this should only be done by the paediatrician when examining him. It is several weeks before a baby is aware of light and dark colours and of moving objects, and it is several months before he responds to seeing things without hearing them.

New-born babies often appear to be cross-eyed purely because they are unable to focus on anything and their eyes wander wherever the muscles wish them to go. Gradually, as the eyes begin to focus and the child begins to see, they line up and become parallel, although the baby's ability to do this is at first limited to only a few seconds after which the eyes again diverge and become cross-eyed. Complete co-ordination of the eyes may not develop until after 6 or even 12 months.

Tears. The tear gland which produces a fluid that lubricates the eye, is buried deep beneath the outer part of the upper eyelid. Under normal circumstances this fluid is carried away from the eye in a duct known as the tear duct which opens at the inner edge of the eye and runs downwards and inwards to open into the back of the nose. If produced in excess, the liquid flows over the edge of the eyes as tears. In a new-born baby the tear duct successfully carries away any excessive amount of tear solution which might be produced by his tear glands. It is uncommon for a young baby to produce tears, even when he is crying. Tears do not form until a baby is about 4 months old and no matter how much a baby may cry in early life no tears will be present unless the tear duct is temporarily blocked.

Breathing

Once a baby is breathing satisfactorily after his delivery he continues to breathe fairly regularly at the rate of about 40 breaths per minute for the first 1 or 2 days. The rate of breathing then falls to about 25 breaths per minute. A child who is resting or sleeping breathes quietly and evenly through his nose and continues to do so while suckling, whether it is at the breast or bottle. Any obstruction of the nose may therefore cause a baby distress during feeding.

Babies do not continue to breathe evenly and smoothly throughout 24 hours of each day. They make marvellous snuffling, grunting and simpering noises which indicate that they are breathing satisfactorily and also arouse the greatest depth of parental instinct and emotion.

Sneezing

New-born babies and young babies frequently sneeze, some more than others. The reason for this is not known but is probably to clear the air passages of the mouth and nose. It does not mean the baby has a cold.

Crying

All babies may have a good cry once every day. There is no golden rule as to how long a baby should cry but he should not be allowed to cry for such a long time that he becomes too tired to take his food. A few minutes of good hearty screaming never did any child any harm.

Hearing

There is no doubt that most new-born babies are able to hear. They respond to sudden noises such as clapping and this is one way of provoking the Moro reflex.

Most babies can certainly hear before they can see and it is probably true that babies can hear noises of low tone before they hear noises of a high tone and therefore are more likely to respond to their father's voice before recognizing their mother's. This is often a great source of amusement to Dad and frustration to Mum. A baby will certainly recognize his mother's voice long before he can visually distinguish her features.

A baby's ears do not need any special cleaning and on no account should cleaning sticks or other objects be pushed into them.

Birthmarks and naevi

Most birthmarks consist of an abnormal collection of small blood vessels just underneath the skin. They may be present on any part of the baby and while the majority of them disappear, some remain and others even increase in size. There are four main types of naevi, or birthmarks.

Temporary birthmarks are mild discolorations of the skin, usually present on the face and neck and noticed shortly after birth. They are most frequent around the eyes, especially on the upper eyelids, and around the nose and the upper lip. They can be recognized as temporary if the baby also has a similar reddish mark on the back of his neck just below the hairline. These will certainly disappear within a few days.

Port-wine stains are brightish red or even purple marks found anywhere on the body, frequently on the face and neck. They may occasionally be quite extensive and even unsightly and the skin is usually of different texture. This type of birthmark does not usually disappear and may even increase in size. It can sometimes be removed by special treatment.

Spider naevi are relatively small marks that appear shortly after birth in the form of a network or cobweb of dilated vessels. They generally disappear after the end of the first or second year.

Pigmented naevi are brownish patches occurring anywhere on the body. They are usually pale and nearly always enlarge as the child grows but seldom become any darker. They are not unsightly.

The treatment of a naevus depends upon its nature as well as its situation. Transient, or temporary, naevi obviously disappear on their own. Spider naevi may respond to special treatment.

The stool

The first stool passed by a baby is meconium, the sticky dark green substance present in his intestine. This is passed during the first 2 days of life. When feeding begins the colour and character of the stools change from dark green to greenish brown and then to a yellowish brown. After the fourth day there may be four or five motions each day, and they are yellow and semi-solid in character. The stools should be watched carefully as they give an important indication of the baby's health. Blood in the stools is abnormal and should be reported to the doctor even though it may be due to nothing more serious than constipation.

35 Prematurity

By medical definition a premature baby is one that is delivered before 37 completed weeks of gestation. Previously the definition of prematurity was based on the weight of the infant, namely any infant less than 2.5 kg. Weight, however, does not always accurately reflect the duration of pregnancy. A diabetic baby, for example, may be quite heavy even at 34 weeks of gestation and suffer all the problems of a premature baby. A growth-retarded baby, on the other hand, may only weigh 2 kg at 38 weeks and not suffer the same problems as a premature baby of only 2 kg.

In the United Kingdom each year about 7 per cent of all pregnancies end in premature delivery. Over two thirds of these occur in babies who are older than 34 weeks and generally weigh about 2.5 kg or more. It is the other third of babies which poses the great problems for paediatricians and obstetricians; these babies are responsible for about 70 per cent of all perinatal deaths, and in fact half the babies born under 1 kg in weight will die.

The dramatic improvement in neonatal mortality in the last ten years is not simply through better antenatal care and socio-economic conditions, but it is a reflection of the great advances made in caring for very small babies. Neonatal intensive care units are established in many parts of the country and act as regional centres for large areas of the population.

The main causes of prematurity are not understood. In 40 per cent of cases, there is no obvious maternal or fetal cause. Socio-economic conditions, however, play an important role. Premature delivery is more common in the lower income groups than in the professional and salaried classes. Other related factors are inadequate or lack of antenatal care, poor living standards, anaemia and pregnancy in the unsupported woman. The woman less than 20 years, who is single, smokes heavily, is undernourished and less than 50 kg in weight, or who must work at a heavy job throughout her pregnancy, is particularly at risk.

Complications of pregnancy may lead to premature delivery of the baby, simply because continued intrauterine existence would be a greater risk to the baby. This group of women includes those who are diabetic, have renal diseases or hypertension or pre-eclampsia, Rhesus disease or ante-partum haemorrhage.

Over-distension of the uterus may precipitate premature labour, and in fact 50 per cent of twin pregnancies deliver before 36 weeks. Polyhydramnios and uterine abnormalities also predispose to premature delivery. Previous damage to the cervix from a termination of pregnancy may weaken the cervical fibres so that they begin to dilate earlier than normal.

Finally, there is a group of women who seem to rupture their membranes prematurely, and in most cases delivery follows. It has been suggested that these women have some inherent weakness of the amniotic membranes, or that a little focus of infection sets up inside the cervix and weakens the membranes at that point. In some women the uterus appears unusually irritable throughout pregnancy, and any infection, especially a urinary tract infection, can precipitate labour.

Premature labour usually begins without any previous warning, the first sign being either premature rupture of the membranes, the onset of uterine contractions or some vaginal bleeding. Premature labour frequently occurs in what has been an otherwise normal pregnancy in a woman who is pregnant for the first time. Once labour has started, there is little that can be done, or indeed probably little that should be done, to stop its progress. However, in about 10 per cent of cases there is a place for inhibiting labour.

One of the problems in the management of a woman who complains of painful contractions before term is to diagnose whether she is really in labour or not. If the cervix is thin (effaced) and dilated to more than 3 cm, the diagnosis is very clear, and it is unlikely that any drugs will stop the progress of labour. However, in the woman whose membranes are intact, and whose cervix is undilated, strict bed rest and an injection of pethidine or Omnopon may well be all that is required to stop the contractions.

Most obstetricians feel that with a fetus less than 34 weeks in gestation, or 1.5 kg in size, very active attempts to stop labour should be made if contractions persist. Most drugs that do this work by relaxing the uterus and need to be given intravenously. The commonest ones are Salbutamol or ritodrine, but even alcohol has been used! Unfortunately the woman tended to become intoxicated unpleasantly with alcohol, and it is no longer used. Salbutamol can cause the mother's heart to race and make her feel very shaky, but it is usually safe for the fetus. Once contractions have stopped, the drip can be taken down and tablets given instead.

Very small babies have immature lungs and lack a substance called surfactant which coats the lungs and prevents them collapsing when the baby breathes out. Breathing difficulty, or respiratory distress, is a major cause of death in very tiny babies. In the early 1970s it was shown that lung maturity could be improved and respiratory distress decreased, if steroids were given to the mother some 24 to 48 hours before the birth of a premature baby. In many hospitals injections of steroids are given if the baby is less than 34 weeks old.

Sometimes it is not possible to stop labour continuing, or to do so would put the mother's life at risk, for example, a woman with very high blood pressure. Where possible, and safe for mother and child, transfer to a hospital with a neonatal intensive care unit is organized. In this way the baby has the best possible paediatric care as soon as he is born.

If labour progresses it is usually shorter and easier than labour at term. The skull of the premature baby is softer than that of a mature baby as the skull bones have not completely developed, with the result that the premature skull is liable to injury at the time of delivery. It is, therefore, common practice to perform an episiotomy and protect the head from excessive pressure changes by a forceps delivery. Epidural anaesthesia may be recommended so that gentle forceps delivery can be painlessly performed and so that no drugs that might depress the baby's respiration need be given.

The earlier the onset of labour, the more likely that the baby will be in the breech position. Many studies from this country and America suggest that the most atraumatic way of delivering a tiny breech baby less than 1.5 kg in size is by Caesarean section.

The premature baby

The premature baby's skin is red, wrinkled and covered with fine hair. His head is small but appears large in proportion to his body and the skull bones are soft. His eyes stay closed; his sucking reflex is poor. His heat regulating mechanism is poorly developed so that he can easily become chilled. The development of the respiratory centre in the brain is immature and the respiratory muscles are not well developed so that premature babies are liable to have difficulty in breathing. They have poor resistance to infections and these are easily contracted. The premature baby sleeps more or less continuously and his cry is infrequent and feeble.

Care of the premature baby

Premature babies are usually nursed in a thermostatically controlled incubator to maintain their body temperature. The baby can, in these ideal circumstances, be nursed without clothes, making observations of colour and breathing more easy for the nursing staff. Oxygen can be administered more easily should it be necessary. Infections can be avoided by isolation and to a certain extent this is achieved by the incubator itself. The premature baby is handled as little as possible and therefore he is not bathed after delivery until his condition is satisfactory. Feeding is always a problem because premature babies require a high protein and a high carbohydrate intake if they are to gain weight adequately and because they lose quite a lot of weight in the first week of life. It is common practice to start feeding as early as possible. The method of feeding depends on the baby's condition. If he is very small and feeble he may be fed small amounts every 2 or 3 hours by means of a special fine plastic tube passed down his throat into his stomach. The tube causes the baby no discomfort. Larger premature babies may be able to suck from a special bottle fitted with a soft teat, and babies over 2 kg can usually feed from the breast. Small feeds are given frequently to reduce the risk of regurgitation during the first week or two of life and then the amount is increased gradually.

A strong bond develops between a mother and her baby even before birth and this takes the form of mothering which is so important after delivery, and even more important for the premature baby in an incubator. The mother sees her baby at the earliest opportunity and handles him as soon as his condition permits. The separation of the premature baby from his mother is unavoidable and although it may cause some heartache the normal physical and emotional relationships rapidly develop as soon as she is allowed to look after him.

Complications of the premature baby

The principal handicaps that the premature baby has to overcome at birth are respiratory difficulties and temperature control. He is also liable to infection, jaundice, anaemia and feeding problems.

Respiratory difficulty is due to the individual organs of the premature baby being immature in comparison to those of the normal full-term infant. Difficulty in respiration, causing shallow, irregular, rapid breathing may develop into a condition known as 'respiratory distress syndrome' to which, unfortunately, premature babies are particularly prone. Treatment of respiratory distress syndrome is supervised by the paediatrician and may require that the baby is mechanically ventilated until he can breathe satisfactorily on his own. As mentioned before, giving steroids to the mother in premature labour may enhance surfactant production and so help the baby's breathing.

Temperature control of the premature baby is difficult and a relatively uniform body temperature is achieved by placing him in an incubator. This is because the baby has very little insulating body fat, and the head provides a very large surface area from which heat can be lost.

Feeding and adequate nutrition are vital in these tiny babies who are capable of more rapid growth than at any other time in human life. Difficulties arise because the baby's nutritional needs are very high, yet the baby is too weak to feed himself and his gut is very immature and may be unable to absorb nutrients properly. Furthermore, tiny babies can lose up to 50 per cent of their energy requirements in their bowel motions. Most babies can be given small and frequent feeds through a nasogastric tube passing into the stomach, but sometimes feeding may be required through an intravenous drip. Breast milk, expressed by the mother, is the best source of fats which the baby can absorb and certain substances important for protein formation. It is also very rich in antibodies and substances which have a protective effect on the baby against infection. If the mother cannot express her milk, the baby may be fed with human milk from a 'milk bank' or artificial formula milk especially designed for the premature baby.

Infection. The premature baby is very susceptible to infections because his resistance is extremely poor. Breast-feeding plays an important part in protecting the baby and, therefore, breast milk is particularly beneficial to the small, feeble, premature baby. Everyone who handles the baby should have clean, washed hands. This has an enormous effect on lowering the incidence of infection in the new-born, and cannot be over-emphasized.

Jaundice appearing in the premature baby at any time during the first week or two of life is fairly common. The baby is frequently examined so that he can be treated if the jaundice becomes too severe.

Anaemia. Iron deficiency anaemia may develop in premature babies, or those of low birth weight. New-born babies, whatever their maturity, have reasonable iron reserves. However, the small baby grows more rapidly in proportion to his birth weight than does the large baby so that he exhausts his store of iron quite quickly and is liable to iron deficiency anaemia. To prevent this the premature baby is given iron by mouth from the age of 4 weeks. In the full-term infant an iron deficiency anaemia is best prevented by the introduction of mixed feeding with foods rich in iron at the age of 3 months.

Progress of the premature baby

Most premature babies progress normally and after a few weeks no one would know that they had been born prematurely. Because their needs are so urgent, it is sometimes easy to forget that the parents too have special needs at this time. It can be very frightening for a mother to see her baby for the first time after a premature birth. The tiny form lies quietly in his incubator, covered in wires which lead to pulse recorders, ECG machines, breathing rate recorders, temperature recorders. The baby's head may be covered with a little cloth cap and be in a large plastic head-box. He may be on a ventilator, with a tiny tube inserted into his lungs.

Not only may it be difficult for parents to accept that this tiny little baby is theirs, in all its strange and alien appearance, but they may feel guilt or a sense of failure because he was born prematurely. They may not yet have had time to complete all their preparations for the birth. The enforced separation of parents and their child adds to their feeling of confusion and anxiety. There may be unspoken fears that the baby will grow up to be abnormal in some way, and in the case of the very premature baby there may be the gradual and sad realization that the baby is dying.

The staff on a neonatal intensive care unit also become very attached to the babies in their care and are usually the people who give most support to parents in these dark hours. It is very important that parents be involved with the day-to-day care of their child, even though physically they may be separated. Yet parents can sit and gaze at their baby, talk to him, even sing to him, to compensate for the lack of cuddling. Gradually they can hold the baby for longer periods of time, feed the baby and see the amazing improvement from day to day.

Follow-up of prematurely born babies is very important and is arranged by the paediatrician before the baby is discharged home. Most children catch up to be similar in size to children born at term.

36 The Abnormal Baby

Congenital abnormality is not only a difficult subject to discuss but it is almost impossible to consider the problem in its correct perspective. It is probably true that every, or nearly every, expectant mother or father is either anxious about, or secretly afraid of, the possibility of their child having some form of congenital abnormality.

It is comparatively easy to talk about the percentage of this and that and indeed percentages of congenital abnormalities are presented later in this chapter, but for those who may either suffer from a congenital abnormality or for the parents of a congenitally abnormal child there is little satisfaction or help to be obtained from a table of statistics and what is meant by normality should be considered before contemplating what is considered abnormal.

Outside the theoretical realms of the Deity the perfect human being does not and cannot possibly exist. There are several reasons for this. Ideals of perfection differ from person to person, making it impossible to create, even in theory, a perfect human who would satisfy everybody's preconceived criteria and, even if each one of us were to consider creating a model of our own ideal person, either he or she would have to combine within one mind and body so many different and yet powerful attributes that it would be an impossibility.

Even though we cannot achieve perfection we can achieve normality. But is this really true? When we look at ourselves, our friends or members of our family, we have come to accept our minor imperfections as being part and parcel of a normal person. Some of us have either big ears or little ears, big noses or little noses, big teeth or crooked teeth, or too much hair or too little hair or a crooked toe, a wart, a mole or even perhaps a small birthmark. No one would suggest that these are really gross imperfections and yet they are congenital abnormalities. Furthermore, the intellect and personality present in a new-born baby are subject to so many external influences and environmental variations that it is small wonder that some of us have bad tempers, fail to pass exams or fail to develop our full potential ability in some particularly valuable artistic or creative attribute.

From a purely medical point of view a congenital abnormality is an abnormality that will, if untreated, adversely affect a person's normal role in society, but to a mother or father the term congenital abnormality means something much more simple and straightforward. The child is either mentally and physically normal or it is not. The incidence of congenital abnormality is approximately 4 per cent, which means that 96 out of every 100 babies are normal while 4 in every 100 suffer from some type of congenital abnormality which may require medical or surgical treatment. These abnormalities can be divided roughly into four groups, of which one quarter are mild, one quarter moderate, one quarter severe and one quarter incompatible with life.

Mild congenital abnormalities

These are present in approximately 1 per cent, or 1 in every 100 of all births, and include such minor abnormalities as extra fingers and toes, large birthmarks, skin tags attached to the ear, or hernias at the umbilicus. Some of these require no treatment while others are very easily corrected by minor operations without leaving any permanent defect.

Moderate congenital abnormalities

Approximately 1 in every 100 babies suffers from a congenital abnormality of moderate degree, although it is realized that in the eyes of the parent they appear to be very severe. Although they are serious, they can be either totally or partially corrected by medical or surgical treatment to such an extent that a normal life is confidently anticipated. They include congenital dislocation of the hip, club foot (which is usually completely cured if treatment begins in the first few days of life), hare lip and cleft palate (for which surgical correction is now well acknowledged), congenital abnormalities of the heart (for which modern surgery can almost work miracles), and blockage or stoppage in the intestine (which can also be corrected surgically).

Severe congenital abnormalities

Approximately 1 per cent of babies suffer from abnormalities of such severity as to influence their lives. These abnormalities cannot be corrected and include mongolism, spasticity, blindness, deafness, absent limbs and congenital lesions of the heart and intestine for which there are no satisfactory surgical solutions.

Congenital abnormalities incompatible with life

Severe abnormalities which are usually incompatible with life affect 1 in every 100 babies delivered. These include hydrocephalus, where the head is grossly enlarged by an excess amount of water, anencephalus, where the skull is not properly formed, and instances when babies have multiple congenital abnormalities. There is usually little or nothing that can be done to correct such abnormalities. Modern medicine and surgery may achieve minor miracles in saving or prolonging life but it cannot perform the impossible.

Abortion

It is undoubtedly true that nature has its own defence mechanism and eliminates some grossly abnormal fetuses at a very early stage of their development, which means that a number of abnormal pregnancies are miscarried early in pregnancy. These include the blighted ovum (see Chapter 18). It is generally accepted that approximately 10 per cent of all human pregnancies are sufficiently abnormal to result in early abortion. Other factors are responsible for the remainder of spontaneous abortions.

Diagnosis of congenital abnormality

It is very difficult to diagnose congenital abnormality during pregnancy but it can nevertheless be done if there is any reason to suspect that any abnormality may be present.

A sample of amniotic fluid can be removed from around the baby by amniocentesis at about the 16th week of pregnancy. This test shows the sex of the child and may demonstrate a mongol abnormality. It is performed for a genetic predisposition to mongolism and the diagnosis at this early stage is essential if there is to be a termination of pregnancy. There are several rare diseases that may be diagnosed by such tests. A diagnosis of Rhesus incompatibility is usually made by testing the blood, and the effect on the baby is judged accurately by taking several samples of amniotic fluid later in pregnancy. Similarly, some hospitals can offer screening for spina bifida babies by testing the mother's blood, suspicious results being confirmed by amniocentesis.

Ultrasound is used to establish a diagnosis of spina bifida, hydrocephaly or anencephaly as well as to show the presence of multiple congenital abnormalities.

When a diagnosis has been made of a congenital abnormality incompatible with normal life it is usual for termination of the pregnancy to be considered. The pregnant woman and her husband are told all the facts and these are discussed fully with them. If the pregnancy is to be terminated the woman is admitted to hospital and premature labour induced.

One particular type of congenital abnormality known as phenyl-ketonuria, if untreated, causes a child to become mentally defective. The disease can be detected by examining the blood of the baby shortly after delivery and can be completely treated. This is a routine test taken on the seventh day after delivery.

Cause of congenital abnormality

Genetic cause

The cause of most congenital abnormalities is not really known, simply because there are so many factors involved. Many abnormalities are hereditary but the reason why they suddenly affect a particular child is not known, although a greater understanding of the science of genetics will eventually provide the answer. Some abnormalities are transmitted only through the female while others are transmitted solely by the male. Others can result only if a specific genetic abnormality is present in a latent or previously unrecognized form in both parents; the presence of such a latent abnormality in one parent alone will not result in an abnormal child, although the child itself may be capable of transmitting the condition if it should marry a person with a similar genetic abnormality.

Just to make life more difficult and the whole subject more complex, a congenital abnormality of genetic nature may also occur either spontaneously or as an inherited abnormality. One such condition is congenital dislocation of the hip which is known to be hereditary in large areas of Northern Italy where it is fairly common, and which also occurs as an isolated abnormality in this country, not usually associated with a family history or with an increased liability of being transmitted to the next generation.

It is impossible here to deal comprehensively with the whole complicated subject of genetics or with the extensive science of chromosomal abnormalities that are known to cause congenital abnormalities. If necessary, further advice should be sought from the family doctor and perhaps from a specialist in genetic diseases.

Age

Congenital abnormalities occur more frequently in babies of women who are under the age of 16 at the time of delivery and in those who are over 40. It is not known why children of very young mothers suffer from a higher than average incidence of severe congenital abnormality. There is an increased incidence of mongolism in a woman having a baby when she is over 40. If there is any family history, near or far, of a mongoloid child, then any woman over 40 years of age should consult her doctor, or a genetic specialist, before starting a pregnancy, especially if it is her first.

Acquired causes

Acquired factors, such as drugs or diseases, account for less than one-third of the total number of congenital abnormalities but they are believed to be responsible for some of the more severe types of abnormality.

Virus diseases, such as rubella (German measles), may result in a congenital abnormality. If a woman has German measles during the first 12 weeks of her pregnancy then she has a 10 to 30 per cent risk that her child will be affected. For other virus diseases the risk is very much less.

X-rays. High levels of irradiation may cause congenital abnormalities. Routine X-rays do not generally cause any harm or damage. X-rays of the unborn baby may predispose to the development of leukaemia before the child has reached adulthood, and are certainly damaging to the unborn baby's genes and chromosomes so that the incidence of congenital abnormality in subsequent generations may be increased. X-rays are thus better avoided during pregnancy unless they are necessary to provide essential information.

Oxygen lack. Deprivation of oxygen during the first 3 months of pregnancy predisposes to congenital abnormality. The two main causes of this—flying in unpressurized aeroplanes and inadequate general anaesthesia—have long since been removed. Passenger aircraft are now pressurized and there is no danger to a pregnant woman from flying in modern aircraft during early pregnancy, providing of course that everything else is normal.

General anaesthesia is now so skilled that people receive more oxygen when they are anaesthetized than when they are awake. However, since it involves the administration of drugs which, although harmless, are better avoided during pregnancy purely as a matter of principle, general anaesthesia should be delayed if possible until after the first 3 months. There is no reason why local anaesthesia should not be administered, provided that the correct dose is properly given.

Drugs are better avoided in the first 3 months of pregnancy and the majority of doctors and midwives even refrain from giving simple iron and vitamin tablets until after the end of the third month. Today all drugs are very vigorously tested to see if they exert any adverse influence on pregnancy or cause any congenital abnormality, and most are completely safe. Some drugs, however, are still under suspicion and only those specifically prescribed by a doctor should be taken.

Maternal health before the onset of pregnancy has a great effect on the pregnancy itself, but babies have a habit of surviving quite happily even in the most extraordinary circumstances—women who are suffering from extreme degrees of starvation will give birth to absolutely normal babies of almost normal weight. Maternal disease, however, such as diabetes, abnormalities of the thyroid, abnormalities of the kidney and raised blood pressure do require careful management. Uncontrolled diabetes can cause congenital abnormalities in the baby and, besides making absolutely certain that her diabetes is properly stabilized before she becomes pregnant, a diabetic woman must be meticulous about its management throughout her entire pregnancy. If she does so, she has no reason to worry.

Prevention of congenital abnormality

Health. General health should be as good as possible and any tendency towards anaemia should be corrected before the onset of pregnancy. Vitamin B deficiency may predispose to spina bifida.

Infection. Any possible infection should be cured before the onset of pregnancy and every effort should be made to avoid any form of infection or infectious disease during pregnancy.

Drugs. No drugs should be taken other than those prescribed by a doctor (see Chapter 14).

X-rays should be avoided in pregnancy unless they are necessary for its management or for the control of disease

Maternal disease. If the mother is subject to chronic illness, especially diabetes, it must be carefully and vigorously controlled before and during pregnancy.

Genetic counselling

There are some diseases which clearly have a dominant or recessive mode of inheritance, such as some forms of eye tumours or deafness or skin disorders. In other cases of congenital abnormality one affected child increases the risk to the parents of having another affected child. Referral to a geneticist is very helpful so that the risks to the parents can be determined and, in some cases, attempts at antenatal diagnosis made.

37 Feeding

Breast or bottle?

Successful nourishment of the newly born baby aids his healthy growth and development and provides contentment to both mother and baby. Breast milk is the ideal food for the baby in the first few months and breast-feeding should be easy and pleasurable to the mother and her child.

If you have decided for one reason or another that you do not want to breast-feed, or if you cannot do so for medical reasons, there is no cause to reproach yourself. Your baby will not be deprived of anything vital and, providing you handle the bottle-feeding in the right way, a very warm and close relationship develops in just the same way as if he were breast-fed. Tests have shown no difference between the rates of progress or development of babies fed naturally or artificially.

Breast-feeding is a wonderful experience for both mother and baby, but it is not by any means the *only* wonderful experience, and just as good a relationship can be established with a bottle-fed baby. If a mother is worried about any of the difficulties in breast-feeding she will be tense and this will be communicated to the baby so that the difficulties are increased. If the mother's milk supply is not adequate, feeding the baby may be more difficult than simply settling for the bottle. If there are any difficulties she should consult her doctor, or her health visitor who can be contacted through any maternity or child welfare clinic if she has not already called at the house.

Breast-feeding

A baby should be put to the breast very soon after his birth, unless there has been some complication in which case he may rest quietly in his cot or incubator for 24 to 48 hours, where he will be fed by bottle with glucose water. The first feed is supervised and the mother is helped and advised by the midwife. These notes are a general guide; you should follow your midwife's instructions.

One most important aspect of breast-feeding is a relaxed and affectionate atmosphere. The baby can sense if this is lacking and may become fretful so that he will not feed satisfactorily. If a mother *wants* to breast-feed, she is far more likely to succeed than if she is reluctant. Indeed, a mother who is reluctant to breast-feed her baby rarely succeeds and both she and her baby benefit if artificial feeding is begun from birth. Breast-feeding is a technique which has to be learned; there are bound to be some difficulties at first and it is essential to persevere for a while rather than give up in despair at the first obstacle.

The incidence of complete breast-feeding is distressingly low for a variety of reasons. Some mothers do not want to breast-feed, whereas others give it up because of inadequate lactation, pain during feeding or difficulty in getting the baby to suck satisfactorily. For any but the most natural mother, the first 3 or 4 weeks may be a rather worrying and difficult time, but the mother who does feed her baby gets her own reward.

The advantages of breast-feeding are many:

1 It provides a happy relationship between the mother and child.
2 It provides the baby with milk of suitable composition and the correct temperature.
3 There is little risk of contamination of the milk or of infection during feeding.
4 It is easier than artificial feeding since there is no mixing of feed and sterilizing of equipment.
5 It is cheaper.
6 Infections, particularly gastro-enteritis, are less frequent in breast-fed babies.
7 It aids involution of the uterus.

Preparations for breast-feeding must begin in early pregnancy, and it is discussed either at the booking clinic or shortly afterwards. For the mother who is breast-feeding, cleanliness is the first essential. A daily warm bath is ideal; hot baths are exhausting and may cause fainting. The mother's hands must be washed before each feed and the nails should be short and clean. The modern tendency is to wash the nipples as little as possible, washing the whole breast only before feeds, using a minimum of soap. Lanolin or other suitable ointment, such as Massé cream, may be applied to the nipples at the end of each feed. A good supporting brassiere should be worn and washed each day. Nightdresses should have shoulder straps that slip off or untie, so that they need not be pulled up over the breasts from below.

The baby obtains milk from the breast on suckling and this experience ought to be a pleasure as well as a necessity for him and the mother. Both should be relaxed and comfortable. The baby must not be tightly wrapped in clothing; let his hands be free to touch the breast if he wants to. The baby may require a few moments to waken up before being put to the breast, and this is an ideal time for a little love and play. When feeding in bed the mother should be supported with pillows so that she leans slightly forward, holding the infant in the crook of one arm. The palm of her other hand supports the breast at which the baby is suckling and the index finger is above the nipple so that it can be guided into the baby's mouth

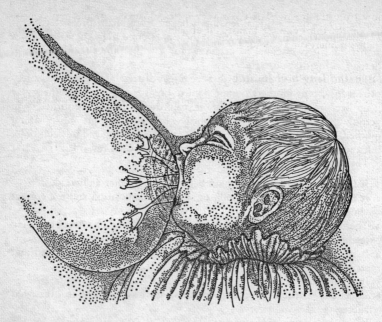

Fig. 38 Breast-feeding

and the breast held back from his nostrils so that he can breathe properly. At first he may need a little help in finding the nipple and if you touch his cheek with the breast he will turn towards it. When he sucks be sure that he takes in his mouth not only the nipple itself, but most of the coloured area around it. Cradle the baby in the right arm while feeding at the right breast, and use the left hand to manipulate the breast. Use the opposite arm and hand for the left breast. If there is soreness from perineal sutures it is more comfortable to lie in bed, first on one side and then on the other. Comfort for the baby and mother is always essential when feeding and a low nursing chair is especially valuable when the mother is out of bed.

At first a baby usually does no more than nuzzle the nipple and lick it, and he should not be forced to suck; he will when he is ready to do so. It may take a few days before he masters the art of sucking and meanwhile he is given a small amount of boiled water between feeds. Since this does not satisfy his appetite he will be hungry when put to the breast, and this encourages him to learn to suck properly. A new-born baby does not require much food for the first 3 days because he is born with an excess of fluid in his body. Loss of this fluid as urine and sweat causes the loss of weight which all babies suffer during the first 2 or 3 days of life. This lack of appetite usually lasts until the time at which the milk begins to flow from the breast. There is a very little colostrum for the first 2 days and on the third day the breasts fill up and proper milk begins to flow in gradually increasing amounts.

Time and length of feeding

It is important to avoid getting sore nipples. For this reason, put the baby to each breast for only 1 minute on the first day, 2 or 3 minutes on the second and third days, and so on up to 10 minutes each side by the end of the first week. It is most important that these times should not be exceeded. Sore nipples are caused by the baby chewing the nipple. This can only happen if the whole nipple and the surrounding areola are not placed properly in the baby's mouth. A baby will suck, chew or rest; a woman knows if her baby is actively sucking at the breast and he must not be allowed to chew or bite the nipple. Ten minutes at each breast is the maximum time allowed when full feeding is established. A hungry baby empties the breast in less time and, as he takes nearly two thirds of his feed in the first 5 minutes, he should be put to alternate breasts at the start of each feed.

The majority of babies of 3.2 to 3.4 kg and over will be contented on feeds at approximately four-hourly intervals—five to six feeds daily. Smaller babies are often happier on three-hourly feeds—six or seven feeds daily. Night feeds should not be forbidden. If a baby will not settle after being made comfortable and given a little water, he is probably hungry and should be fed. Water does not pacify a hungry baby and he will not learn to sleep at night by screaming for hours. There is no danger of the baby forming a habit of waking to be fed in the night. When he gets enough food during the day he will sleep for longer periods at night until eventually he sleeps from 10.30 p.m. until 5 a.m.

Some mothers may wish to demand feed their babies, and providing this is carried out in a sensible fashion there is nothing wrong with it and it gradually resolves into a regular feeding routine which is acceptable to mother, baby and the rest of the family. It is often more relaxing and successful than sticking to a rigid timetable.

Breaking the wind

Most babies bring up wind once during the feed, usually when they are being changed from one breast to the other. To 'wind' the baby he is held upright against the left chest and his back gently patted or rubbed. This slight movement releases the air in his stomach. If the baby is held upright no milk will come up with the air. He should be 'winded' again at the end of the feed. If the baby is laid in his cot without first bringing up wind, he will bring it up later with part of his feed, or it will pass into his intestine and cause colicky pain.

Complete emptying of the breasts

The breasts should be completely empty after feeding and until breast-feeding is fully established they should be expressed after each feed, thus stimulating lactation and avoiding engorgement. A few minutes spent expressing milk after feeds can make the difference between successful and unsuccessful lactation, and the art is quickly learned.

Maintenance of breast-feeding

Continual breast-feeding should present no difficulty providing that lactation has been properly established. Lactation usually falls off a little during the first few days at home when the mother has the baby on her own and is busy doing all the housework and shopping. For a few days, therefore, the baby may be fretful and less contented but with a little patience and understanding he will settle down. Good health, plenty of rest and nutritious food are essential for the mother if breast-feeding is to be continued successfully. Spicy foods and stoned fruit should not be eaten because they can affect breast milk and upset the baby.

Test weighing should never be undertaken unless there is reason to suspect that the baby is underfeeding. A single test feed is of little value; the results of two or three feeds may be useful, but test weighing should ideally be continued over 24 hours. The baby should be weighed on accurate scales in his clothes before being fed and again in the same clothes after the feed without changing his napkin even if it is dirty. The difference between the two weights is the amount of milk he has taken from the breast.

Overfeeding. It is impossible to overfeed a baby on the breast; he will take what he needs and no more. But underfeeding *is* possible and if the baby is obviously hungry he can occasionally be given a bottle after his breast-feed. The holes in the bottle teat must not be too large or he will get milk more easily than from the breast which may make him prefer the bottle. Apart from this there is no truth in the old wives' tale that once a baby has been on a bottle he will not return to the breast.

Complementary feeding is a temporary measure when the supply of breast milk is not sufficient. The baby is given additional milk immediately after an inadequate breast-feed; this should be done when it is hoped to establish satisfactory breast-feeding in the near future. The last feed at night may be complemented to make sure the baby, and therefore the mother as well, have a good night's rest.

Supplementary feeding consists of giving bottle milk in place of a breast-feed and should not be done when the breasts do not contain enough milk since their production of milk is stimulated by suckling. Occasionally it may be used if breast-feeding is well established and the mother wishes to be absent at feeding time.

Will breast-feeding affect your figure?

Having a baby has some effect on the breast outline. The breasts are inclined to lose some of their firmness, though this is usually not very marked after the first or even second baby, but is more common after breast-feeding and especially if the breasts are allowed to become engorged. Once the breasts have sagged nothing can be done to restore their shape except plastic surgery. Hot and cold sponging night and morning is often advised, but does not usually help. Simple windmill exercises are useless because the breasts do not contain muscle. Exercises to improve posture or strengthen the muscles of the arms may help the appearance of the breast outline. Creams are of no value. Wearing a good brassiere is more important than anything else.

Some women who breast-feed find that their breasts become smaller.

Difficulties in breast-feeding

Engorged breasts. If the breasts are not prepared for feeding they commonly become heavy and hard on the third and fourth day of the puerperium. This is painful and should be treated by:

1 Bathing the breasts in warm water before feeds and gently stroking the breasts firmly towards the nipple for a few moments.
2 Expressing some milk, putting the baby to the breasts for a few minutes and then expressing the remaining milk.
3 Applying lanolin to the nipples and wearing a firm supporting brassiere.
4 Paracetamol tablets can be taken to relieve discomfort.

Cracked nipples. If cracked nipples are treated promptly they will heal rapidly. The baby should be taken off the breast for 24 hours if the nipple is tender and 48 to 78 hours if cracked. The milk should be expressed from the breast manually or by breast pump. Ointments soothe the nipple but must be applied sparingly. Lanolin or Massé cream may be used; Betnovate is the most efficient treatment but must be prescribed by your doctor.

Difficulties in breast-feeding due to the baby

1 Premature babies may be too weak to suckle at the breast and should not be taken out of the warm nursery.
2 Congenital abnormalities such as cleft lip or cleft palate prevent the infant from sucking.
3 Thrush infection of the mouth may make the baby disinclined to feed.
4 Snuffles, usually due to nasal infection, interfere with breathing during suckling.
5 Mentally subnormal babies do not use their tongues effectively for successful breast-feeding.
6 Jaundice causes lethargy and disinclination to feed.

Reasons for not breast-feeding

If there is a severe psychiatric disorder of the mother, breast-feeding may be inadvisable because of the possibility of the mother doing harm to her child.

Some of the drugs used to control epilepsy are excreted in the milk in which instance the mother must not breast-feed. Each woman however must be assessed individually and attention given to her condition and to the safety of her child.

A mother suffering from active pulmonary tuberculosis must not breast-feed, both for her benefit and the safety of her baby. Mothers whose chest infections have healed are usually allowed to breast-feed, but only on the advice of the chest physician.

Breast-feeding is seldom allowed in women who suffer from chronic nephritis or who have had malignant diseases of any kind.

A baby with Down's syndrome (mongolism) is usually difficult to feed and he should then be artificially fed. If, however, breast-feeding can be established easily it should be encouraged.

There are diverse opinions about breast-feeding of babies who are to be adopted. Each of these mothers and babies are dealt with as an individual problem.

Artificial feeding

A baby is bottle-fed when breast-feeding is impossible or impracticable, or if the mother does not want to breast-feed.

New-born babies cannot easily digest plain fresh cows' milk because it contains more protein, fat and mineral salts, but less sugar than human milk. Furthermore there is considerable variation in the chemical structure of these elements, especially the protein, so that cows' milk must be slightly modified to make it suitable for human infants.

Dried milk

Dried or powdered milk is made by heating cows' milk to a specific temperature and removing the fluid by evaporation. To reconstitute the milk, water is added by the mother as instructed on each individual packet. Dried milk suitable for baby feeding is prepared in two forms: half-cream and full-cream. Some brands of dried milk are already sweetened while others are not and sugar must be added to these.

The advantages of dried milk are:

1 It is already sterilized and does not easily become infected.
2 The method of preparation is simple, each packet giving full instructions.

3 It is convenient, easily transported and a constant supply can be easily stored.

Its main disadvantage is that it has to be reconstituted with sterilized water in sterilized utensils.

Liquid artificial milk

Previously prepared milk in sterile disposable bottles is available, although it is more expensive than dried milk.

Arrangement of feeds

Bottle-feeds are usually given approximately every four hours but some babies prefer a three-hourly regime. Times should not be rigid but a scheme should be worked out which satisfies both the baby and the particular routine of the home and family. A baby does not always accept the same quantity of milk mixture at each feed. The breast-fed baby, regulating his own feeds, seldom takes exactly the same amount at every feed and the artificially fed child must therefore be allowed to decide to a certain extent upon the volume of his feed. He may want an extra ounce or two at his last feed at night and he may want a larger early morning feed.

Choice of bottles and teats

Feeding bottles with a wide neck are easier to fill and clean. They are also better for travelling because the teat can be kept clean and protected by reversing it inside the bottle.

The teats should be carefully chosen and the same type used throughout bottle-feeding. The plain-ended teat is the most satisfactory though certain babies prefer the bulb-ended type. A teat with a flange at the base is easier to put on the bottle. The holes in the teat should be of such a size that the milk drips from the upturned bottle at the rate of 12 to 20 drips a minute. The rate of flow must be adjusted to meet the needs of the individual baby so that he can feed easily without choking.

The most important aspect of bottle-feeding is hygiene. A baby can get an upset tummy or even a severe infection from his bottle if it is not properly sterilized. One of the simplest and most reliable methods of sterilizing all bottle-feeding equipment is by using sodium hypochlorite (Milton).

The equipment required for feed preparation is several bottles, teats, measuring jug, spoon to mix the powdered milk, knife for levelling off, cleaning brush, large container for sterilizing, the powdered milk and boiled water.

To make up the feed make a smooth paste with a little of the previously boiled water and powder and then add the correct amount of water, the exact amount of which is clearly set out in the instructions on the milk packet. If you leave any lumps of powdered milk during the mixing which cannot pass through the holes in the teat, your baby won't get his full ration of milk because the lumps will stick in the teat and block the flow of milk. This will cause the baby great frustration and also let him suck in air which will give him wind.

To test the temperature of the feed shake a few drops on the back of your hand and feel the bottle with the inside of your arm to make sure the milk is not above body temperature.

The amount of the feed. It is important to know how much to offer your baby at each feed and as a rough guide, since babies vary so much in their needs, 90 ml should be given for every pound of your baby's weight every 24 hours. A complete table is usually printed on every tin or packet of dried or powdered milk. For example: a baby weighing 4.5 kg will need 10×90 ml = 900 ml each 24 hours and if he is on six feeds a day each can be 140 g. If he finishes the bottle, try making up an extra ounce each time. It is easy to underfeed a baby but contrary to general belief it is virtually impossible to overfeed a young baby as he simply brings it back if his stomach is full.

A baby can swallow a great deal of wind during bottle feeding so it is important to make sure that the holes in the teats are the correct size.

If you have a refrigerator you can make up all the feeds you need for the day provided they are cooled quickly and always kept refrigerated until needed. You should warm the bottle to the correct temperature either in water in a suacepan or in an automatic bottle warmer. Make sure the milk is the correct temperature. If you do not have a refrigerator then it is probably best to make up each feed separately.

Evaporated milk

Evaporated milk is made by removing about half the water. The treatment of the milk during evaporation leads to physical changes in the protein which result in better digestibility. It is unsweetened and sugar must be added. It is easy to make up a feed by pouring the milk directly from the punctured can and adding sugar and water as required. The usual basic formula for feeds is 1 part of milk and 2 parts of water, with half a teaspoonful of sugar to every 85 g of mixture. This mixture is well tolerated by all babies, including premature babies, although minor alterations may be necessary on special occasions.

Cleaning. After the feed the bottle and teat must be well washed in cold water. This cleans the bottle and does not coagulate the milk proteins which could otherwise adhere in a film to the bottle. A bottle brush can be used to complete the cleaning, and then hot water used to remove the fat.

Sterilization of bottles and teats

Bottles and teats may be heat-sterilized or treated in sodium hypochlorite solution. The latter method is preferable. It is simple, less dangerous, more efficient, easier; it preserves the teats well and the bottles do not get furred, cracked or damaged. It can be used for plastic bottles.

Heat sterilization. The bottle and teat are completely immersed in cold water in a saucepan, boiled for 10 minutes and left in a covered pan to cool until the feed is required. After preparing the feed and filling the bottle, the teat is placed on the bottle and covered with a beaker or egg-cup to keep it clean. If the bottle is sealed with a valve, the teat is left covered in the boiled water until the feed is ready to be given.

Cold sterilization. The bottle and teat are completely immersed in a solution of sodium hypochlorite in which they are left until the next feed is due. The solution is changed each day.

Mixed feeding

Opinions vary widely on the advisability of adding cereal to a baby's diet. Each baby is an individual. Like all of us, he or she has different and individual tastes. There is no fixed time to introduce mixed feeding.

Vitamins

All babies must have a good supply of vitamins A, C, and D, whether in solid foods or in a concentrated form. Vitamin A helps prevent infections and helps normal growth. Vitamin C ensures healthy blood vessels and helps to prevent anaemia. There is not enough vitamin C in either bottle or breast milk but it is present in orange juice which can be given after a few weeks. Vitamin D is found with vitamin A and is essential in the formation of good, strong bones. Cod liver oil is rich in vitamins A and D and is most often prescribed for babies when they are a few weeks old. When your baby does start taking vitamins it is best to give them to him just before you bath him so that the oily preparations cannot stain his clothes.

38 Common Complications Affecting the Infant

The vast majority of babies are normal at birth and remain so. If you were delivered in hospital, you should take advantage of the opportunity to learn from the maternity staff as much as possible about baby care. The more you handle and look after your own baby while you are in hospital the sooner will you gain confidence in his management and the ability to recognize anything abnormal or unusual.

Crying is part of a normal baby's natural daily life. It is good exercise and causes no harm. Frequently, however, it may indicate hunger, thirst, temper, cold or heat or that the baby requires attention. Most mothers soon learn to recognize the meaning of these various cries.

Sore buttocks. Nappy rash is probably the most common condition affecting healthy babies. A substance called urea, always present in the urine, is turned into ammonia by bacteria that are normally found on babies' skins and also on wet or soiled napkins. Ammonia is very irritant to the skin causing redness and soreness where it has been in contact with the baby's skin for any length of time. This can be overcome in four ways, all of which are necessary if treatment is to be successful. Firstly, napkins should be changed frequently and as often as necessary to avoid leaving the baby wet or soiled. Secondly, wash the baby carefully, paying particular attention to the skin folds, rinse away all soap and dry thoroughly. Thirdly, apply a good cream such as zinc and castor oil, petroleum jelly or a reliable proprietary cream. Fourthly, only really clean napkins should be used.

Skin rashes. In the first few months of life a baby sometimes develops a reddish rash on the neck and face. This is due to overheating, either as a result of too high a room temperature or because the baby is wearing too many warm clothes. Perspiration indicates that clothing is too heavy and too warm. A similar rash caused by excessive dribbling may accompany teething.

Ear infections. An indication of earache is fretfulness and a tendency for the baby to hold and pull his ear. Earache sometimes accompanies teething, but at an earlier age any discharge from the ears is an indication of an infection and your doctor should be consulted.

Vomiting is usually of no significance. All babies vomit a little; this is called positing or regurgitation and happens during or shortly after a feed A slight adjustment to feeding routine may cure it although some babies continue to vomit regardless. Regurgitation after feeds accompanied by wind is fairly common in normal babies. The appearance of the vomit varies considerably. Fluid returned soon after a breast-feed usually has the appearance of unaltered milk. If there is some delay before vomiting takes place, the vomit contains curdled milk. The presence of mucus suggests irritation of the lining of the stomach. Vomit of any kind has an unpleasant sour but not foul odour. The management of vomiting should be to treat the underlying cause which is usually a simple feeding problem. If the vomiting becomes serious consult your doctor at once.

Constipation. The baby's motions change their colour and consistency during the first few days of life. They are greenish-black for the first two days and gradually change to a light yellow colour always being soft in consistency. There may be as many as two or three motions in a day although some breast-fed babies may go for two or three days without passing a motion. Provided the baby does not have to strain unnecessarily and the motions are a normal colour, and are soft, then there is no need for concern. Misunderstanding about constipation in infants frequently occurs. If a baby's stools are infrequent but of normal colour and texture, then the baby is not constipated. If the motions are infrequent and hard then he is constipated. This may be corrected by the addition of a little sugar to feeds.

Sticky eyes are not uncommon and not serious if treated promptly. A sticky eye as an indication of infection is recognized by a yellowish discharge at the inner corner of the eye. The doctor should be informed and further treatment will be prescribed by him if the discharge is heavy and the eyes become red and swollen.

Watering of the eyes is also quite common in infancy and should clear up without treatment between the sixth and eighth months.

Colds and snuffles are troublesome but not always serious in young babies. The baby is irritable and his difficulty in breathing caused by a blocked nose interferes with his feeding. Colds in babies should not be neglected and the advice of a doctor should be sought. Colds apart, some babies get snuffles resulting in an increase in the natural secretion of the nose. Nothing need be done unless, as on rare occasions, it interferes with feeding, and the doctor may then prescribe treatment.

Thrush is a common cause of slow feeding. It is a fungus infection recognizable as small white patches on the inside of the cheeks, on the tongue and palate. It may be confused with curds adherent to the mouth immediately after a feed. Gentle swabbing of the mouth will remove any curds but not the white patches caused by thrush. Treatment is simple: the baby's mouth must be kept very clean and his feeding equipment meticulously sterilized. Nystatin suspension, prescribed by a doctor and given every 4 hours, results in a rapid cure. Fungus infections in a baby's mouth are nearly always caused because the baby is infected from his mother's vagina at delivery, so she will also require treatment.

Engorged breasts are fairly common in babies of both sexes during the first few days of life. It is not a serious condition, requires no treatment and disappears within a few days or may rarely continue for a few weeks. The enlargement is due to activity of the glandular part of the baby's breast immediately after birth, since there are no longer maternal oestrogens in the circulation. In male infants the testicles are also sometimes slightly enlarged.

Menstruation is sometimes seen in a new-born baby girl. It is caused by the sudden stopping, after delivery, of maternal hormones passing to the baby, and is usually noticed on the 3rd or 4th day of life. A small area of the napkin may be stained with bright red blood. No treatment is required since the condition is self curing and is present for only about 48 hours.

Jaundice occurring in the new-born infant about the 3rd day of life is very common and need cause no anxiety. This is called physiological jaundice and is due to the baby's blood having a high content of red cells which are rapidly broken down after birth. One of the end products of the breaking down of red cells is the yellow pigment called bilirubin which increases in the circulating blood to cause the jaundice. The liver of the baby at birth is unable to excrete the bilirubin sufficiently rapidly to prevent jaundice appearing. The jaundice should fade after the first week.

There are some serious causes of jaundice in the new-born baby such as Rhesus incompatibility. Most of these affect the baby within a few hours of birth so that he is yellow by the end of the first day of his life. If jaundice becomes very severe a condition known as kernicterus may develop in which the baby's brain cells may be damaged. Because of the recognition by paediatricians of the dangers of severe jaundice, kernicterus is rare today. The bilirubin level in the blood can be partly controlled by drugs and by exposing the baby to a special light. An exchange transfusion will always be used to lower the bilirubin level if the more simple methods fail.

Gastroenteritis is a serious condition in babies and should have immediate medical attention. Gastroenteritis is an infection which is transmitted to the baby via his food usually because his feeding utensils have not been kept hygienically. It cannot be stressed enough that high standards of cleanliness must be observed when dealing with babies.

Acute gastroenteritis can develop from a mild 'tummy upset'. Vomiting, frequent, loose and watery stools are followed by dehydration. Medical aid must be sought immediately. The baby must be isolated and given adequate fluid either by mouth or intravenously depending on medical instructions. When the infection has been treated, the vomiting and diarrhoea cease and the baby can again start to take fluid by mouth.

Haemorrhagic disease of the new-born baby is rare. When it does occur it starts about the 3rd day of life. The cause is not fully understood. Bleeding comes from the stomach and bowel and also from other organs. It is treated by giving an injection of vitamin K to help blood coagulation which is often deficient in the first few days of life. Most maternity hospitals arrange for all babies to have an injection of vitamin K shortly after birth to safeguard against this disease.

39 Birth Injuries

Bruises. The normal pressures exerted on the baby's head during normal labour are such that some bruising will nearly always be present over the face or scalp of a baby. These marks rapidly disappear during the first 24 hours. A cephalhaematoma as well as the caput are bruises on the head as a result of normal labour. The size of the bruises may vary according to the difficulty and length of labour.

Bruising may also be caused by forceps or the vacuum extractor (ventouse). Bruises or marks made by the blades of the obstetric forceps disappear after 2 or 3 days and do not leave any permanent injury or damage.

Facial palsy is the name of a particular condition where the nerve supplying the lower half of one side of the baby's face is temporarily paralysed. This nerve is particularly unprotected just beneath the ear, and during a forceps delivery it may be bruised or damaged so that one side of the baby's face fails to move properly shortly afterwards. The movement and tone in the face return to normal spontaneously after a few days or a few weeks at most and the baby is not left with any permanent injury or deformity.

Fractures. The majority of babies' bones are very soft but occasionally they may be particularly brittle so that fractures of bones in the legs, arms or a collar bone may occur at birth especially if delivery is difficult. Even so, these fractures do not often require any specific treatment and the bones heal spontaneously leaving no permanent effect. Fractures may occasionally happen in the skull bones if the labour has been very difficult but are now rare.

Intracranial haemorrhage is bleeding that occurs into the brain and is nearly always the result of a premature or difficult labour. The condition is serious but is becoming increasingly rare. Unfortunately haemorrhage into the brain is particularly liable to happen in premature babies and it is for this reason that many doctors prefer to deliver premature babies by forceps which protect the baby's skull from any injury.

The eyes. Haemorrhage may occasionally be present in the white part of the new-born baby's eye. The bruising is a result of pressure on the baby's head as it passes through the pelvis and it always clears up spontaneously without any treatment or permanent defect.

40 Circumcision

Circumcision is the operation of removing the prepuce, or foreskin, of the male. There are three reasons for performing the operation:

1 Religious.
2 Because it is medically advisable.
3 Because the parents wish it to be done.

Circumcision for religious reasons is usually performed on or about the eighth day amongst Jews, either by a doctor or by a lay person who has been specially trained to do the operation. If the baby is premature, not gaining weight, is jaundiced or for any medical reason is considered unfit for the operation, then this is postponed until he is fit enough for circumcision to be performed.

Medical indications for circumcision are very few. The foreskin may be very tight with only a tiny pinhole opening at its end so that it is impossible to draw the skin back. Paediatricians in Great Britain are reluctant to advise circumcision without any real medical indication because they do not consider that there is any advantage to be gained and the operation, like any operation, always presents a certain hazard. The arguments that the foreskin is dirty, that it has to be kept clean, that infection can occur underneath it and that circumcision in later life is a most uncomfortable and unpleasant procedure are not considered very substantial by most paediatricians. There are opposing arguments that the foreskin must have been provided for a purpose, that it should be washed and cleaned like any other part of the body, that in childhood a mother should teach her child to retract the foreskin and wash beneath it as a normal part of body hygiene and that if these simple rules are obeyed then infection should not occur in later life.

If circumcision is not necessary for medical or religious reasons it may not be obtainable in the National Health Service. In some countries, especially in the United States, Canada and Australia, circumcision has become almost a routine operation to be performed by the obstetrician at or within a few hours of delivery. It is certainly true that if the operation is going to be performed then it should be performed as soon after delivery as possible or on about the eighth day when the baby has established himself in a feeding routine and is gaining weight satisfactorily. Many doctors believe that operations should not be performed on the third, fourth or fifth days of life because not only is haemorrhage more likely during these days but the general effect of the operation on the baby is upsetting at a time when feeding is being established. Very few doctors or paediatricians in Great Britain would agree with, or even permit, circumcision to be performed at or immediately after birth and therefore the operation, if it is going to be undertaken, has to be deferred until the eighth day or thereabouts.

If you want to have your baby circumcised you must discuss it with the paediatrician or with your own doctor, but do not be surprised if your request does not meet with the approval you had hoped. Some doctors do agree with it and some do not.

If the operation is performed then one of several techniques may be used. It is important to keep a very careful watch during the first few hours after the operation to make certain that the penis is not bleeding. If no dressing has been applied you will be told how to bath the baby and about the special care of the penis. If a dressing has been applied you will probably be told that this should be soaked off in the bath one or two days after the operation. A plastic device may be used to perform the operation and you may find this device tied on to the end of the child's penis. The device will drop off after three or four days. Whatever type of operation is done the penis is nearly always swollen and slightly inflamed for a few days but if you treat it as you are told everything will gradually settle down satisfactorily. If you are at all worried you should call your doctor or if the operation has been performed in hospital you should telephone the hospital and ask their advice.

41 Perinatal Death

It is commonly thought that the safest and best time to have a first baby is between the ages of 16 and 20. The first report of the British Perinatal Mortality Survey (published by E. & S. Livingstone Ltd, 1963) showed that this is not true. It is safer, so far as the baby is concerned, for the first baby to be delivered when the mother is between the ages of 20 and 24. The next safest age group is when she is between 25 and 29, and the third safest when she is under the age of 20. The table below indicates the relative danger or safety of producing the first, second, third or fourth child during the various age groups, from which it will be seen that, from a purely statistical point of view, it is better to have first, second, third and fourth children between the ages of 20 and 24, or the second, third and fourth child between the ages of 25 and 39, or the second child between the ages of 30 and 34. Most obstetricians nowadays, therefore, no longer advise that teenage is the ideal time for pregnancy and they would advise that, if it is reasonably possible, a married woman should have her first child before she reaches the age of 30.

Age of mother	1st baby	2nd baby	3rd baby	4th baby
under 20	106	101	382	
20–24	98	69	77	84
25–29	100	62	91	98
30–34	132	77	102	111
35–39	168	120	108	128
40–44	312	179	220	157

The table shows the average risk of death to a baby depending upon the mother's age and size of family, when it is compared to an average risk of 100. Those figures below 100 are the most favourable whereas those above 100 are least favourable, e.g. the risk to the first-born baby of a woman of 42 is 3 times greater than if she were 32, and is 5 times greater than that to a second child of a 27-year-old woman.

The term perinatal death is a fairly recent concept and it includes all those babies who are stillborn or born dead as well as all babies who die during the first week of life. The incidence of perinatal death has fallen greatly over the past 50 years. In 1979 the figure was 14.8 per thousand which means that out of every thousand deliveries, over 15 babies were either dead at birth or died during the first week of life. Quite a large number of these babies were premature while others suffered from severe congenital abnormalities that were not compatible with their continued survival. The other side of the coin shows that 98.6 per cent of all pregnancies that reach the 28th week do result in delivery of a live baby who survives beyond the first week of life, after which the chances of anything adverse happening to him are very small indeed. Extensive enquiries are carried out and detailed surveys made by the authorities whenever a baby fails to survive.

While no one would dream of being complacent, it must nevertheless be admitted that quite a large proportion of the 15 babies per thousand who die shortly after birth (neonatal death) do so because of some factor that is entirely unpreventable. This does not stop every effort being made to increase the overall survival rate of every baby but it has resulted in a greater realization that not only must babies survive but they must also be healthy. The three major causes of perinatal death are prematurity, congenital abnormalities incompatible with life, and asphyxia when the supply of oxygen to the fetus is inadequate. This happens with a sudden antepartum haemorrhage such as abruption. These three conditions all have a socio-economic variation, and perinatal mortality is three times greater in social classes IV and V than in social class I. The unsupported woman is particularly at risk, especially if she is a young teenager.

The decline in the perinatal death rate over the years has been due directly or indirectly to improvements in antenatal care. The whole range of improvements for maternal welfare have exerted an influence upon the production of a greater number of live healthy babies. The advent of antibiotics in the control of infection, the understanding of blood groups and blood transfusion, the better treatment of anaemia, heart disease, diabetes, lung disease and kidney disease, together with the control of pre-eclampsia and eclampsia, are all major factors in the reduction of the perinatal death rate.

Probably the most important step that will be taken over the next few years will be a greater understanding of the causes of prematurity and improved care of the premature baby who really does require very expert nursing. Improved care with more rigid and better antenatal supervision is certainly the most potent factor in the prevention of prematurity, stillbirths and neonatal death.

It is an unpalatable and unfortunate fact that babies do occasionally die but it is also true that behind the scenes the authorities devote very considerable time, trouble and money in research to find out why these catastrophes occur. All doctors and midwives are keenly aware of the problem and do their utmost to ensure the welfare of those under their care

Indeed one might reasonably suggest that this book has been written as a contribution towards the next logical step in the health and welfare of the pregnant women of this country and their babies—better and more complete cooperation in antenatal care. If pregnant women are to be asked to accept more stringent supervision during their pregnancy then they must understand the reasons for any inconvenience which they may undergo and they must realize that everything they are asked to do is for their own and for their babies' benefit. Above all, the mother and all the members of her family must realize that they must accept the final responsibility for her welfare and that of the unborn child. The care of the baby throughout its intrauterine existence is the major factor in determining its future life.

42 Fertility

Normal fertility

What is normal fertility? This is a very simple question which is frequently asked but to which there is no simple and straightforward answer. It depends upon many factors and is essentially a very personal question to which the answer is different for every individual according to her history, age, physique, symptoms as well as her psychological background, the fitness of her husband, the frequency of intercourse and the stresses and strains of everyday life.

Broadly speaking, fertility varies with age, upon which usually depends such factors as the frequency of intercourse and health. The normal healthy young woman in her early twenties who is having intercourse three or more times per week has a chance of becoming pregnant according to the following:

One month	30 per cent
Two months	45
Three months	55
Six months	65
One year	80
Two years or longer	85

The above figures refer to an apparently fit, healthy young woman married to a fit and apparently healthy man, but of course, while most people tend to consider fertility or infertility to be a female problem, the male is totally responsible in 30 per cent and partially responsible in about 50 per cent of instances of infertility.

Age of the woman

Age is undoubtedly linked to fertility. There are many reasons why this is so and in a modern civilized society the age at which pregnancy is desired is usually somewhat different from the age at which marriage takes place. Nevertheless, if a woman wishes to become pregnant, the table below gives a rough idea of her chances of success depending on her age:

Under the age of 20	95 per cent
20–25	94
26–30	89
31–35	83
36–40	76

Fertility begins to fall after the age of 25, but the decline is comparatively slow until the age of 30, when it accelerates and increases quite rapidly from the age of 35 onwards. There is a strange phenomenon associated with the fertility of women which has long been known as the 'last fling of the ovary'. This is a sudden and unexplained rise in fertility at about the 39th year of life, which accounts for many an unexpected pregnancy in the late thirties and is usually the reason why the mother of teenage children, or even the young grandmother, suddenly finds herself in a state of unexpected pregnancy.

Age of the man

The effect of age upon male fertility is not well understood, but it does not appear to obey the same dramatic changes that affect women. There seems to be a gradual decline in the fertility of the male from a fertility rate of 95 per cent or more at the age of 20, to a 10 per cent fertility rate at the age of 60. Insufficient attention has been paid, especially in Great Britain, to the part that the male may play in infertility and, whereas until fairly recently it has been accepted that the male may be either fertile or infertile, it is now recognized that degrees of fertility in the male may play a much more important part than has been considered in the past.

Frequency of sexual intercourse

The ease with which a woman becomes pregnant is generally related directly to the frequency of sexual intercourse. There are, of course, many factors which influence the frequency of intercourse. Firstly, age, in so far as the young have intercourse more frequently than the old; then pregnancy is more likely because the young are more fertile than the old. Also there is the simple fact that if sexual intercourse occurs four times a week, sperms will almost always be present in the outer part of the Fallopian tube waiting for ovulation to occur, whereas if sexual intercourse occurs only once a week, the exact date of ovulation may be missed for several consecutive months.

It has often been suggested, and it is probably true, that a man's seminal count and also his potency will vary according to his general health as well as the number of times he has intercourse. If he is fit and well intercourse will certainly be more frequent than when he is ill or tired.

Emotional factors

Emotional factors, psychology and personality all play a large part in the process of conception. Psychological factors, stress, strain, tiredness and overwork can all lead directly or indirectly to unsatisfactory intercourse. These factors, of course, are more obvious in the male who may be either unwilling to have intercourse or may be incapable of maintaining a satisfactory erection.

It is when normal and satisfactory intercourse is taking place and all investigations have failed to reveal any abnormality that the really unknown psychological and emotional factors are evident. It is quite common for a couple who, having tried desperately to become pregnant over a number of years, have eventually decided on adoption and the wife has then become pregnant even before the adoption papers can be finally signed. These and many other examples do indicate that a relief from mental strain, anxiety and worry can occasionally play a vital part in conception.

Old wives' tales about fertility

Painful periods. It has often been stated that painful periods may give rise to infertility later in life and the more painful a girl's periods, then the greater the difficulty will she have in becoming pregnant and the more likely is she to miscarry. Nothing could be further from the truth. The spasmodic pain of which so many women complain on the first or second day of their normal period shows that their ovaries are working normally and there is no truth whatever in the suggestion that they will have any difficulty either in conceiving or in retaining a pregnancy. One might add here that the converse of the above is not true. Women can ovulate quite normally without having painful periods and, while painful periods are a sign of ovulation, 95 per cent of the women who do not have pain with their periods are, in fact, ovulating perfectly normally.

Irregular periods. Some women always have and always will have irregular periods. The only problem posed by an irregular menstrual cycle is the difficulty in deciding the exact date of ovulation. If sexual intercourse is occurring more than twice a week the exact time of ovulation is immaterial anyway. People who always have irregular periods are just as fertile as those who always have regular periods.

Infrequent periods. Women who have infrequent periods are just as fertile as those who have regular periods, the only disadvantage being that the woman who has only three or four periods a year has only three or four chances a year of becoming pregnant instead of thirteen as in the woman who has a period every 28 days.

Retroversion of the uterus. Approximately 17 per cent of girls are born with their uterus in a tilted or backward position. This is perfectly normal for them and their uterus will remain in this position for the whole of their lives. It is not associated with any difficulty in becoming pregnant nor is it associated with any increased tendency to miscarry. This so-called congenital type of retroversion is different from the acquired type of retroversion in which the uterus is tilted backwards as a result of disease or infection in the pelvis. It is then the disease or infection which limits the fertility and not the retroversion. The position of the uterus does not matter.

Family history. There is no truth in the stories that just because your mother had some difficulty in becoming pregnant or that she miscarried frequently, you are likely to do so, nor is there any truth in the suggestion that because your sisters have suffered from problems then you are likely to as well.

Advice

When should you see your doctor to ask him about your fertility? If you have any reason whatsoever to doubt your own fertility, or if you have any gynaecological symptoms that you consider to be abnormal, such as discharge, pain, irregularity or heavy bleeding, then you should consult your doctor about these.

If you do not have any abnormal symptoms, opinions on seeking advice about fertility are divided. The traditional school of thought that advice should not be sought until pregnancy has failed to occur after two years of normal intercourse without any attempts at contraception, is the answer that will be found in most medical textbooks. A lot of young people today, however, are not satisfied with this for two very good reasons. Firstly, they consider that if pregnancy has not occurred, two years is too long to wait before seeking advice and, secondly, they believe that there is always a chance that some abnormality may be present of which they are unaware because it is not causing them any symptoms and that this should be treated sooner rather than later. They also argue that since all women are supposed to have regular gynaecological check-ups and cervical smear tests, surely it is logical for them to ask about their own fertility. These arguments carry a great deal of force and there is no reason why a woman or even a couple should not seek advice regarding their fertility even before they plan to establish a pregnancy. This does not mean that extensive investigations should be undertaken, but a simple check-up to exclude any general disease, such as anaemia or any local condition within the reproductive tract, is certainly advisable. Any abnormality can then be treated or corrected rather than waiting for two years before its discovery.

When does infertility exist?

Infertility is something that is entirely relative depending as it does on age and circumstance. No one would pretend that a young woman of 18 who already has one child should seek advice about her inability to become pregnant again with the same urgency as a woman of 39 who married for the first time only six months previously. There are therefore two different aspects with regard to the advice that should be sought about fertility or infertility:

1 A routine general examination and examination of the pelvic organs to make certain that everything is normal.
2 Specialized examinations when a couple have failed to establish a pregnancy after a period of time which may vary from two years in the young to as little as three months in a woman who is older.

Investigation of infertility

Medical history

The first and most important aspect in the consideration of fertility is the past medical history of both the woman and her husband. The woman's past history will give many small indications about her fertility and normality. The age of onset of her periods, the regularity of her menstrual cycle, the duration and character of the flow, any pain and the time it occurs, evidence of ovulation pain or discomfort in the middle of the menstrual cycle, premenstrual tension, pain or other symptoms during the week or 10 days before the onset of the period, are all important. The doctor will ask about a past history of any generalized medical disease, especially those that might affect the liver, kidneys, heart or lungs, as well as any infection of the urinary tract (cystitis), or vaginal discharge; any abdominal operations, especially acute appendicitis, or any history of pelvic infection (especially gonorrhoea), previous pregnancy, miscarriage or abortion. The doctor will also want to know some details about sex life, especially the frequency of sexual intercourse and whether there is any pain or discomfort. The answers to all these simple questions, as well as to others concerning general health, are essential as a basis for a medical record.

A similar history is taken to obtain a record of the husband's past and present medical health. Mumps is of particular importance, because it can affect the testicles.

Examination

The wife. A general examination confirms that the general health of the woman is satisfactory and pelvic examination excludes any local abnormality. Good general health improves fertility and some very simple advice such as reduction of weight, relief of anxiety, stress and strain, understanding of over-tiredness and perhaps just simply a good holiday may go a long way towards correcting any latent or potential infertility that may exist.

The husband or partner has a general physical examination which will discover any obvious abnormality. The commonest problem is overweight and a simple weight-reducing diet should deal with it. Other factors such as over-tiredness, overwork, anxiety, too much alcohol and too many cigarettes, while they may be considered of little significance, can in fact exert quite a marked effect on fertility. Examination of the genitalia excludes local abnormality.

Any obvious abnormalities that may be present in either partner should be corrected. Advice will be given regarding the exact time of ovulation and the fact that pregnancy is most likely if intercourse takes place in the 2 or 3 days immediately preceding ovulation.

The doctor may refer the couple to an infertility clinic or to a specialist if a pregnancy is not established in what is considered a reasonable length of time.

Tests for the male partner

The most important test for the husband or partner is an examination of the seminal fluid to ascertain the sperm count and other details about the semen. The specimen of seminal fluid must be obtained in a clean, sterile jar by a process of masturbation. Seminal fluid collected in a condom during intercourse is not satisfactory because the condom may contain chemicals that destroy or damage the sperms. Also it is of paramount importance that the entire ejaculate should be obtained. The specimen may be produced at home and taken to a laboratory, but care must be taken that the jar or bottle is kept at body temperature and it should arrive at the laboratory within an hour of ejaculation. The exact time of ejaculation should be noted on the bottle.

The investigations performed upon the seminal fluid and an example of normal results are:

> Consistency: gelatinous
> Colour: opaque, white
> Volume: 2–5 ml
> Number of sperms: 60–150 million per ml
> Motility: 80 per cent motile after one hour
> Abnormal forms: less than 10 per cent
> Pus cells: 0–1
> Agglutination: nil

It is obvious that the motility of the sperms as well as their normality is just as, if not more, important than the total number of sperms present. A reduction in the total number of sperms usually indicates that there is some suppression in the formation of sperms, the commonest reason for this being abnormal temperature regulation in the testicles. The testicles are meant to function at a temperature less than that of the body temperature and any factor or factors which tend to raise the temperature of the testicles will suppress or diminish the normal formation of an adequate number of sperms. Items such as jockstraps, close fitting underpants, repeated and prolonged hot baths, electric blankets and, especially, overweight, are all factors which tend to raise the temperature of the testicles and thus seriously diminish the manufacture of sperms. If any of these factors are applicable they should be eliminated. A cold bath twice daily or bathing the testicles in cold water twice daily helps to improve sperm formation. Overindulgence in alcohol or tobacco further diminishes the production of spermatozoa.

The other main group of sub-fertile men are those in whom the testicles produce an adequate number of sperms but infection or inflammation in the prostate and seminal vesicles results in inadequate storage and maintenance of the sperms and a rise in the number of pus cells present.

Agglutination means that the sperms are adhering to each other, or in groups, with either the heads or the tails stuck to the adjacent sperm.

If there is any abnormality in the seminal count this is repeated on one or perhaps more occasions. If the abnormality persists, further investigation is undertaken in order to ascertain the cause of the deficiency before deciding on the necessary treatment.

Tests for the female partner

A very extensive and exhaustive series of tests has been designed for the infertile woman, but since these can only be undertaken in highly specialized gynaecological departments they have not been included here, especially as their value remains unproven.

Five main questions are asked:

1 Is normal sexual intercourse occurring?
2 Are the cervix and cervical canal healthy?
3 Is normal ovulation occurring?
4 Are the Fallopian tubes normal and functioning satisfactorily?
5 Is the uterus normal and is the lining of the uterus properly prepared?

Normal sexual intercourse

It is surprising how often sexual intercourse is, in fact, either unsatisfactory or occurring at the wrong time in the menstrual cycle or is so infrequent that the chances of conception are unlikely.

The cervix and cervical canal

The mucus within the cervical canal is an essential part of the whole process of conception and if the cervix is infected or in any way abnormal, then the mucus within the canal may also be abnormal. The normality of the cervix together with the mucus are determined by simple clinical examination.

Post-coital test. This extremely simple test reveals a great deal of information. It is very probable that the mucus in the canal of the cervix will only permit the passage of spermatozoa at or about the time of ovulation and it is therefore important that this test should be undertaken at this particular time in the menstrual cycle.

Mucus from the canal of the cervix is very gently aspirated about 6 or 8 hours after intercourse and is then examined under the microscope. Under normal circumstances many active and normal spermatozoa will be present in the specimen. A complete absence of sperms in the specimen may mean an absence or reduced number of sperms in the seminal specimen, so that the husband or partner must be retested. The presence of dead sperms in the cervical mucus even at the time of ovulation is a relatively common finding among women who are suffering from infertility and has given rise to the idea that some women will kill sperms in the cervical mucus. This apparent hostility of the cervical mucus to spermatozoa is inadequately understood but it may be the result of infection within the cervix and cervical canal, or of a very complicated immune reaction where the woman makes antibodies against her husband's or partner's sperms.

Ovulation

Several methods can be used to find out if normal ovulation is taking place. Perhaps the simplest and the easiest is the daily recording of the basal body temperature. The temperature is taken each morning immediately on waking, which means that it must be taken before getting out of bed and also before having a drink. It is recorded on a special piece of graph paper provided for this purpose. The basal body temperature remains at a fairly constant level during menstruation and after menstruation until the 13th or 14th day of a regular 28 day cycle. The temperature may dip slightly when ovulation occurs and then immediately rise by anything from 0.5 to 1°F above the level of the temperature in the first half of the cycle. This temperature level is maintained until just before the next menstrual period when, if conception has not occurred, the temperature falls dramatically, followed by menstruation within 12 to 24 hours. The rise in basal body temperature is caused by the action of progesterone secreted from the corpus luteum during the second half of the menstrual cycle, so that if the body temperature does go up during the second half of the cycle, this is strong evidence that ovulation has occurred.

Proof of ovulation can also be obtained by examining the mucus from the canal of the cervix, the characteristics of which change at the time of ovulation.

The hormone progesterone affects the whole of the reproductive tract and the result of its activity on the vagina can be observed by taking vaginal smears during the first and second part of the menstrual cycle. If ovulation has occurred (and therefore progesterone is being produced), specific changes can be seen in the vaginal smears during the second half of the cycle.

Endometrial biopsy is a particular test in which a small portion of the lining of the inside of the uterus is removed during the second half of the menstrual cycle. This small operation is performed without any discomfort either in the out-patient department or as part of a more complicated and extensive investigation. If ovulation has occurred it is obvious from the lining of the uterus.

Ovulation should not only occur regularly, but must be associated with adequate production of the corpus luteum. Where ovulation fails or is inadequate, extensive testing may show a reason and may lead to the use of fertility drugs (such as clomiphene or gonadotrophins) which stimulate the ovary to produce mature follicles. In the more recently recognized condition of raised pituitary prolactin, bromocryptine allows natural ovulation (suppressed by prolactin) to occur and the corpus luteum to function properly. The investigation of ovulatory failure is a highly complex affair and should be conducted by a specialist unit. From such a unit fertility drugs may be prescribed but their effect will be closely observed.

Oral contraceptive pills. Fertility is not increased after a course of oral contraceptive tablets. There is no truth in the belief that a short course of oral contraceptive tablets results in a 'fertility rebound' during which fertility is increased. Even so, it is nevertheless true that pregnancy does occasionally follow a course of oral contraceptive tablets given to a woman who has previously proved to be infertile. The exact reason for this is not known, but it may have something to do with the reduction in emotion and tension which occurs when a woman is taking an oral contraceptive, knowing that pregnancy cannot occur. When she stops taking the pill she becomes pregnant before the tension has had time to build up again. Stopping the oral contraceptive tablets may also be carefully timed to coincide with a holiday which may therefore be the deciding factor together with an increase in the frequency of intercourse.

Tests of the Fallopian tubes

If all the other tests have so far proved normal, then the state of the Fallopian tubes is assessed. If the Fallopian tubes are open they are said to be 'patent' and if they are not open they are said to be 'blocked'. Tests of tubal potency are: insufflation, hysterosalpingography and laparoscopy. These three tests should be performed during the first half of the menstrual cycle as soon as possible after the end of the menstrual period.

Insufflation, which may be performed either as an out-patient or an in-patient, is a procedure for testing the Fallopian tubes by passing carbon dioxide through a special applicator into the uterus. If the Fallopian tubes are patent the gas will flow into the peritoneal cavity at a normal pressure. If the Fallopian tubes are blocked, then the carbon dioxide will not pass along them even if the pressure is raised to its highest permissible limit.

The information provided by a positive insufflation is that at least one Fallopian tube is functioning normally. It does not, however, give details of both Fallopian tubes, simply because the passage of gas along one tube will provide a normal tracing. If the carbon dioxide does not escape from the uterine cavity this does not necessarily mean that the tubes are, in fact, blocked. The muscular coat of the Fallopian tube may have gone into spasm which may be sufficient to prevent the passage of gas along the tube. Insufflation, therefore, does have certain limitations, although the ease with which it can be performed and the lack of discomfort, as well as the fact that it does not require extensive equipment, combine to give it a useful place in the investigation of infertility.

Insufflation does have one further main advantage, in that occasionally the carbon dioxide may dislodge a mucous plug from the cavity of the Fallopian tubes. The frequency with which conception follows insufflation in a woman who has previously been considered infertile would indicate that this particular advantage occurs much more frequently than is generally appreciated.

Hysterosalpingography is an investigation similar to insufflation, except that X-ray opaque dye is injected into the uterus instead of gas. X-rays are taken which reveal details of the size of the cavity of the uterus, together with any possible congenital abnormality, or distortion of the cavity. They also provide information about the condition of the cervical canal, a factor that may be important in women who suffer from recurrent abortion. The shape, outline and position of the Fallopian tubes are demonstrated as the dye passes along them. As dye spills from the tubes into the abdominal cavity further information about the tubes and ovaries is obtained. This test is more reliable than insufflation particularly with new X-ray techniques and the use of the image intensifier.

Laparoscopy. This technique has become very popular for the investigation of infertility. Under general anaesthesia a half-inch incision is made in the umbilicus and the laparoscope (a narrow telescope-like instrument) is passed into the abdominal cavity. It contains its own light so that the surgeon can inspect the pelvic organs checking the uterus, tubes and ovaries for evidence of past or present disease. A harmless blue dye introduced into the uterus through the cervix will be seen to spill out into the pelvic cavity if the tubes are patent. Laparoscopy will enable the surgeon to decide if surgery to the tubes is necessary to help restore fertility.

Artificial insemination

Artificial insemination is used to describe the technique whereby seminal fluid, previously produced, is placed at the top of the vagina or in the canal of the cervix. The seminal specimen may be produced by the husband, in which case it is known as 'artificial insemination husband' (AIH) or by a donor especially selected for that purpose, in which case it is known as 'artificial insemination donor' (AID). There are many ethical and legal arguments surrounding both AIH and AID. Obviously artificial insemination by a donor is a much more drastic step than artificial insemination by the husband or partner, but artificial insemination in any circumstances should not be undertaken without very careful consideration and discussion of all the available facts with the family doctor. Before artificial insemination can be considered, the wife must be very carefully examined to ensure that she is capable of having a normal pregnancy and a normal baby and also to ascertain accurately the time of ovulation.

Artificial insemination by a husband or partner is only performed where normal intercourse is either not possible or not practicable, or where a specialist might consider that the amount of seminal fluid is so small that there is an advantage to be gained by artificial insemination. AIH can be performed by the woman herself by the use of a special cervical applicator, in which the seminal fluid is placed and which she then puts in the vagina and over the cervix. In this way there is a maximum possibility of the sperms entering the cervical canal.

Donor insemination is usually restricted to those instances where it has been conclusively proved that the husband or partner has no sperms or that his sperm count is so low as to render pregnancy either very unlikely or actually impossible. Artificial insemination by donor is not normally available as part of the National Health Service. A donor is very carefully selected because his height, colouring, physique and intelligence are similar to the husband's or partner's, and his seminal count is tested. If it is found to be normal, artificial insemination with a specimen of the donor's seminal fluid is performed by the doctor, who places the semen at the top of the vagina close to the cervix by means of a special syringe and cannula. It is obvious that the donor and the recipient should not meet, nor be aware of each other's identity.

Some couples seek artificial insemination donor as an alternative to adoption. Since the introduction of the Abortion Act the number of babies available for adoption has been drastically reduced and it is, therefore, possible that the demand for artificial insemination donor may increase in the future.

Rhesus incompatibility. Some women became sensitized before anti-D immunoglobulin was available and have suffered from several disastrous and unproductive pregnancies as a result of Rhesus incompatibility. If such a woman has a homozygous Rhesus positive husband or partner the couple may have considered the possibility of artificial insemination with a Rhesus negative donor. Such artificial insemination would give rise to a Rhesus negative baby who would not be affected by the mother's antibody.

In-vitro **fertilization ('test-tube babies').** In recent years hope has been given to a small number of couples, in whom normal pregnancy is prevented by irreparable damage to the woman's Fallopian tubes. This often occurs as a result of pelvic infection, and tubal surgery may not always be successful. It is now possible to collect an egg at the time of ovulation, by using a laparoscope to visualize the ovary. The egg is then fertilized in the laboratory with the husband's or partner's semen, and grown in very sterile and controlled surroundings. The resulting fertilized egg, if healthy, is then re-inserted into the woman's uterus a few days later.

As yet, this is not a facility that is universally provided by the National Health Service, and as with artificial insemination there are many ethical arguments about the creation of life outside the human body.

43 Family Planning

This book is designed primarily as a guide to pregnancy, together with its associated aspects and problems. Family planning, or the control of conception, is an essential part of the subject of reproduction since ideally a child should be born because it is wanted, not because it cannot be prevented. This ideal is made possible by the intelligent understanding of conception and the use of modern contraceptive methods whereby conception can be controlled satisfactorily and safely. The majority of marriages are more satisfactory when there is a good sexual relationship, and this can be achieved more easily by the confident use of conception control than when there is a constant fear of unwanted pregnancy.

That contraception is entirely for the prevention of conception is a rather outdated idea which must be replaced by the more modern view of the control of conception: that a couple may produce the number of children they desire at a spacing they consider to be expedient, according to their social and economic circumstances. The natural desire to exercise this voluntary control is rapidly increasing with the result that more frequent demands are made for advice and discussion on the available methods of contraception. For various economic and social reasons, the limitation of family size and the optimal spacing of children are a necessity for most married couples.

The National Health Service in Great Britain is in the process of accepting responsibility for the provision of a comprehensive service to advise on the control of conception, mainly because of popular demand and public pressure. Meanwhile, the Family Planning Association, who have more than one thousand clinics throughout the United Kingdom, provide an excellent service. This association is entirely voluntary and its ability to cater for the entire population is, therefore, somewhat restricted. Most local authorities now provide a rather limited family planning service, and the number of family planning clinics in hospitals is gradually increasing, although the majority only provide this service for their own postnatal or other patients.

From a medical point of view certain conditions may provide a temporary or permanent threat to the health of a woman should she become pregnant. These are surprisingly few and far between but pregnancy must be satisfactorily controlled. Pregnancy may be permanently advised against in the presence of a few rare conditions such as advanced heart disease, advanced renal disease, previously treated and cured malignant disease, and some other rare illnesses seldom seen in the United Kingdom. Limiting the number of pregnancies may be necessary in a woman suffering from severe Rhesus incompatibility, although this is becoming an increasingly rare condition. Temporary postponement of pregnancy is advisable after an operation or debilitating disease, or after severe pre-eclampsia in a previous pregnancy, or as a result of recent 'mental breakdown', or for social reasons such as caring for elderly relatives or children who are unwell.

From a purely scientific point of view, the medical reasons for limiting or spacing pregnancies must have a very elastic interpretation. Fear of an unwanted pregnancy may have very serious effects on the mental and physical health of a woman. It can limit or stop her desire for sexual intercourse, so that her relationship with her husband may become strained or even break down, and this has far-reaching effects on the health and welfare of the whole family.

Any reliable method used for the control of conception depends for its efficiency on its correct and proper application. Most couples practise some form of conception control without ever having any knowledge, consideration or discussion of all the techniques available to them. It is strange how the most enlightened woman, or even doctor, becomes biased in an opinion of one or more contraceptive methods. The reliability of the different methods must always be considered before a decision is reached and it must be remembered that published figures are often prejudiced by vested interests or by personal enthusiasm.

The choice of contraceptive method depends upon the particular requirements of the couple concerned. It is of paramount importance that if a woman is going to use a contraceptive it must be acceptable to herself as well as to her partner. Her sex life is her own affair and it should not be influenced by elderly relations, neighbours or girl friends. If the method chosen is not acceptable to her mentally, psychologically or aesthetically, then it is bound to have a deleterious effect upon her normal and harmonious sex life. She can only reach a satisfactory decision as a result of enlightened and frank discussion after all the facts have been placed at her disposal.

The methods available are:

1 *Abstinence*
 Total abstinence
 Abstinence during the fertile phase
2 *Female contraception*
 Spermicidal substances in the vagina
 Douching
 Occlusive diaphragm
 Intrauterine contraceptive devices
 Suppression of ovulation

     Altering cervical mucus
     Surgical sterilization
3 *Male contraception*
     Withdrawal (coitus interruptus)
     Condom or sheath
     Drugs
     Surgical sterilization

Abstinence

Total abstinence

Total abstinence is the only absolute and certain method of preventing conception. It must be remembered, however, that sperms deposited at the vulva or at the entrance to the vagina can migrate up the vagina and may therefore result in conception. This can happen in a woman who still has an unruptured hymen and has never had complete sexual intercourse. Sperms can also be transferred after ejaculation by a finger inserted into the vagina.

Abstinence during the fertile phase

This is known as the 'rhythm method', involving the use of the 'safe period' which depends on avoiding sexual intercourse during the days when conception is likely to occur. It is a method of control of conception accepted by the Roman Catholic Church. The use of the safe period depends on certain basic principles which must be properly understood if it is to be used as an efficient method of conception control.

The normal menstrual cycle lasts for approximately 28 days, but the duration of the menstrual cycle varies from woman to woman and a regular 28 day cycle is by no means an absolute rule. The importance of this point is that ovulation occurs *14 days before* the next menstrual period and *not* 14 days *after* the previous period. At ovulation the egg is shed from the ovary and unless it is fertilized within 18 hours it dies. It necessarily follows, therefore, that fertilization must occur within 18 hours of the time of ovulation. Counting the first day of the period as day 1 of the menstrual cycle, ovulation occurs on the 14th day of a 28 day cycle, but since it also occurs 14 days before the next period, it will be on the 15th day of a 29 day cycle, the 13th day of a 27 day cycle, the 20th day of a 34 day cycle, or the 21st day of a 35 day menstrual cycle.

The exact timing of ovulation may vary even in a person who has a very regular menstrual cycle, although not usually for more than 24 hours on either side of the 14th day before the next period. It may occasionally vary by as much as 3 days, especially as a result of stress, strain or shock. Thus, although ovulation usually occurs 14 days before the next menstrual period it may frequently occur anywhere between the 13th and 15th day of a regular 28 day cycle, and can, on rare occasions, take place anywhere between the 11th and the 17th day (or between the 18th and 24th day of a 35 day cycle).

Newly ejaculated sperms are contained within the semi-gelatinous seminal fluid which is slightly alkaline. The vagina is acid and the cervix alkaline. Unless sperms can gain access to the cervix within 15 or 20 minutes following ejaculation they are killed by the acid medium of the vagina. Those that gain access to the alkaline environment of the canal of the cervix rapidly swim up the uterus and along the Fallopian tubes. This journey takes approximately 45 minutes. These sperms survive and remain capable of fertilization for approximately 2 days, but may occasionally live for as long as 7.

By adding together the extremes of sperm survival on the one hand and the range of ovulation on the other, it can be seen that *in a normal 28 day menstrual cycle* it is possible for conception to occur if intercourse takes place at any time between the 9th and the 17th day inclusive. This is the 'dangerous period'. The safe period is divided into two parts: the first 8 days of the menstrual cycle, counting from the onset of menstruation and from day 18 to day 28 inclusive, providing the woman has a 28 day cycle. If the menstrual cycle is regular and these rules have been carefully applied conception is unlikely to occur, but a warning must be given that there are plenty of instances of women becoming pregnant following intercourse even as early as the second or third day of a regular 28 day menstrual cycle. This conception results either because sperms have survived for a particularly long time, or, more likely, because of so called 'spurious ovulation' at an unusually early day in the cycle. Such a pregnancy is quite normal. Ovulation in the human female, unlike some animals, is not dependent on either sexual intercourse or orgasm but spurious ovulation is a rare phenomenon which may be provoked by sexual stimulation.

The safe period must be very carefully calculated if the usual cycle is not a 28 day cycle. For instance, in a 35 day regular menstrual cycle the dangerous time is from day 15 to day 25 inclusive, so that under these circumstances the safe period is from the first to the 15th day and from the 25th to the 35th day. If the menstrual cycle is irregular, the time of ovulation is correspondingly irregular and it is difficult to calculate the expected safe period. Added safety may be provided if the woman checks her own cervical mucus, which becomes very watery at ovulation (Billings method).

A previously regular menstrual cycle may become irregular in the immediate postnatal months, or as a result of travel, strain or illness, and also in the late thirties or early forties, and it is during these times that the safe period is unreliable.

Female Contraception

Spermicidal substances in the vagina

Chemical spermicides are available as soluble pessaries, creams, jellies or foaming tablets which are inserted into the vagina before intercourse. Spermicidal substances used alone are not recommended because they are not completely reliable and should be used with some form of occlusive device or diaphragm. Spermicidal substances themselves contain chemicals which kill sperms very rapidly, but if ejaculation occurs directly into the canal of the cervix there is no opportunity to kill the sperms before they gain access to the cervical canal. It is for this reason that spermicides only constitute a reliable contraceptive when used with some form of occlusive device. A list of efficient chemical spermicidal preparations which have been tested may be obtained from the Family Planning Association or any of their clinics.

Sponges or tampons soaked in a spermicidal chemical and placed in the upper vagina prior to intercourse are designed to prevent direct ejaculation into the cervical canal. These are relatively inefficient, however, since they are frequently displaced during intercourse and are now little used.

Douching

Douching the vagina with a spermicidal or antiseptic solution immediately after coitus in order to wash away the sperms that have been implanted in the upper vagina is a fairly common method of attempting to achieve contraception. It can only be effective if done immediately after sexual intercourse and before any spermatozoa have managed to reach the alkaline medium of the cervical canal, whence they cannot be dislodged. This method has very obvious aesthetic disadvantages as well as being highly inefficient and occasionally dangerous.

Occlusive diaphragm

An occlusive diaphragm is a rubber or plastic diaphragm which is placed in the vagina, either over the cervix alone or over both the cervix and the anterior vaginal wall, and forms a barrier to the direct passage of sperms into the cervical canal. Sperms can, theoretically, pass round the edge of such a diaphragm and it is therefore only completely effective when used with a chemical spermicidal agent. Sufficient time must be allowed for complete destruction of the sperms before the diaphragm is removed. In actual practice the diaphragm is liberally covered with spermicidal cream or jelly and inserted at any convenient time before intercourse. It should remain in position for a minimum of 6 hours after intercourse. A properly fitted diaphragm causes no discomfort and neither the owner nor her partner should be aware of its presence. Because an occlusive diaphragm is always used with a spermicidal cream, douching is unnecessary either after intercourse or after the diaphragm has been removed.

Since it is essential that a diaphragm should fit properly your doctor or the local family planning clinic should be consulted if this method of contraception is contemplated. The technique of inserting an occlusive diaphragm is very simple and although its removal may sound complicated, it is also extremely simple, and the proper use of a diaphragm can be mastered very quickly and efficiently by most women. When a diaphragm is first fitted complete instructions are given for its use. A second visit after a few days shows the doctor whether the diaphragm is being inserted correctly and placed in the proper position.

The size of the diaphragm should be checked regularly since the size and shape of the vagina may change, especially if there is a marked change in weight, or as a result of illness or the formation of vaginal prolapse, or following pelvic operations. In any event, every woman should have a routine vaginal examination, together with a cervical smear and discussion of her contraceptive technique every one or two years. A diaphragm always needs refitting after childbirth and this is usually done at the postnatal clinic.

There are three main types of occlusive diaphragm: the Dutch cap, the cervical cap and the Vimule.

The Dutch cap, or vaginal diaphragm, is a dome-shaped diaphragm made of thin rubber with a rubber covered metal rim containing a spring. The sizes vary from 60 to 95 mm in diameter. The diaphragm fits on the anterior vaginal wall stretching from the posterior fornix of the vagina, just behind the cervix, downwards to rest just behind the symphysis pubis. It thus covers the cervix, and during intercourse the penis is introduced into the vagina between the diaphragm and the posterior vaginal wall, so that ejaculation occurs in a position where the sperms cannot gain direct access to the cervix. The diaphragm itself is held in position by the tension of the gentle spring in the rim. It is unsatisfactory when the vaginal tone is lax, or when a considerable degree of prolapse is present, since it cannot then be retained easily, and it may also be unsatisfactory after repair operations on the vaginal wall.

The correct size of diaphragm is extremely important because a properly fitting diaphragm is both efficient and completely comfortable so that the woman is not conscious of its presence. A diaphragm may be inserted either by compressing it between the fingers or by introducing it into the vagina on a special applicator. When a diaphragm is fitted, instructions are given about the type of spermicidal cream or jelly that should be used and the amount that should be placed upon each surface.

The majority of women who use a diaphragm find it is satisfactory, especially if it is inserted every night as a matter of routine. Most women

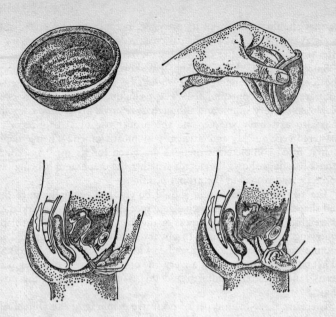

Fig 39 The Dutch cap

remove it the following morning about 8 hours after intercourse although at least 6 hours is generally stated to be sufficient. The main reasons for pregnancy occurring when this method is used are that the woman has been careless or has a retroverted uterus. If the uterus is tilted backwards it is very easy to insert the diaphragm so that its upper margin lies in the anterior vaginal fornix thus leaving the cervix exposed. If a woman has a retroverted uterus then special care must be taken in fitting the diaphragm and in its subsequent use.

The cervical cap is a rubber device shaped rather like a thimble with a solid rolled rubber rim. It is available in five sizes and fits snugly to the column of the cervix where it is held by suction. Since it is only reliable if the cervix has parallel sides, is healthy and not lacerated by previous deliveries, the cervical cap is not as popular as the vaginal diaphragm. However, when the uterus is retroverted, the cervix points downwards and forwards into the vagina and the cap is then more easily manipulated onto and off the cervix. Some women prefer a cervical cap to a diaphragm, despite the fact that it is more difficult to manipulate, mainly because it is smaller, covers less of the vaginal wall and may allow more satisfaction during intercourse. Contrary to general belief it is seldom dislodged during intercourse. Very accurate initial fitting as well as careful instruction in its use are essential. It should always be used with a spermicidal cream or jelly and removed about 8 hours after intercourse.

The Vimule is a cross between a diaphragm and a cervical cap and, like these, has to be accurately fitted and careful instruction given to the woman before its use. It remains in place by suction and must be used with a spermicidal cream or jelly.

Intrauterine contraceptive devices

Intrauterine contraceptive devices are made of metal or plastic and placed within the cavity of the uterus. They became popular in the 1930s when Grafenberg developed a silver coiled wire ring which was inserted into the cavity of the uterus and left there undisturbed for approximately one year before being removed or changed. Its major disadvantage was that it required an anaesthetic for both insertion and removal. Before this, various types of intrauterine and intracervical contraceptive devices had been used though the majority had, for various reasons, been found unsatisfactory.

The Grafenberg ring earned an undeservedly bad reputation, not only because it was said to be inefficient and ineffective, but also because it was supposed to cause infection in the uterus and the pelvic organs and predispose the woman to cancer of the uterus. In fact from about 1930 to 1950 it was one of the most efficient forms of contraception available. It certainly never caused infection, or the likelihood of cancer of the uterus, but if a woman using a Grafenberg ring developed pelvic infection the symptoms were aggravated by its presence in the uterus.

It must always be remembered that the whole problem of contraception or the control of conception is bedevilled by bigotry and prejudice, and many doctors and scientists have condemned the Grafenberg ring and other intrauterine contraceptive devices because of supposed complications that never existed in reality. After the Second World War the pressing need for population control on a scale not previously envisaged resulted in a more critical examination of these methods, as a result of which plastic devices were introduced. They varied in shape and size, as well as in the type of plastic used and eventually replaced other materials such as tantalum, steel, stainless steel and nylon, partly because of their reliability and flexibility, but also because of the ease and cheapness with which they could be produced. The Lippes Loop, Margulies Spiral, Birnberg Bow, Saf-T-Coil and Dalkon Shield became very popular. More recently devices incorporating copper elements which increase their efficacy by a local effect have been introduced and have gained widespread acceptance. The development of safe intrauterine devices has led to their acceptance in most communities.

These devices are flexible so that they can be straightened and fitted into introducers which are then passed gently into the canal of the cervix, after

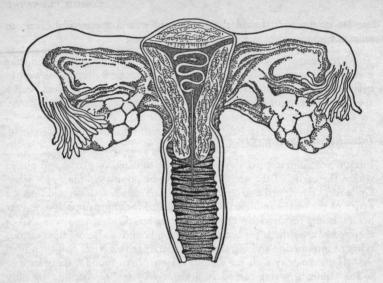

Fig. 40   An intrauterine contraceptive device

which the device itself is released within the cavity of the uterus to take up its previous shape. The majority have fine nylon threads that hang down through the cervix into the upper vagina, and can be felt by the woman herself or by an examining doctor to make sure that the device is in a satisfactory position.

The threads are so fine that they do not interfere with normal intercourse and neither partner is aware of them. The technique of insertion of a plastic device is simple in any woman who has had a baby or even a miscarriage, and is also painless, or associated with only mild discomfort. It is possible to insert one without any pain or discomfort into some women who have never been pregnant, but the majority, as well as all unduly nervous women, do require an anaesthetic. The removal of the device by pulling gently on the threads is simple, easy and painless.

Intrauterine devices (including the more recently introduced metal and plastic ones) are now previously sterilized by a special irradiation technique which makes their insertion even more simple than before. Some women experience minor degrees of uterine cramp, rather like period pains, immediately after insertion but this is generally relieved by codeine or a similar drug. The device should be inserted either during or immediately after the period to ensure that the woman is not pregnant. Slight continuous or intermittent bleeding may occur for a few days and the first few periods may be unduly heavy or prolonged. Not all women can tolerate these devices and approximately 20 per cent have to be removed within 3 months because of discomfort, actual pain, continuous and heavy bleeding or vaginal discharge.

The exact mechanism whereby an intrauterine contraceptive device works is not known. The following suggestions have been put forward:

1 The presence of a device alters the chemical composition of the fluid within the uterus and the mucus within the canal of the cervix so that the sperms cannot penetrate through either the cervix or the uterus.

2 The presence of the device within the uterus makes the migration of sperms more difficult.

3 The device provokes increased contractions of both the uterus and the Fallopian tubes, so that the fertilized ovum is propelled towards the uterus far more rapidly than is normal and reaches the uterine cavity before its chorionic villi have developed, or before the lining of the uterus is ready to receive it. This is the most probable factor. This is caused by increased prostaglandin release.

4 The normal preparation of the endometrium is prevented by the presence of the device.

5 The device increases the contractions of the uterus, so that it expels the newly fertilized ovum.

It must always be remembered that the majority of people have very definite views about contraception, particularly about the method of contraception which they themselves should adopt, and despite what anyone may say they will use the contraceptive of their choice. If they are forced to use a contraceptive they do not like or in which they have no confidence, it can quite easily exert a deleterious effect upon their sex lives. One of the strongest indications, therefore, for the use of an intrauterine device is for those people who request it because they do not wish to take hormones nor do they wish to use any mechanical form of contraception, or to practise coitus interruptus or the safe period. It is undoubtedly a relatively efficient and acceptable contraceptive for those women who can tolerate it, although a woman who is happy using a simple mechanical contraceptive correctly, or safely taking an oral contraceptive, gains nothing by using an intrauterine device. Their ideal use and their main value are in the population control of a whole community but there is no reason why they should not be used by particular individuals who so desire.

The contra-indications for intrauterine contraceptive devices are:

1 If a woman has pain with her periods (especially if she has never been pregnant) then an intrauterine device is likely to make it more severe. A small amount of pain may not matter, but fairly severe menstrual pain should be discussed with a doctor or at the clinic before the device is inserted.

2 If the periods are unduly heavy or prolonged then very careful thought

must be given before a device is inserted, because they always have a tendency to increase both the amount and the duration of bleeding. This does not matter if the period is short or the amount of bleeding very little, but if the periods are prolonged or the bleeding profuse then a device should not be inserted until these symptoms have been eliminated.

3 An intrauterine device should not be inserted if there is pelvic infection but can usually be inserted with complete safety after this has been cured.

4 Intrauterine devices used not to be inserted unless a woman had been pregnant as it was technically difficult and rather painful unless performed under anaesthetic. With the introduction of the newer and smaller devices this is no longer true and the patient who has never been pregnant can usually have a device fitted with minimal discomfort. This possibility may be ascertained by a simple examination.

5 Intrauterine devices are not usually inserted until several weeks after delivery and during this time some alternative method such as a diaphragm or sheath should be used.

Suppression of ovulation

If ovulation, or the production of ova, is stopped the woman cannot become pregnant.

Oral contraceptive pill

The two main hormones produced by the ovary are oestrogen and progesterone. The administration of both of these hormones in the correct dose will suppress ovulation, but if either progesterone or oestrogen are given alone it requires a relatively high dose to prevent ovulation. A combination of the two hormones is therefore used in the majority of oral contraceptive tablets. The amount of oestrogen which each tablet may contain is limited in Great Britain to 50 micrograms per day, because higher doses than this have been shown to increase the incidence of clotting disorders in the blood.

Small doses of some progesterone preparations will also act as quite efficient contraceptive agents by altering the constituents of the mucus in the cervical canal as well as the contractions and secretions of the Fallopian tubes, but the contraceptive pills in general use in Great Britain are limited to those which suppress ovulation, although they may also have some of these effects. A great deal of money is being spent on research into the causes of side effects of the contraceptive pill and undoubtedly improved pills and completely new contraceptive agents will be available in the foreseeable future.

Oral contraception by the suppression of ovulation is the most efficient of all contraceptive methods yet available. Approximately one million women in Britain take an oral contraceptive. The tablets are taken for 20 or 21 days in each menstrual cycle, starting on the 5th day after the onset of the period. (Some brands are marketed in packets of 28, containing the 21 tablets with active ingredients followed by 7 tablets containing sugar, or a similar substance, so that one tablet is taken every day.)

The exact mode of action of oral contraceptives is still in doubt. Although their efficiency is accepted and has been widely exploited in their favour, the exact reason for this efficiency is not precisely known. The administration of a small quantity of a mixture of oestrogen and progesterone certainly exerts an influence upon the delicate mechanism of ovulation and seems to hoodwink the body (especially the pituitary gland) into believing that ovulation is not necessary and, therefore, the production of an ovum is suppressed. The mechanism is very similar to that which causes the suppression of ovulation during pregnancy.

The enormous controversy that exists concerning the administration of the contraceptive pill for contraceptive purposes is clouded by many irrelevant issues. It has both good and bad aspects and its advantages and disadvantages are an individual matter for every woman.

The hormones, progesterone and oestrogen, used in contraceptive pills are accepted in much larger doses by doctors and scientists as being satisfactory for the treatment of gynaecological disorders and threatened abortion in early pregnancy. Any drug carries certain dangers, however slight, just as there are dangers in crossing a busy street. From a purely medical point of view, the controversy over the use of oral contraceptives is whether it is justified to administer drugs for contraceptive purposes when there is no medical reason to prevent a pregnancy. An injection of morphine may be given to a man who has just broken his leg in a car accident, but no one would give this to a man if he was not in pain. While some people believe that oral contraception is justified by virtue of its very high rate of efficiency, others, who accept the principle of the control of conception, are incapable of objective evaluation of the methods available. Oral contraceptive agents may contain hidden and as yet unknown dangers, but at the present stage of our knowledge it is surprising how many intelligent and well-meaning people have a genuine opinion against their use. Some doctors feel very strongly about these views, especially if they are asked to perform abortions on patients whose 'boy friend did not like the idea of the pill' or whose mother 'could never agree to it anyway'.

Oral contraception is by far the most efficient contraceptive available. The pregnancy rate is virtually nil amongst those who take the tablets conscientiously and regularly. It is easy, simple and aesthetically acceptable. It does not interfere with sexual intercourse and there are no mechanical devices involved. It controls the menstrual cycle to a regular 28 days and reduces the amount of menstrual loss, as well as controlling or eliminating pain with the periods. There are many other minor advantages.

The modern contraceptive pill contains approximately 10 per cent of the dose of hormone administered in oral contraceptive tablets 20 years ago. The side effects are, therefore, less severe and fewer in number than those previously encountered, but, as the dose of hormone in oral contraceptives has gradually been reduced, the incidence of 'break-through' and intermenstrual bleeding has increased. This is related to hormone imbalance and may occur during the first few days of taking a contraceptive pill, or even the first few cycles. This 'spotting' between periods varies considerably but affects about 5 to 10 per cent of women who take the pill. The blood loss usually begins on or about the 17th day of the cycle and continues for 1 or 2 days, or, on occasions, lasts until the next period. Rarely is the bleeding sufficiently heavy to be like a period itself. If spotting alone occurs the tablets should be continued for the remainder of the cycle. Your doctor should be told if this type of bleeding recurs, as it is possible to change the type of pill to one with a higher progesterone or oestrogen amount in order to prevent further bleeding.

Some people are unduly sensitive to specific drugs and this is as true of hormones as it is of antibiotics or aspirin. It is very difficult to assess the other side effects of oral contraceptive agents. Most people, especially women, are either 'pro-pill' or 'anti-pill' while a few are neutral.

Nausea is usually a transient symptom beginning shortly after the first tablet is taken and lasting for only a few days. It may, however, continue for much longer and become increasingly severe. Actual vomiting is unlikely with modern low-dose contraceptive tablets but does occasionally happen in women who are hypersensitive to hormones.

Fluid retention within the body may produce the rather annoying group of symptoms of which some women complain for a few days before their period: breast enlargement and tenderness, nervousness, irritability, depression, a general sensation of lethargy, headache or even migraine, swelling of the fingers and ankles and a generalized feeling of being waterlogged or bloated. Most women retain fluid for a few days before a period but the severity of the symptoms of premenstrual tension is not always related to the amount of fluid retained. Some women who gain 1.8 or 2.2 kg in weight have quite severe symptoms while others have no symptoms at all. This applies to women taking oral contraceptives and it is made even more difficult to understand since one of the more successful treatments for premenstrual tension is to give a woman a low-dose oral contraceptive.

Weight gain. Most women undoubtedly gain weight while taking the pill just as some women gain excess weight when they are pregnant. There is a factor in the oral contraceptive agents which causes some fluid retention and may even cause some weight increase but the majority of women gain weight while taking contraceptive pills because they are eating more. Women with a weight problem must be even more careful if they take oral contraceptives. Uncontrolled weight gain is obviously undesirable.

The breasts may increase in size if there is development of breast tissue This is usually considered an advantage, although the increase is sometimes sufficiently marked to be unwelcome. Breast enlargement may cause discomfort and occasionally pain which is so severe that the pill has to be stopped.

Menstruation itself is normally very much shorter, the loss reduced and the blood darker; actual cessation of periods may occur while taking an oral contraceptive, but this should not give rise to concern, because they will nearly always begin shortly after the pills are discontinued. Only on very rare occasions is a drug, such as Clomiphene, necessary to restore the normal menstrual rhythm after a long course of oral contraception.

Sexual behaviour. The psychological effect exerted by the oral contraceptive pill is virtually impossible to predict. Some women have an increase of libido and others undoubtedly have a suppression of sexual desire, but whether these changes in sexual behaviour are psychological or a result of the hormones themselves is not certain.

The dangers of oral contraception have been very much over-stressed but should nevertheless always be considered with its advantages and the requirements of the woman concerned.

The genital tract. There is no evidence that oral contraceptive tablets predispose to cancer of the uterus or the cervix; in fact it is just the opposite. The mucous secretion from the cervix may be increased causing a certain amount of whitish vaginal discharge. The continuous administration of oral contraceptives undoubtedly predisposes some women to fungus infections of the vagina. An isolated attack can be easily cured by a fungicidal agent and recurrent attacks prevented by treatment on one night each week for an indefinite period. These infections, however, while they are not dangerous, may cause such irritation and annoyance that a woman will change her contraceptive technique.

The breasts. Oral contraceptives do not cause cancer of the breast or even make it more likely to develop, but their use is not advised in any woman who has suffered from malignant disease and this is especially applicable to those women who have suffered from cancer of the breast itself.

The liver. Oral contraceptives may alter the function of the liver but not to a degree that can be recognized clinically. They are not given to a woman suffering from severe liver disease, or to anyone who has been recently jaundiced.

Carbohydrate metabolism. A great deal of publicity has been given to changes which may occur in the carbohydrate (or sugar) metabolism in women taking oral contraceptives. Whilst they do not cause diabetes, they do alter a woman's tolerance to glucose and should be used with care in diabetics.

Heart disease. Expert advice should certainly be obtained by any woman who suffers from any form of heart disease before embarking on a course of oral contraceptives, although they are not necessarily forbidden.

Varicose veins. A number of women who take oral contraceptives complain that varicose veins in their legs become more prominent, or that actual varices have developed while they have been taking the pill. It is not known if contraceptive pills exert any influence on the formation or increase of varicose veins.

Thrombo-embolic disease. Both oestrogen and progesterone cause changes in the clotting mechanism of the blood, but the clinical importance of this has been difficult to assess. Undoubtedly, oestrogen causes the greater changes and it is for this reason that the amount of oestrogen has been restricted in oral contraceptives available in Great Britain.

The main problem with regard to alterations of the blood clotting mechanism is that clots which form in blood vessels may then circulate to the lungs and cause what is known as a pulmonary embolus. If the pulmonary embolus is sufficiently large, then sudden and dramatic death may occur. It is estimated that about 1 in every 2,000 women who are taking the pill is admitted to hospital each year for treatment of a venous thrombosis associated with an embolus, whereas in women who are not on oral contraceptives the figure is about 1 in every 20,000. There is also a strong relationship between the use of oral contraceptives and deaths from pulmonary emboli. Deaths occur in approximately 1 in every 100,000 women taking the pill each year. This risk of death is about seven times greater in women who are taking the pill than in women who are not on oral contraception.

The risk of thrombo-embolic disease to a woman on an oral contraceptive is definite although difficult to assess, but it is certainly less than the risk of thrombo-embolic disease during pregnancy.

Cardiovascular disease. The pill may also affect the metabolism of fats in the body, and predispose to the formation of arterial fatty clots, which may lead to a stroke or heart attack. It should not be prescribed in the woman over 35 years of age, especially if she smokes, is obese or has high blood pressure.

Pure statistics show that oral contraception is not only the most efficient but is also the safest method of control of conception, since alternative methods, being relatively inefficient, lead more frequently to abortion or pregnancy where the dangers are greater than the intrinsic dangers of the pill itself. There are risks in every form of medication and the risk inherent in taking oral contraceptive pills must be weighed against the known hazards of pregnancy or abortion. Contraceptive pills are not prescribed for any woman who has suffered from malignant disease, liver dysfunction, cardiac disease, renal disease, diabetes, mental depression, epilepsy or who has a history of thrombo-embolic phenomena or thrombophlebitis.

The contraceptive pill can be taken after delivery. Women who are not breast-feeding should start the pill on the 21st day after delivery regardless of the amount of vaginal bleeding still present, so that the first period will begin approximately 6 weeks after confinement. A woman who is fully breast-feeding will not usually ovulate, so she will not menstruate or become pregnant. When weaning begins ovulation recommences and since a woman is unaware of exactly when it occurs, she may conceive. If she is breast-feeding she should start the pill about 21 days before she plans to start weaning her baby. If a period does not come after the first course of tablets she should wait 7 days and start the next course of tablets. A period will arrive after weaning has been completed.

The pill is often prescribed for women who are breast-feeding although lactation is occasionally affected.

The 'once only' pill (post-coital pill). It has been known for many years that the administration of high doses of oestrogen within 48 hours of coitus causes failure of implantation, and then abortion. In Great Britain this form of contraception may only be prescribed by doctors in certain family planning clinics, and close follow-up of the woman is required. Although congenital abnormality has not been reported in pregnancies which continue, this is a theoretical risk and the woman should be offered a therapeutic abortion. This form of contraception is restricted to situations of unexpected coitus, including rape. An intrauterine device fitted within 72 hours of coitus may also have the same effect.

Long-acting injections

Long-acting hormone preparations were originally used in developing countries where the regular use of contraceptives could not be guaranteed. The popularity of such injections is growing in this country and they are particularly useful where combined oestrogen–progesterone pills are contra-indicated or where it is essential that a woman runs no risk of pregnancy, such as in the 3 months after rubella vaccination.

The injection consists of a progesterone derivative which is slowly released from an oily medium over the course of 3 months. Although the injection suits the majority of women who try it, the occurrence of annoying side effects such as the cessation or irregularity of periods or spotting of blood has prevented its widespread use as a routine contraceptive.

Altering cervical mucus

Sperms are deposited at the top of the vagina during ejaculation. The semi-gelatinous seminal fluid protects them from the acid of the vagina for about 15 or 20 minutes, after which they are killed unless they have managed to enter the canal of the cervix. The cervical canal is filled with slightly alkaline mucus which allows them to live. It seems, however, that this mucus is only able to keep the sperms fit and alive when the oestrogen and progesterone which normally circulate through the female body are at a particular level and in a precise balance. These conditions only occur immediately before and during ovulation when the cervical mucus under-goes characteristic changes and there is rapid sperm penetration and easy access to the upper genital tract. It is now believed that sperms are almost completely incapable of penetrating through the barrier of the cervical mucus at any other time during the menstrual cycle.

It should be theoretically possible to alter the hormone balance only very slightly but nevertheless sufficiently to prevent these characteristic changes in the cervical canal at ovulation. The cervical mucus would thus be permanently impenetrable to sperms. Small doses of some progesterone-like substance administered each day will, in fact, have this contraceptive action while being too small to suppress ovulation. Several substances that have been marketed have proved quite effective and in Britain are used in women who are lactating or who cannot take the oestrogen-containing pill for a medical reason (for example, the older woman).

Surgical sterilization

Surgical sterilization of a woman involves blocking the Fallopian tubes which are the passages from the ovaries to the uterus so that neither sperms nor ova can travel along them. Generally speaking, before this is done the written consent of both partners must be obtained. Sterilization of a woman must always be considered as an irreversible procedure, although a few operations to repair Fallopian tubes that have previously been divided or tied have been successful. Reconstruction is impossible if the tubes have been removed.

Sterilization is performed by making a small incision in the lower abdomen and tying, dividing or removing the Fallopian tubes. The opera-tion is today considered less hazardous than the removal of the appendix, but it does require admission to hospital that varies from 3 to 7 days, and a general anaesthetic.

Sterilization by laparoscopy has grown in popularity in recent years. The laparoscope, a very thin telescope, is inserted through the umbilicus and used to visualize the Fallopian tubes. A second small instrument is used to occlude the tubes by diathermy to destroy small segments or by the application of clips or rings to a loop of Fallopian tube. This operation also requires a general anaesthetic but the stay in hospital is reduced to 2 or 3 days.

Sterilization by removal, cutting or diathermy of the Fallopian tubes has no untoward effects after the immediate convalescence from the operation. The periods, the menstrual cycle, menopause, sexual intercourse, sexual satisfaction, and libido are completely unchanged.

It is important that the irreversible nature of the operation of female sterilization is properly understood by any woman and her husband or partner before it is undertaken. A final word of warning is that in very rare instances pregnancy has been known to occur in women who have had their Fallopian tubes either tied or divided.

Male contraception

Withdrawal

Coitus interruptus is an extremely common practice to which people usually refer when they say that pregnancy has been avoided by 'being careful'. Sexual intercourse takes place in a normal manner but the penis is withdrawn immediately before ejaculation. The unreliability of this method is obvious, but it nevertheless has general advantages. It costs nothing and it requires no equipment. It has a high failure rate. The obvious cause of failure is when ejaculation occurs within the vagina, but even if this is avoided the prostatic fluid secreted prior to ejaculation may contain active sperms. Also it is possible for sperms ejaculated at the vulva to migrate up the vagina and enter the uterus.

Coitus interruptus not only imposes a strain upon the man but is also a common reason for the failure of the woman to achieve an orgasm and therefore she does not enjoy intercourse fully. It can thus cause an anxiety state in both partners and the possibility of an unwanted pregnancy adds a further strain. It is not a method that can be recommended but, despite this, is widely used with a high degree of success by a large number of people who make no complaints. It must be repeated, however, that basically the method is unreliable and that people who practise it would probably enjoy their sexual intercourse more frequently and more fully if they used an adequate contraceptive.

Condom or sheath

In this method the penis is completely covered by a sheath made of very thin rubber (the condom) which is used only once, or a thicker material (washable sheath) which can be used repeatedly. A lubricant is advisable, although the majority of sheaths are already lubricated with a spermicidal jelly or cream. The condom is a fairly reliable method of contraception.

Its failure rate depends on the care with which it is used so that the sheath does not break or slip. Some women prefer to use a soluble spermicidal pessary as an additional precaution. It can, however, cause psychological disturbances sufficient to interfere with the potency of some men and many couples object to it because of the impairment of sensation or because of the inevitable interruption when the sheath is put on, since it can only be placed on the penis during an erection.

Drugs

Several drugs have been developed which either suppress formation of sperms or reduce their speed and energy. These are efficient contraceptive agents because they render fertilization impossible but have, so far, proved either too toxic or have caused impotence. An acceptable male contraceptive pill will undoubtedly be perfected in the near future.

Surgical sterilization

Surgical sterilization of a man is known as vasectomy. Sperms travel along a small duct called the vas deferens from the testicle to the prostate and thence eventually to the penis. The operation, designed to cut and tie the vas as it passes along the inguinal canal in the groin, is a comparatively minor surgical procedure which can be performed under a local anaesthetic in a few minutes. Some surgeons prefer to operate under general anaesthesia, but even then the patient need stay in hospital no longer than a day. The advantage of male sterilization is the ease with which it can be accomplished, and that it is reversible by a further operation in more than 70 per cent of men. (In the woman, operation for reconstruction of the Fallopian tubes is much less satisfactory.) The operation should, nevertheless, be regarded as irreversible.

Following vasectomy, sperms are still present in the seminal fluid for a considerable number of weeks and sexual intercourse need not be avoided but adequate contraception must be used until all sperms are known to have disappeared. This is done by performing seminal analyses. Two consecutive analyses showing a complete absence of sperms must be performed before contraceptive-free intercourse is allowed, and this may take as long as 3, or even 6 months.

There is no evidence that male sterilization by vasectomy has any deleterious effect upon either the psychology or the sexual activity of the male although it is still believed that this could easily occur, especially in a man who is particularly sensitive.

If sterilization is considered, then a decision as to whether the man or the woman should be sterilized can only be reached after a full discussion between the couple and their doctor.

44 The Abortion Act 1967

An abortion is the termination of a pregnancy before the end of the 28th week of pregnancy. Such a termination is against the law if it does not come within one or more of the four categories mentioned in the Abortion Act 1967 (published by Her Majesty's Stationery Office) and if the termination is not carried out under the conditions mentioned in the Act. In other words, if the Act is obeyed, then a pregnancy may be terminated lawfully, but if the Act is not obeyed then it is still unlawful, or criminal, to procure an abortion before the end of the 28th week of pregnancy.

According to the Act it is not a legal offence for a registered medical practitioner to terminate a pregnancy if 'two registered medical practitioners are of the opinion, formed in good faith' that

1 the continuance of the pregnancy would involve risk to the life of the pregnant woman greater than if the pregnancy were terminated; or
2 the continuance of the pregnancy would involve risk of injury to the physical or mental health of the pregnant woman greater than if the pregnancy were terminated; or
3 the continuance of the pregnancy would involve risk of injury to the physical or mental health of any existing children of the family of the pregnant woman greater than if the pregnancy were terminated; or
4 there is a substantial risk that if the child were born it would suffer from such physical or mental abnormalities as to be seriously handicapped.

It is also specified that an abortion must be performed in a National Health Service hospital or an approved place, with the provision that an emergency operation might have to be performed elsewhere.

All abortions that do not conform with the Abortion Act 1967 are illegal. Although the number of illegal or backstreet abortions has been drastically reduced since the Act came into force, there are undoubtedly some illegal abortions still being performed.

The question of abortion has always given rise to a great deal of social, religious and legal differences of opinion and while the Abortion Act 1967 may have legalized abortion when it is carried out under special circumstances, it certainly does not lessen the magnitude of the problems that surround the whole subject. The Act itself has clarified the legal position of the termination of pregnancy, but it has already caused a certain amount of criticism as well as an increasing number of medical and legal problems.

Methods of inducing abortion

The damage or destruction of the fertilized ovum even before implantation is theoretically an abortion. Intrauterine contraceptive devices may cause this to happen and it is likely that the so-called 'morning-after' (or 'once only') pill does lead in many instances to the destruction and loss of a fertilized ovum. The possible use of large doses of hormone during the second half of the menstrual cycle to induce abortion means that these must be taken before any possibility of pregnancy can be proved and also before the suppression of the first menstrual period.

There are no drugs that can be administered to cause abortion safely and certainly. The prostaglandin group of hormones is now in common use for abortion. They are used for abortion between 14 and 24 weeks when they are given either by an abdominal injection into the uterus or by a catheter inserted through the cervix. It is likely that in the near future prostaglandins will be given as vaginal pessaries for abortion in the earlier weeks of pregnancy. Other drugs may be used as abortifacients but generally have serious side effects.

Operation

The safest method of inducing early abortion is by operation, of which there are several types.

Dilatation and evacuation was the accepted method of abortion before the 14th week of pregnancy. It was popular for many years. The cervix was dilated to an appropriate size and the products of conception were removed by curettage.

Vacuum aspiration has taken over from dilatation and evacuation, since it is considered to be more efficient and to give rise to fewer complications. The cervix is dilated and the products of conception are then removed from the cavity of the uterus by suction using a special aspiration curette.

Hysterotomy (abdominal). Most gynaecologists would agree that a pregnancy can only be terminated from below (that is via the vagina) up to the end of the 13th, or perhaps the 14th, week of pregnancy. Thereafter the vaginal route is increasingly dangerous and where prostaglandins are not available, or there is another complication, abdominal hysterotomy is indicated. This means that a miniature Caesarean section is performed and an incision is made in the uterus, the products of conception removed and the uterus repaired. Following this operation the patient has to recover as though from any other major abdominal operation, and since a scar is now present in the uterus this will need close observation in future pregnancies.

Hysterectomy means the removal of the uterus (or womb). This particular operation is seldom performed to terminate a pregnancy.

The dangers of abortion

The dangers of abortion are still seriously underestimated. Deaths following abortion form one of the major factors among the causes of death during pregnancy in Great Britain. Abortion accounts for 8.1 per cent of the number of pregnant women who died in Great Britain in 1976, when there were 6 deaths following abortion, but this is only one particular aspect of the dangers of the operation. The other dangers are:

Injury or damage to the uterus or other organs at the time of operation. This particular danger should occur infrequently but it must be remembered that the termination of a pregnancy is a particularly difficult operation and such injuries are bound to occur occasionally even in the most skilled hands.

Retained products of conception. If a small portion of the pregnancy remains within the uterus, then retention of part of the products of conception may, and probably will, give rise to two further complications, those of haemorrhage and sepsis. Haemorrhage is heavy bleeding following soon after the operation. The first sign of sepsis is usually the onset of pain. If the sepsis becomes severe or if it remains untreated then the future fertility of the woman may be jeopardized.

The long-term effects may be numerous and they may be either mild or dramatic. Recurrent abortion may occur as a direct result or indirectly due to damage to the upper part of the canal of the cervix. Infection may give rise to pelvic pain and discomfort, and may spread to the Fallopian tubes causing infertility. Caesarean section may have to be performed because the uterus has been previously scarred. Postpartum haemorrhage may occur if the placenta becomes unduly adherent to the inside of the uterus over an area from which the endometrium has been completely removed.

Psychological ill effects. Very little is yet known about the psychological ill effects of termination of pregnancy. Such ill effects, however, do have to be weighed against those of allowing a pregnancy to continue.

Glossary

Technical words and terms are defined in this book when they occur for the first time. A glossary is however included for simple and easy reference.

accidental haemorrhage premature separation of a placenta which is normally implanted (abruptio placentae)

aerophagy swallowing air

amenorrhoea absence of menstrual periods

amino acids organic chemicals, many of which are always linked together in the formation of a protein molecule

amniocentesis an operation to remove a small quantity of amniotic fluid

amniotic fluid the fluid surrounding the baby in the amniotic cavity

anaemia a low haemoglobin level of the blood

anaesthesia loss of sensation

anaesthesia (general) loss of sensation accompanied by loss of consciousness

anaesthesia (local) anaesthesia of a part of the body created by means of injection

analgesic a drug used to kill pain

anatomical changes changes in the structure of an organ

antenatal the time during pregnancy prior to delivery

antepartum haemorrhage haemorrhage from vagina that occurs after the 28th week of pregnancy and before delivery

antibody a substance manufactured by the body to counteract the effects of antigen

antibodies special substances made by the body to protect it from specific disease or infection

anticoagulant drugs drugs which reduce coagulation in the blood

anti-D immunoglobin the special Rhesus antibody that destroys Rhesus positive red cells especially in the baby

antigen a substance which, when introduced into the body, often during illness or disease, provokes a reaction and the formation of antibody to destroy it

asphyxia lack of oxygen

atrophy degeneration or wasting away

basal body temperature the body temperature whilst sleeping

binovular twins non-identical twins

blastocyst the early developing ovum

blighted ovum a pregnancy in which the fetus does not develop satisfactorily

blood pressure the pressure created by the heart within the major blood vessels in order to force blood round the body

Braxton Hicks' contractions painless uterine contractions which occur about every 20 minutes throughout pregnancy

breech presentation a baby presenting buttocks first

bronchi the larger tubes within the lungs

brow presentation the position of the baby when his head is very poorly flexed so that the brow lies over the cervix

caput succedaneum a swelling that appears on the baby s head during the process of labour

carpal tunnel a tunnel on the front of the wrist formed by bone and fibrous tissue through which the nerves and tendons run to the fingers

catheter a tube used to drain urine from the bladder

cephalic presentation a baby presenting head first

cervical canal the canal in the cervix from the uterus to the vagina

cervical erosion an ulcer on the cervix

cervix the lower part of the uterus

chorionic gonadotrophin the hormone, formed by the chorionic villi, that is initially responsible for the continuation of pregnancy. Its presence in urine is used to diagnose pregnancy

chorionic villi the sponge-like processes on the outer surface of the developing ovum that enable it to embed in the endometrium on the 7th day

chromosome one of the rod-like structures which occur in pairs in the nucleus of every cell in the body. They are composed of genes. There are 23 pairs of chromosomes in each human cell

chronic illness an illness which has lasted for a long time

circumcision operation for the removal of the foreskin or prepuce

congenital abnormality an abnormality present at birth

corpus luteum the gland formed in the ovary after ovulation. It produces progesterone in the second half of each cycle and this hormone helps to maintain the newly implanted pregnancy

crowning the moment of delivery of the baby's head

decidua the inner lining of the uterus during pregnancy

deep transverse arrest the position of the baby in the uterus when his head faces sideways instead of backwards and becomes stuck in this position

diathermy the use of a special electric current in medical treatment

diuretics drugs that increase urine output

divarication separation of the muscles in the mid-line of the abdomen

Doptone an ultrasonic fetal heart detector

dura the layer of tissue immediately surrounding the spinal cord

dysmature 'small for dates'. This refers to a baby that is smaller than would be expected for the duration of pregnancy

ectopic pregnancy a pregnancy situated outside the cavity of the uterus

embolus (pl. emboli) blood clot

endocrine relating to hormones

endometrium the lining of the inner surface of the uterus

epididymis a network of connecting tubes adjacent to the testicle in which the sperms are collected before their passage along the vas deferens to the seminal vesicles

epidural anaesthetic an anaesthetic given into the epidural space surrounding the spinal cord

episiotomy incision into the perineum

ergometrine a drug used to make the uterus contract

external cervical os the opening at the vaginal end of the cervix

face presentation the position of the baby when his head is extended so that his face is delivered first

Fallopian tube the tube that connects the ovary to the uterus

fascia a thin, tendon-like sheath surrounding muscles

fertilization the union of the ovum and the sperm

fetal distress a shortage of oxygen in the fetus

fetus the baby while still in the uterus

fimbriae the finger-like processes at the

ovarian end of the Fallopian tube

fluid balance chart a chart showing all fluids taken by mouth or given intravenously together with all fluids leaving the body as urine or vomit, etc.

fontanelles the small areas in the skull not covered by bone at birth

FSH (follicle stimulating hormone) hormone secreted by the pituitary that causes ovulation to occur

fundus the upper part of the uterus

gamma globulin a special protein extracted from the blood that contains a high quantity of antibody

gene a member of any of the pairs of physiological units which control the development of certain characteristics in the fetus, one gene from each pair being transmitted from each parent. The genes are in a unique pattern in the chromosomes of each person

genetics the science of the study of genes

gonads ovaries or testicles

Graafian follicle a developing ovum within the ovary

gynaecologist a doctor who specializes in diseases peculiar to women (contrast with **obstetrician**)

haemoglobin the protein present in red blood cells responsible for their colour and for carrying oxygen

hiatus hernia a hernia in the diaphragm that allows the stomach to partially extend into the cavity of the chest

human placental lactogen (HPL) a placental hormone useful for assessing feto-placental health

hyaluronidase an enzyme carried by sperms, that liquefies mucus, in particular the protective mucus surrounding the new ovum

hymen the fold of skin that partially covers the lower vagina and is ruptured during first intercourse

hyperemesis excessive vomiting

innominate bone the bones at the side of the pelvis, beside the sacrum

insemination deposition of sperms in the female genital tract

internal cervical os the opening of the upper end of the cervical canal

intervertebral disc the small cartilaginous disc which separates the bony segments of the spine

intravenous given into a vein

involution the natural process whereby the uterus returns to normal size after delivery

ketones acids present in the urine as a result of excessive vomiting or starvation

labour the process of delivery of the baby

lactation the process of milk production

levator ani the main muscles in the pelvic floor

LH (luteinizing hormone) hormone secreted by the pituitary gland that stimulates the formation of the corpus luteum and therefore ensures the secretion of progesterone

libido sexual desire

lie the longitudinal axis of the baby within the uterus

lightening this is the term describing the relief from pressure on the upper abdomen and diaphragm when the baby's head drops into the pelvis and the upper part of the uterus descends 8 or 10 cm. This happens at the 36th week of pregnancy in a primigravida

linea nigra the pigmentation along the mid-line of the abdomen during pregnancy

liquor amnii the fluid surrounding the baby in the uterus

lithotomy position the position in which obstetric and gynaecological operations are performed with the patient's legs supported in stirrups

lochia blood-stained discharge from the vagina after delivery

lower uterine segment the lower part of the body of the uterus

mastitis neonatorum enlargement of the breasts of the newly born infant

meconium thick, sticky greenish material present in the baby's rectum before and after birth

metabolism the burning of food by the body to create energy and warmth

micturition passing urine

monilia (thrush) infection by candida albicans of the vagina and of the new-born baby's mouth

morula the developing ovum when it has divided into about 32 different cells

moulding alteration in the position of the bones of the baby's skull during labour

mucus a sticky substance secreted by special glands which usually has a protective function

multigravida a woman during her second or subsequent pregnancy

mutations variations in the pattern of genes that might produce congenital abnormalities

myomectomy the removal of a fibroid from the uterus followed by reconstruction of the uterus to allow subsequent pregnancy

neonatal death death within 28 days of birth

obstetrician a doctor who specializes in pregnancy (contrast with **gynaecologist**)

oedema swelling of the tissues of the body caused by fluid

oesophagus the food pipe or tube that connects the throat to the stomach

oestriol an oestrogen estimated during pregnancy to assess the function of the placenta

oestrogen female hormone formed by the developing ovum

operculum the plug of mucus that fills the cervical canal throughout pregnancy

organism a bacterium or virus

ovulation the production of an egg or ovum from the ovary

ovum the female egg cell

oxytocic drug a drug which makes the uterus contract

paediatrician a specialist doctor who looks after children and especially new-born babies

perinatal death still-birth or neonatal death

perineum the area between the anus and the vagina

persistent occipito-posterior position the position of the baby when his head does not rotate during labour and continues to face forwards, even in the second stage of labour

physiological changes changes in the function of an organ

pigmentation discoloration of the skin

placenta the afterbirth. It is responsible for transferring the baby's vital requirements from the mother to the baby in the uterus and for transferring the baby's waste products to the mother

placenta praevia a placenta implanted over the lower uterine segment

polyhydramnios an excessive amount of amniotic fluid

polyps benign overgrowths of, or from, a mucous membrane

postnatal after delivery

pre-eclampsia a condition specific to pregnancy, characterized by a raised blood pressure, swelling of the fingers or ankles and protein in the urine

premature baby a baby that weighs less than 2,500 g

premature labour labour before the 38th week of pregnancy

presentation the part of the baby that is lying over the cervix and will therefore be delivered first

primigravida a woman having her first pregnancy

progesterone female hormone secreted by the corpus luteum

prostate a gland at the base of the bladder in the male

psychology the science of the nature and phenomena of the human mind and conduct

psychoprophylaxis a method of preparation for childbirth

puerperium the 28 days immediately after delivery

pulmonary embolus a blood clot in the lungs

quickening feeling fetal movements for the first time

Rhesus disease the destruction or damage of the red blood cells of a Rhesus positive baby while it is still in the uterus of a Rhesus negative woman who has developed Rhesus antibodies

Rhesus factor a special factor in human red cells, the absence of which may predispose to Rhesus disease

sacrum the lower part of the spine

seminal count examination of the sperms in the semen

seminal vesicles small organs at the base of the prostate that store sperms prior to ejaculation

sinus a small hole or canal

Sonicaid an ultrasonic fetal heart detector

sperm the male reproductive cell

spermatogenesis the formation of sperms

sphincter the circular muscle controlling the opening of a tube or canal

still-birth the birth of a dead baby after 28 weeks of pregnancy

stress incontinence involuntary leakage of urine on exertions such as coughing, straining or sneezing

subcutaneous fat the layer of fat that lies immediately beneath the skin

sulphonamide an anti-bacterial drug similar to an antibiotic

symphysis pubis the joint in the front of the pelvis where the pubic bones meet

Syntocinon a drug that makes the uterus contract

testicles male reproductive organs where sperms are formed

thoracic cage the rib cage

thrush (monilia) a fungus infection

tone the tension that is present in muscle

trimester one third of pregnancy

    first trimester 1 to 14 weeks

    second trimester 14 to 28 weeks

    third trimester 28 weeks to term

trophoblast the cells on the outer edge of the chorionic villi

ultrasound very short waves which can detect movement. It is used in midwifery to detect the fetal heart

umbilical cord the cord connecting the baby's umbilicus to the placenta and containing two umbilical arteries and one vein

uniovular twins twins developed from one egg. They are identical

urethra the tube that leads from the bladder to the vulva

uterus womb

varices dilated veins

vas deferens the tube that links the testicle to the seminal vesicles

vascular containing many blood vessels

vernix the greasy white material which covers the baby in the uterus

vestigial glands glands not necessary to the body

viability the ability of a baby to exist after birth

virus an organism or micro-organism smaller than a bacterium

vulva the external part of the female reproductive organs

Wharton's jelly the jelly-like substance that surrounds the blood vessels in the umbilical cord

Conversion Tables

The bold figure in the centre represents whichever unit is to be converted:
e.g. 1 *cm* = 0.4 *in* and 1 *in* = 2.5 *cm*

cm = centimetre   *kg* = kilograms   *l* = litres
in = inches   *lb* = pounds   *pt* = pints
                      g = grams   *ml* = millilitres
                     oz = ounces

	Length			Weight			Volume	
cm		*in*	*kg*		*lb*	*l*		*pt*
2.5	1	0.4	0.4	1	2.2	0.6	1	1.8
5.1	2	0.8	0.9	2	4.4	1.1	2	3.5
7.6	3	1.2	1.4	3	6.6	1.6	3	5.3
10.2	4	1.6	1.8	4	8.8	2.3	4	7.0
12.7	5	2.0	2.3	5	11.0	2.8	5	8.8
15.2	6	2.4	2.7	6	13.2	3.4	6	10.6
17.8	7	2.8	3.2	7	15.4	4.0	7	12.3
20.3	8	3.1	3.6	8	17.6	4.5	8	14.1
22.9	9	3.5	4.1	9	19.8	5.1	9	15.8
25.4	10	3.9	4.5	10	22.0	5.7	10	17.6

1 *kg* = 1,000 *g*
10 *g* = 0.35 *oz*
1 *l* = 1,000 *ml*

Index

Bold references refer to illustrations.

body, male/female 35
bone: deformities 230, 231
  marrow disease 231, 297
bottle-feeding 141, 237
  v. breast-feeding 484, 485, 489–90
  milk used 490–1, 492
  routine 491–2
  equipment and
    sterilization 492–3
bowel regulation 162–3, 186–7
  difficulties after childbirth 407,
    412, 440, 448
brassiere, importance of
  suitable 141, 157–8, 238–9
  and for nursing 158, 401, 485,
    489
Braxton Hicks' contractions *see*
  uterine contractions
breast-feeding **486**, 128, 141, 237,
  251, 417, 440, 484–9, 531
  drugs and 235–6
  effect of mother's diet on 488
  and cardiac patients 293–4
  and tuberculosis patients 303,
    490
  effect on uterus 400, 401
  condition of breasts during 401–2
  and lactation 406
  fluid intake necessary 409, 410
  need to stop in event of
    infection 419, 420
  anti-coagulants and 426
  in case of twins 435
  effect on uterine bleeding 442
  duration of 444
  slimming inadvisable during 447
  effect on figure 450, 489
  protection by 476
  v. bottle-feeding 484, 485,
    489–90
  difficulties during 489
breasts **56**, 49, 55–7
  changes in during pregnancy 21,
    47, 96, 99, 112, 118, 119, 128,
    119–200, 450

and after delivery 401–2
  care of 57, 128, Chapter 15 417,
    441, 443, 450, 498
  infection in 418–20
  effects of contraceptive pill 529
  see also brassiere; engorgement
breath, first, of baby 339, 341,
    453–4
  and resuscitation
    procedures 457–9
  and the establishment of
    respiration 461, 469–70
  fetal lung maturity and 312
breathing, maternal 108–9, 127,
    129, 190
  and heart conditions 292
  and in twin pregnancies 432–3
  and in multiple pregnancies *see*
    also inhalation analgesia 437
breech presentation **319**, 133, 183,
    316, 317, 387, 395–6, 474
  delivery of 320, 366, 368,
    Chapter 27, 401
  in twins 397, 434–5
bromocriptine 236
brow presentation 379
bruising, on baby's head 498
'butterfly mask', pigmentation on
    mother's face 201

Caesarean section 21, 266, 328,
    374, 382, 422, 464
  when necessary 252, 271, 274,
    276, 277, 294, 306–8, 314, 381,
    386–8, 395, 396, 474
  anaesthesia during 234, 358–60
  history and techniques 385–6,
    30–2
  pregnancies following 388–90
  convalescence following 392
  and liability to cystitis 420
calcium, importance in diet 160,
    221, 224, 234, 410
calculation, of delivery date 22,
    133–19